CLINICAL APPLICATION OF
CARCINOEMBRYONIC ANTIGEN ASSAY

CLINICAL APPLICATION OF CARCINOEMBRYONIC ANTIGEN ASSAY

Proceedings of a Symposium, Nice,
October 7-9, 1977

Editors:

B.P. Krebs, C.M. Lalanne and
M. Schneider

Centre Antoine Lacassagne
Nice, France

 1978
Excerpta Medica Amsterdam-Oxford

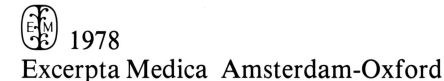

International Congress Series No. 439

ISBN 0-444-90028-4

Library of Congress Cataloging in Publication Data

Main entry under title:

Clinical application of carcinoembryonic antigen assay.
   (International congress series ; no. 439)
   1. Cancer--Diagnosis--Congresses. 2. Carcinoembryonic antigens--Analysis--Congresses. I. Krebs, B.P. II. Lalanne, Claude M. III. Schneider, Max, 1904- IV. Series (DNLM: 1. CEA--Analysis--Congresses. 2. Carcinoembryonic antigen--Analysis--Congresses. 3. Gastrointestinal neoplasms--Diagnosis--Congresses. 4. Lung neoplasms--Diagnosis--Congresses. 5. Bronchial neoplasms--Diagnosis--Congresses. 6. Breast neoplasms--Diagnosis--Congresses. W3 EX89 no. 439 1977 / QZ310 C641 1977]
RC270.C49   616.9'94'0792   78-4111
ISBN 0-444-90028-4

Publisher:
Excerpta Medica
305 Keizersgracht
Amsterdam
P.O. Box 1126

Sole distributors for the USA and Canada:
Elsevier/North-Holland Inc.
52 Vanderbilt Avenue
New York, NY 10017

Printed in The Netherlands by Krips Repro, Meppel

CONTENTS

II. Bronchus carcinoma

IV. Breast cancer

V. Gynaecological cancer

VI. Urological and head and neck cancers

VII. Monitoring — Screening and diagnosis

VIII. Other markers

X

INTRODUCTION

The development of techniques for measuring the serum levels of carcinoembryonic antigen (CEA) has raised great hopes. Its usefulness in diagnosis, in monitoring of treatment and perhaps in early detection of cancer is shown by many studies, which ranks this antigen as a model for other markers.

However, some apparent discrepancies have at the same time clouded the originally promising prospects. The doctor, facing these conflicting reports is meeting great difficulty for introducing CEA measurement in daily routine practice. Even more so because this test is expensive and cost of Health steadily rising.

As a consequence, the CEA assays are at the present time used in too few patients and not always for those who would most benefit of it.

The Nice Symposium aimed at changing this situation by establishing how it will be possible and wise to enlarge the application of the test. This search is based on all the data already accumulated in the world. The variations of CEA have been studied in various sites of cancer and in different situations. The results, in some cases positive and in othersnegative, delineate the field of the practical application and the role of the test in clinical work.

One may hope that wide detection of cancer by routine laboratory methods will be achieved. It will be especially important in the case of occult cancer, which escapes diagnosis by reason of its small size or deep-seated position. This achievement will promote earlier and more active treatment. It will also promote the use of chemotherapy and immunotherapy in the case of preclinical disseminated disease, where the chance of cure is increasing with new drugs and new methodologies. Therefore, it could help to reach better survival rates in the near future.

C.M.LALANNE
Director of the Centre Antoine Lacassagne

SOME REMARKS FOR THE SYMPOSIUM

A.I. GOUSSEV*

I should like to thank Dr.C.M. LALANNE, President, and Dr. B.P. KREBS.

WHO gives great importance to the problem of cancer, especially early diagnosis and standardization of diagnostic reagents ; therefore it was decided that WHO should be represented at this Symposium , especially for the Workshop on Assay Methods to plan out future collaboration programmes. I wish to take this opportunity to convey, on behalf of Dr. MAHLER, Director-General of WHO, our best wishes for success in your work here in NICE. Being an intergovernmental organization with a membership of more than 140 countries, both developed and developing, WHO's aim is the improvement of national health services and the implementation by Member States of the most recent scientific achievements.

Let me tell you something about activities of the Immunology unit of WHO.

Immunology has several programmes related to public health practice. Some of these activities are :

1. Training of post-graduate students in both basic and applied immunology by means of a network of Immunology Research and Training Centres, which now cover all regions. These centres carry out training in immunology and conduct research related to diseases prevalent in their particular areas. Only two weeks ago an advanced course on the immunology of infectious diseases was organized by the Centre in Lausanne, Switzerland. Fifteen students from developing countries took part in the course, and all of them practised modern immunological techniques, such as solid phase radioimmunoassay and enzyme-linked immunoadsorbent assay.

2. A network of collaborating exists for immunoglobulins, the serology of autoimmune disorders, testing of natural resistance factors, tumour-specific antigens etc, established with the aim of assisting research. Research on many projects is financed, or partially financed, through agreements with institutions in various countries.

3. I would especially like to tell you about our programme for the standardization of immunological reagents and methods, which has

.../...

* Medical Officer Immunology, WHO
  12011 - GENEVE   SWISSLAND

been developed in close cooperation with the International Union of Immunological Societies. The aim is to standardize the reagents required to make immunological techniques available for routine hospital practice. A fluorescein-labelled sheep anti-human immuno-globulin has been accepted as an International Standard and a fluorescein-labelled goat anti-human IgM will be submitted for appro-val as an International Standard in December 1977. Work is continuing towards a standard for fluorescein-labelled sheep anti-human IgG, for an international serum protein standard and on the standardization of reagents used in emzyme-linked antibody test systems in the immunological context. As you know, tumour-associated antigens, alpha-fetoprotein and carcinoembryonic antigen (CEA) were accepted last year as International Standards.

In this connexion, I would like to draw your special atten-tion to the Standard for CEA. This Standard was prepared by the National Institute for Biological Standards and Control (London) and is available to all interested workers for calibrating their own antigenic preparations using different techniques of measurement. Before acceptance, it was tested by several laboratories in collabo-ration with WHO. It is known that a fast immuno-perchloric method of preparation of CEA has been proposed by scientists from France, the Soviet Union and Japan. As a result of this, it appeared possible to prepare monospecific antisera against CEA, NCA and NCA2.

On the basis of these data I should like you to discuss the following :

1) What further steps on the standardization of CEA could be undertaken in the future ? Is there is a need for the preparation of standard mono-specific antisera directed to CEA, NCA and NCA2 ? In my opinion, the preparation of such standards would permit the more precise calibration of antigenic and antibody preparations and could greatly enhance the usefulness of tests in distinguishing between cancer and other diseases.

2) Finally, I would also like to have your opinion as to the immunological and other methodes that could be used in routine clinical practice for the early diagnosis of gastrointestinal and other forms of cancer, in the screening of apparently healthy persons who may possibly be cancer patients (high-risk groups). I also hope you will discuss the means of implementation of methods useful in the field of clinical oncology and the role which WHO could play in it.

THE SPECIFICITY OF THE CEA AND ANTI-CEA REACTION: PROBLEMS AND FUTURE
PERSPECTIVES

J. Shuster and P. Gold

Division of Clinical Immunology and Allergy, Montreal General
Hospital and the Montreal General Hospital Research Institute,
Montreal, Quebec

The existence of unique tumor antigenic constituants was demonstrated uniquivocally by Foley almost 25 years ago, using the
technique of rejection of tumor tissue transplanted between syneneic
rodent species (1). Ethical considerations preclude a similar
experimental approach in man, however, the development of specific
humoral and/or cell-mediated antitumor immune responses on the part
of the tumor bearing host to his own tumor, and to tumors of similar
histopathologic origin and type is indirect evidence for the existence of unique, tumor specific components in the growing tumor (2).
In addition, the immunization of heterologous species with extracts
of human tumor tissue, has resulted, after suitable absorption with
the appropriate corresponding normal tissue, in the development of
antisera that appear to detect tumor associated antigens as judged by
the precipitation reactions observed in agar gel and related media
(3). Among the major tumor markers that have been characterized by
this last approach are the carcinoembryonic antigen (CEA) and α_1-
fetoprotein (AFP). However, with the development of more sensitive
radioimmunoassay procedures, and the analysis of the distribution of
these markers in a variety of normal and tumor tissues, as well as in
the circulation of patients suffering from a variety of benign and
malignant disorders, it has become apparent that the reagents and
methodology currently employed in the measurement of these markers
does not result in data that is truly indicative of tumor specificity
(4). A number of papers in this conference illustrate this point
clearly with respect to the prototype molecule, the carcinoembryonic
antigen (CEA). The vast literature that has accumulated with respect to CEA over the past decade has clearly indicated the inherent
difficulties in developing radioimmunoassays for specific tumor
products.

Criteria for the Ideal Tumor Immunodiagnostic Assay

Ideally, radioimmunoassays for immunodiagnosis should have a
low incidence of false negative and false positive reactions so that
the assay in question will be optimized for both diagnosis and mass
screening of the population at large. Furthermore, the assay itself
should assist in the specific organ localization of the tumor, i.e.
the assay should be both tissue and tumor specific (5). As concerns
all of these parameters, the radioimmunoassays currently in use for
the measurement of circulating CEA are less than optimum, and thus

4

these assays as presently performed cannot be used in isolation for either primary tumor diagnosis or population screening. Instead, the vast literature indicates that the assay has its widest use as a prognostic indicator. Pre-operatively, CEA levels greater than 10-20 ng/ml plasma are strongly suggestive of metastatic tumor dissemination while a post-operative fall in CEA titer to normal is suggestive of a "curative" resection. More important, however, has been the observation that serial CEA measurement in the post-operative period is currently the single most reliable indicator of complete surgical resection of the primary tumor, of early tumor recurrence, and of the response to cancer therapy. More recently, the early rise in CEA levels after initial successful resection of the primary tumor has been used as an indicator for second look surgery (6).

Major Unresolved Questions

While it is true, that for most assays an increase in sensitivity usually results in some loss of specificity, the observed clinical results with the radioimmunoassays currently used to measure circulating CEA were unexpected in view of the initial results obtained with respect to the tissue distribution of CEA as judged by gel diffusion experiments (3,7). It would appear that these differences do not simply reflect the relative sensitivities of the gel and radioimmunoassay procedures themselves. To a large extent the discrepancies between the initial data and the more current clinical data reflect our limited knowledge of the nature of the products that we are measuring and the purity and/or specificity of the reagents that are used in the radioimmunoassay itself. To date, there has been little standardization of the radioimmunoassays for CEA with respect to both the antigen and the antisera that are employed. It is for these reasons that there are several major unresolved questions that remain with respect to the molecular biology of CEA and the clinical significance of the measurement of levels of CEA. These questions persist because: (1) The structure of the CEA molecule is still largely unknown; (2) The number and nature of the antigenic sites (epitopes) on the CEA molecule have not yet been definitively established; (3) It is not clear if CEA is really a tumor specific marker or if its presence in the circulation merely reflects the increased secretion, during malignant transformation, of a molecule that is normally present in trace quantities in normal tissue; and (4) The physicochemical nature of "CEA-like" molecules has not yet been defined.

Physicochemical Properties of CEA

CEA consists of a single chain structure, cruller in shape, that has a molecular weight of about 200,000. The CEA molecule is glycoprotein in nature and has a CHO:protein ratio that varies from 1:1 to 6:1 in preparations obtained from different individual tumors (4,8). This heterogeneous composition is reflected by the observed intramolecular and intermolecular heterogeneity that has been found both in a given preparation of CEA and between different CEA preparations obtained from different individual tumors. Although the varying sialic acid content of individual CEA molecules probably accounts for a good deal of the polydisperse mobility of CEA on alkaline polyacrylamide gels, this parameter does not account for all of the <u>intramolecular</u> heterogeneity of CEA. The major monosaccharide residue in the CEA molecule is N-acetyl glucosamine. Trace quantities of N-acetyl galactosamine usually indicate the presence of a low molecular weight contaminant that co-purifies with the CEA molecule. Initial chemical degradative studies have demonstrated that the oligosaccharide side chains of the CEA molecule have a sequence that is not unique, but appears to be quite similar to that reported for a variety of circulating glycoproteins (9). Aspartic acid or asparagin, glutamic acid or glutamine, as well as threonine and serine represent the major amino acid residues present in CEA. The absence, or the presence of trace quantities of methionine, may simply reflect the technical difficulties in the measurement of this amino acid residue. The intrachain disulfide bonds present in CEA appear to be necessary for optimal reactivity in the CEA radioimmunoassay, indicating that the protein, rather than the carbohydrate moiety, may represent the major antigenic determinants of the CEA molecule, although this still remains to be clearly demonstrated.

Antigenic Heterogeneity of CEA

In view of the size and molecular complexity of CEA, it is not surprising that CEA should consist of multiple antigenic determinants (10). Thus, antisera raised against CEA would be expected to react with several distinct sites on the surface of the molecule. Heteroantisera produced against CEA have been shown to react with 12 cross-reacting antigens which have been given various alphabetical designations. Recent studies, however, have shown that the CEA cross-reacting materials, variously normal NCA, NGP, CEX, CCEA-2, CCA-III and β_E are probably immunologically identical (11). It is evident from these studies, that if the antisera to CEA are not truly "monospecific", a variety of cross-reacting glycoproteins may interfere with the specificity of the CEA radioimmunoassays. Thus, both chemical and immunochemical analyses of cross-reacting and "CEA-like" substances will be of some importance. It should be noted, in this regard, that an antiserum directed primarily towards the common antigenic portion(s) of two distinct macromolecules, one of which is tumor specific while the other is not, will result in a complete reaction of identity in agar gel leading to rather erroneous conclusions concerning the macromolecular antigens in question.

CEA-like Molecules

As previously noted, the circulating products from a wide variety of tumors and other diseased tissues may inhibit the CEA radioimmunoassay, depending upon the reagents employed. Several of the circulating products that inhibit the CEA radioimmunoassay are in contrast to CEA, more labile to perchloric acid (4,12). Furthermore, a recent study that employed a battery of standard CEA molecules and anti-CEA antisera indicated that the CEA extracted from a metastatic colonic tumor and from the plasma of the same patient were antigenically different based on the capacity of these two products from the same patient to inhibit the various CEA radioimmunoassays that were established using different CEA molecules and different batches of anti-CEA antisera (13). As a consequence of these and other observations, the concept has arisen that there exists a family of "CEA-like" molecules. Although these molecules may be similar in size to CEA, little is known of their chemical structure. In a number of the CEA radioimmunoassays that have been established, "CEA-like" substances may account for the extreme variability in the values used to distinguish the normal range of circulating CEA from that found in patients with neoplastic conditions (14).

Increasing the Specificity of the CEA Radioimmunoassay

In theory, the specificity of the CEA radioimmunoassay can be enhanced by either using a more homogeneous antigen preparation and/or more highly specific antisera. Sub-fractions of CEA prepared by lectin (Con A) affinity columns apparently demonstrate increased CEA immunoreactivity, but as yet large scale clinical studies with this material have not been performed (8). A preparation of CEA, designated CEA-S was prepared using cesium chloride density gradient centrifugation in addition to the more routine procedures of CEA purification (15). Although initially promising in terms of increased tissue and tumor specificity, more recent studies with a larger population of patients have not shown this to be the case (5,16,17).

As previously noted, the specificity of the anti-CEA antisera currently in use represent a major problem. Recent studies indicate that the majority of the antibodies in anti-CEA antisera react with common antigenic sites on the CEA molecule rather than the unique and putative specific tumor site (18). In the future, in order to develop a "monospecific" antiserum, it will be essential to isolate, in adequate quantities, the "CEA-like" materials from a variety of normal tissues and non-colorectal tumors, and utilize these materials when coupled to solid phase supporting media, to sequentially and selectively absorb the anti-CEA antisera. Crude extracts of normal colorectal mucosa and non-colorectal tissues do not contain significant concentrations of these "CEA-like" materials to serve as adequate vehicles for complete and effective absorption of the anti-CEA antisera in the liquid phase. It is, thus, imperative, that the "CEA-like" molecules be purified, an approach that most likely will require the use of affinity chromatography using unabsorbed or partially absorbed anti-CEA antisera.

A recent publication has attested to the feasibility of the above approach. A "CEA-like" material, called CEA-M, was isolated in pure form from the subcellular membrane fraction of colon tumors (19). This material was used to produce heterologous anti-CEA-M antisera. The resulting antiserum was initially partially absorbed with a variety of normal crude tissue extracts and subsequently completely absorbed with purified CEA-S. Following this absorption, the antisera reacted fully with CEA-M, but failed to react significantly with CEA-S. A radioimmunoassay established with ^{125}I-CEA-M showed a more selective pattern of reactions with a variety of products obtained from both normal and malignant tissues than was observed prior to absorption. This increased specificity

was in turn reflected in the preliminary results obtained with a
limited number of sera obtained from cancer patients (20). This
study indicates that an assay established with highly absorbed antisera appears to be more specific than data reported with a variety
of other assay procedures employing more polydisperse antisera. A
larger scale clinical study of the CEA-M-anti-CEA-M system is awaited
with interest.

It is quite obvious from the foregoing discussion, that
although tumor specificity may be apparent with heterologous antisera
in agar gel reactions, one must view these claims with some skep-
ticism until the ultimate criterion is fulfilled namely, the analysis
by radioimmunoassay of a large number of representative sera obtained
from normal individuals and patients affected with a variety of
benign and malignant diseases. It is only in this fashion can the
true specificity of the reactants used to detect tumor markers in gel
precipitation media   be precisely defined.

Future Perspectives

The prototype clinical studies with CEA indicate that at the
present time, tumor markers may have their greatest clinical role in
the monitoring of patients with established cancer for both early
post-operative recurrence of their disease and for their response to
chemotherapy, radiotherapy, immunotherapy, or a combination of these
procedures (4,12,21). Since not all tumors produce CEA, the clinical
data indicate that it is less than likely that a single marker will
be elevated in all cases of a particular tumor type. It would, thus,
be more expedient to employ a battery of tumor markers to monitor the
sera of cancer patients. These markers need not necessarily be tumor
specific but, in combination, they may accurately reflect the tumor
burden at a given time. A variety of non-specific tumor markers have
already been described, which include a variety of polypeptide
hormones that are produced ectopically in different malignant disorders. Ectopic production of these materials results in certain
well defined paraneoplastic syndromes. The serial measurement of
these polypeptide hormones by radioimmunoassay may adequately reflect
the tumor burden and response to surgery, radiation and/or chemotherapy. Evidence that multiple markers may be required for a given
tumor type is well illustrated in the study of the serum levels of
AFP and HCG in response of germ cell tumors to chemotherapy (22). In
general, the circulating levels of AFP and HCG fall in parallel with
successful tumor therapy. However, several examples have been cited
where the levels of one of these markers decreased appreciably yet
clinically the patient failed to respond to treatment. In many of
these cases, however, the levels of the second marker remained dis-
cordantly high or continued to rise, more accurately reflecting the
true clinical situation. Thus, by simply measuring a single parameter, the true response to chemotherapy may not always be mirrored
in the results obtained.

In conjunction with the use of multiple tumor associated
markers noted above, the search for new tumor specific markers is
essential, for it is likely that these parameters will be most useful
both for tumor diagnosis and screening of the population for malignancy. One particular avenue worth pursuing in this regard is the

analysis of circulating immune complexes that have been shown to be present in the sera of cancer patients. These complexes may well contain both tumor antigen and specific antitumor antibody (23,24) Hence, the isolation of these immune complexes, and the separation of the individual components in these complexes, may, in a single step, provide a source of both specific tumor antigen and specific antitumor antibody. It is likely, that since these products have been defined by the host's own antitumor immune response, that the antigen(s) so detected will, indeed, be tumor specific. If the antigen so defined appears to be one that is common to a variety of tumors of the same histopathologic type, the ideal situation may then arise in which one can measure a tumor product that is specific and that will permit precise tumor localization. Only such a combination of circumstances may allow for specific tumor immunodiagnosis and population screening.

REFERENCES

(1) Foley, E. (1953): Cancer Res., 13, 835.
(2) Hellstrom, K.E. and Hellstrom, I. (1974): Adv. Imm., 8, 209.
(3) Gold, P. and Freedman, S.O. (1965): J. Exp. Med., 121, 439.
(4) Fuks, A., Banjo, C., Shuster, J., Freedman, S.O. and Gold, P. (1975): Biochem. Biophys. Acta, 417, 123.
(5) Herberman, R. (1976): Cancer, 37, 549.
(6) Balz, J.B., Martin, E.W. Jr. and Minton, J.P. (1977): Rev. Surg., 34, 1.
(7) Gold, P. and Freedman, S.O. (1965): J. Exp. Med., 122, 467.
(8) Rogers, G. (1976): Biochem. Biophys. Acta, 458, 355.
(9) Hammarstrom, S., Engvall, E., Johansson, B., Svensson, S., Sunblad, G. and Goldstein, I. (1975): Proc. Nat. Acad. Sci., U.S.A., 72, 1528.
(10) Hammarstrom, S., Svenberg, T. and Sunblad, G. (1976): In Onco-Development Gene Expression (1976), p.559, Academic Press, New York.
(11) Von Kleist, S.: Proceedings of the Symposium on Clinical Application of Carcinoembryonic Antigen and Other Antigenic Markers Assays, Nice, 7-9 October 1977, in press.
(12) Shuster, J., Freedman, S.O. and Gold, P. (1977): Am. J. Clin. Path., Nov.
(13) Vrba, R., Alpert, E. and Isselbacher, K.C. (1975): Proc. Nat. Acad. Sci., U.S.A., 72, 4602.
(14) Lawrence, D.J.R., Stevens, U., Bettelheim, R., Darcy, D., Leese, C., Turberville, C., Alexander, P., Johns, E.W. and Neville, A.M. (1972): Br. Med. J., III, 605.
(15) Plow, E.F. and Edgington, T.S. (1975): Int. J. Cancer, 15, 748.
(16) Edgington, T.S., Astarita, R.W. and Plow, E.F. (1975): New Eng. J. Med., 293, 104.
(17) Herberman R.: personal communication.
(18) Proceedings of the International Research Group for Carcino-embryonic Proteins Meeting, Copenhagen, Aug. 1977, in press.
(19) Leung, J.P., Plow, E.F., Eshdat, Y., Marchesi, V.T. and Edgington, T.S. (1977): J. Imm., 119, 217.
(20) Leung, J.P., Eshdat, Y. and Marchesi, V.T. (1977): J. Imm. 119, 664.

(21) Zamcheck, N., Doos, W.G., Prudente, R., Luri, B.B. and
     Gottlieb, L.S. (1975): Human Pathol., 6, 31.
(22) Braunstein, G.D., McIntyre, K.R. and Waldman, T.A. (1973):
     Cancer, 31, 1065.
(23) Theofilopoulous, A.N., Wilson, C.B. and Dixon, F.J. (1976):
     J. Clin. Invest., 57, 169.
(24) Theofilopoulous, A.N., Andrews, B.S., Urist, M.M., Morton, D.L.
     and Dixon, F.J. (1977): J. Imm., 119, 657.

NORMAL ANTIGENS CROSS REACTING WITH CEA

P.Burtin

C.N.R.S. Villejuif, France

SUMMARY

        Currently three glycoproteins are known to cross-react in the
CEA anti-CEA system : NCA (non specific cross-reacting antigen), NCA
2 and BGP 1 (biliary glycoprotein one). Immunochemical studies allow
a conceptual pattern for the distribution of common and different
antigenic sites in these substances. Histoimmunochemical studies are
described in order to clarify tissular localisations of the different
antigens. These methods require antisera of high specificity, whereas
on the other hand radioimmunoassay requires less specific antisera.

CHARACTERISTICS OF ANTIGENS

        NCA was first described by MACH et al(1) in normal lung extract.
After immunoelectrophoresis of colonic cancer perchloric extract two
precipitin lines are obtained with anti CEA serum, there exists
always two precipitin lines with crude colonic cancer extract. The
presence of NCA in this extract explains this phenomenon. The electro-
phorectic mobility of NCA is quite the same as CEA (β). NCA is a glycoprotein of 60.000 MW, 3.5 S with a glucidic fraction around 30-40%.
There is a specific antigenic site on NCA absent from CEA (2), thus
despite the small size of NCA, it is obvious that NCA is not a fragment from CEA.

        NCA 2 was discovered in our laboratory in perchloric acid ex-
tract from feces and meconium (3). The electrophoretic mobility of
NCA 2 is similar to those of CEA and NCA, but after aging, one obser-
ves an increase in this mobility. The molar weight is intermediate
between NCA and CEA. One of the antigenic sites of NCA 2 is specific,
the others exist also on CEA. The hypothetic pattern of the antigenic
distribution between CEA, NCA and NCA 2, could be described as
follows :
        - one antigenic site is common to CEA, NCA and NCA 2
        - another exists in CEA and NCA 2 but not in NCA
        - we never found a common site between NCA and NCA 2, absent
          from CEA
        - furthermore, each molecule possesses a specific antigenic
          site.

        Nevertheless, this must be complicated after the discovering
of BGP 1 by SVENBERG (4). This glycoprotein is closely related to

11

NCA as far as crossreaction with anti-CEA serum is concerned. Antigenic site(s) common to CEA and BGP 1 are similar to antigenic sites common to CEA and NCA. But BGP 1 has a specific antigenic site with high immunizing power. Therefore, the members of CEA family are at least four, without taking into account a possible antigenic variability of CEA itself.

TISSULAR LOCALISATIONS OF THESE MOLECULES

In colonic cnacer, localisation of CEA and NCA is similar: with both kinds of antibody, the labelling is on epithelial lining and on glandular lumen. In gastric cancer, results are nearly similar. Nevertheless we observe also a slight labelling of intercellular walls with anti-NCA antibodies. But in bronchus mucosa, there is only a poor fluorescence contrasting with many positive cells included in the alveolar wall. In alveolar macrophages in culture (collaboration with Dr. VOISIN, Lille, France), we found also a strong labelling with anti-NCA. In the spleen, many cells are positive : polynuclear and also big mononuclear isolated cells. This lead us to look for leucocytes in peripheral blood. In blood the majority of polynuclear cells present a strong cytoplasmic fluorescence either diffuse or granular. Furthermore immunofluorescence studies show that NCA is also located on the cell surface. In conclusion, NCA is an antigen of the myelomonocytic line. NCA was also observed in some cultured melanoma cells.

In gastric and colonic tumours using specific anti-NCA 2 antibodies, the labelling is similar to the labelling obtained with specific anti-CEA antibodies : i.e. labelling of the epithelial lining and glandular lumen. Cytoplasmic labelling is observed in the peritumoral mucosa and this kind of labelling becomes stronger when the mucosa is taken far from the tumour. In the colon, one notices diffuse labelling of all cells in all colonic glands. Foetal colon presents a strong labelling with anti-NCA 2 antibodies.

PRACTICAL CONSEQUENCES

For histoimmunochemical purposes, anti-sera need to be well absorbed in order to become very specific. For example with anti-CEA antibody absorbed with NCA 2 we found that there is no CEA in gastric metaplasia contrasting with previous published data obtained with a non-absorbed anti-serum. This is also true for some gastric cancers. They contain more NCA and NCA 2 that CEA. So it is important to use highly monospecific anti-CEA sera.

Concerning radioimmunoassay the specificity of antisera does not influence the results in a major way. Absorption of antisera by NCA for example will not modify the results. The explanation for this could lie in the differences of antibody affinity ; affinity for CEA is always much higher than affinity for cross-reacting substances. This is true for NCA, NCA 2 and BGP 1. All reagents must be controlled but generally anti-CEA sera could be used for radioimmunoassay of CEA without previous absorption. In the same way, measurements of cross-reacting substances with radioimmunoassay (for example VON KLEIST et al.(5) for NCA) generally do not need specific anti-serum absorbed with CEA.

REFERENCES

(1) Mach,J.P., Pusztaszeri,G. (1972) : Immunochemistry,9, 1031.

(2) Von Kleist,S., Chavanel,G., Burtin,P. (1972) : Proc.Nat.Acad.Sci., USA, 69, 2492.

(3) Burtin,P., Chavanel,G., Hirsch-Marie,H. (1973) : J.Immunol.,111, 1926.

(4) Svenberg,T. (1976) : Int. J.Cancer, 17, 588.

(5) Von Kleist,S., Troupel,S., King,M., Burtin,P. (1977) : Brit. J. Cancer, 35, 875.

QUANTITATIVE DETERMINATION OF CARCINOEMBRYONIC ANTIGEN BY TWO DIFFERENT METHODS

J. KADOUCHE[1], Y. NAJEAN[1], K. BELDJORD[2] and A. DEPIERRE[3]

1 - Department of Nuclear Medicine, Hôpital Saint-Louis, Paris,

2 - Hematological Laboratory - Centre Pierre et Marie Curie, Hôpital Mustapha, Algiers,

3 - Department of Professor L. Israel, Hôpital Franco-Musulman, Bobigny, France.

COMPARISON OF METHODS

Since Gold and Freedman first discovered carcino-embryonic antigen (CEA), its clinical value for the detection and particularly the follow-up of certain forms of neoplasia has been discussed in numerous papers. The practical value of a method of quantitative determination depends largely on its specificity, sensitivity and reproducibility and on certain technical factors. In France two methods are at present commercially available.

One of these (Roche Diagnostica) derives from Hansen's original technique. The antigen it uses is an extract of hepatic metastases of cancer of the colon, and the quantitative determination is carried out with a perchloric extract of dialysed plasma. Following incubation with an excess of anti-CEA antiserum a second incubation takes place in the presence of labelled CEA, which is followed by the separation of the free and the bound antigen by precipitation of the bound fraction by means of zirconium gel.

The other method (CIS method) uses as the antigen an extract of hepatic metastasis originating from a primary cancer of the colon, the antigenicity of which is similar to that of the CEA first described by Gold and Freedman. The serum to be tested is treated with an excess of anti-CEA antiserum, then with the labelled antigen and, finally, with an anti-gamma-globulin serum bound to a solid phase, by which means the bound and the free antigen are separated from each other.

In the present paper, these two methods are compared. Reproducibility and sensitivity have been determined with the aid of standard antigen samples. 36 simultaneous quantitative determinations by the two methods have been carried out in control subjects and 378 in patients in various stages of cancer.

This paper is concerned with the technological and methodological aspects of the study; the comparative study of the clinical value of the two methods will be the subject of a future publication.

METHODS

Throughout this study we have very accurately followed the technical directions given by the manufacturers of the two batches used (Roche and CIS). All investigations concerning one particular aspect have always been carried out by one and the same technician Counting was always done over a period of time long enough to allow a statistical accuracy of 99%. For the statistical calculation, the standard methods have been used.

RESULTS

Reproducibility of quantitative determination of standard samples

The calibration curve was studied 10 times with a single determination batch, using the same standard sample.

For the double-antibody method (the CIS method) we used the curve in standard veronal buffer, pH 8.4 ± 0.2, containing 0.25% BSA to avoid the protein effect and the coating of the tubes. The results were expressed in % of $\frac{B}{T}$; the standard deviation calculated for each of these 8 experimental points and expressed as percentages from the mean was less than 5.5%.

With the method using zirconium gel (Roche method), the standard deviation at 5 experimental points was less than 4%.

The same standard sample was studied using different batches. This study has been carried out for 10 estimations, using different lots of reagents.

The same antibody was always used; in this manner, combined with inter-system reproducibility, we tested the immunoreactive capacity of the antigen at each labelling.

For each concentration of the curve, the results were expressed as the B/Bo ratio. We calculated a mean B/Bo with variance standard deviation and coefficient of variation in order to trace a median curve with surrounding curves.

With 10 experiments and 7 experimental points, carried out to trace the calibration curve, the coefficient of variation (1 SD.) varied according to the points from 2.5 to 12.32% with the CIS method with CIS antiserum lot No. 04; for the 4 experimental points of the Roche method it varied between 5.2 and 9.5% with antiserum lot No. 01196.

This comparative study was carried out under optimal technical conditions: the same material, the same experimenter and the same technical conditions, which explains the very small deviations obtained compared with other, similar studies and also compared with what would probably be obtained in daily routine application of the methods. Moreover, the calibration curves have been established without the perchloric extraction and dialysis that are necessary when plasma samples are tested by the Roche method.

With both methods studied we have measured, using different batches for each estimation, the Bo/T value, which represents the capacity of the antiserum to bind itself to labelled CEA. For each of the 10 batches studied, the same antiserum was used.

The variation with the Roche method amounted to 11.4% for one standard deviation; with the CIS method, this variation amounted to 20.6%.

Sensitivity of the quantitative determination of standard samples

Sensitivity was studied using the 4 points at the bottom end of the calibration curve, with the corresponding radioactivity of the precipitate and the confidence limits. The smallest amount detectable was determined by direct reading from the graph (Figs. 1 and 2).

In normal human plasma, the limiting sensitivity for confidence limits of 95% amounted to 4.2 ng with the CIS method and to 0.45 ng with the Roche method.

Comparison of the same standard determined quantitatively with both methods

A standard sample of the CIS method was determined quantitatively with successive dilutions by the Roche method. In 39 pairs of values, the correlation was remarkably good (r = 0.98), and the equation of the regression line was Y = 0.24x + 0.34, in which Y is the value obtained by the Roche method, and x is the value obtained by the CIS method. The standard deviation of the curve was p = 0.085. A standard sample of the Roche batch was studied with different dilutions by the CIS method, and here the correlation coefficient for 55 pairs was r = 0.99 with Y = 0.24x + 2.09 in which Y is the result obtained by the Roche method and x is the result obtained by the CIS method. The standard deviation of the curve was P = 0.0026.

Comparison of the methods used to obtain the calibration curve

Roche recommend for their method quantitative determinations of samples in an ammonium acetate medium, 0.01 M pH 6.5 ± 0.2, and quantitative determinations of the standard in EDTA medium containing bovine serum albumin and sodium azide as a preservative. Therefore, we have carried out a comparison of the standard curve obtained in EDTA medium and in ammonium acetate medium, using biological samples for the quantitative determinations.

Figure 3 shows that, in the latter case, the maximal binding obtained is increased from 49.8% to 76%, thus shifting the entire calibration range. The difference leads to an underestimation in EDTA of the amount of antigen by 6.25 ng at point 0, by 7.7 ng at point 2.5 and by 10.75 ng at point 6.25.

For the CIS method it is recommended to establish the calibration curve in the presence of 50 μl of a pool of normal human plasma in order that the small amount of CEA (or other proteins reacting with anti-CEA antibody) which are normally present may be subtracted from pathological readings.

We have compared the calibration curves in normal human plasma. The results show a medium parallelism of the curves, the differences of the values ranging from 20 ng at point 0 to 12 ng at point 80 and to 4 ng at point 320 (Fig.4).

Intra-test reproducibility using control samples of serum or plasma

Although the reproducibility of quantitative determinations of standard samples has by now been demonstrated, it was still necessary to verify the reproducibility of control samples of serum or plasma in an intra-test comparison.

For the 4 Roche controls, determined quantitatively by the CIS method, the variation coefficients for a standard deviation are essentially the same as those observed with the intra-test and the inter-test of the Roche standard.

For the 4 Roche controls, determined quantitatively by the CIS method, the variation coefficients for a standard deviation are essentially the same as those observed with the intra-test and the inter-test of the CIS standard; for these 4 controls determined quantitatively in the Roche system, the variation coefficients were higher than those observed with the intra- and inter-test of the Roche standard.

It is curious to observe that for the 4 Roche controls, the best variation coefficients were obtained when the Roche standard was used in the CIS system (Table 1).

17

Table 1   Intra-test check with the four Roche control sera

Values indicated[*]	Values found using the Roche method	Values obtained after manipulation by the CIS method	
		Calibration curve with:	
		Roche standard	CIS standard
0.7 ± 1	1.27 ± 0.22[**]	2.96 ± 0.28[**] 7 determ.	5
		3 determ.	5-10
4.5 ± 1	6.31 ± 0.88	7.1 ± 0.33	41.8 ± 2.8
8 ± 1	8.92 ± 0.91	11.4 ± 0.9	79.3 ± 7.4
15 ± 3	14.42 ± 2.1	26.66 ± 2.22	182.2 ± 13.1

Values measured by the intra-test check for 10 determinations

* by Roche Diagnostica

** 1 S.D.

Comparison of the results obtained with the two methods in 414 cases (36 normal subjects and 378 pathological samples)

The findings obtained are shown in Figures 5-9.
Comparison of the 36 control values each one measured in triplicate with the CIS method and in duplicate with the Roche method, shows one single case with values higher than normal with the CIS method (average 18 ng) and the Roche method (average 3.2 ng) (Fig. 5).
Three other cases, however, gave abnormal values with the Roche method (averages 9.5, 9.4 and 12.2 ng), whereas there was satisfactory reproducibility between the two or three measurements of each determination. One hundred and sixty-three determinations in patients showed agreement between the values within normal limits or at the limits of normal for the two methods (Fig. 6); in 10 cases the values were higher than the threshold 15 ng/ml with the CIS method, but lower than 2.5 ng/ml with the Roche method (Fig.7). It should be noted, however, that one of these values is distinctly pathological (65 ng) with the former method. On the other hand, 129 cases showed levels between 2.5 and 15 ng with the Roche method and values lower than 15 ng with the

CIS method (Fig. 8). Finally, 76 cases showed distinctly pathological values with both methods (higher than 15 with the CIS method, higher than 2.5 with the Roche method) (Fig. 9a and b).

The correlation of these 76 pairs is:

r = 0.95 with Y = 0.312x + 15.898,
in which y is the value obtained by the Roche method
x is the value obtained by the CIS method. The
standard deviation of the curve is P = 0.012.

DISCUSSION

Most of the papers published in the last few years have been concerned with the clinical usefulness of quantitative determination of serum CEA. However, inter-pretation of the readings is valid only if the relia-bility of a particular test method has been demonstrated, its specificity is adequate, its limits of sensitivity and of error have been determined and its reproducibility confirmed.

In this paper we have compared two methods: that in-troduced by Roche, which is based on the experience gain-ed in over 500,000 quantitative determinations carried out in the U.S.A., and that introduced 3 years ago in France by CIS. Methodologically the two methods differ considerably. A comparative study of this nature was sug-gested as a conclusion at the symposium held in Paris on April 8th and 9th, 1976. It has been carried out with the complete agreement and support of the Roche diagnost-ica houses in Basle and Paris and the Department of Radio Elements of the Atomic Energy Commission (Saclay).

The method of obtaining the antigen (organ used, method of extraction) affects the biochemical charac-teristics of CEA and particularly the immunological reactivity of the antibodies obtained. Moreover, recent studies have led to the isolation of a CEA-S which, compared with the Roche CEA, shows greater specificity in regard to neoplastic conditions. The heterogeneity of CEA's obtained in the traditional manner may have been one of the causes of the differences in the results obtained by different methods, and of the number of false-positive results obtained.

The complicated nature of the Roche method is a possible source of error which might explain the lesser inter-test reproducibility in 'routine' working situa-tions. The value of perchloric extraction and of dialysis has been debated, but it would appear to be useful in that it reduces 10-15% of the false-positive readings to normal values. On the other hand, the omission of this stage from the CIS method has not resulted in such a large proportion of excessive readings in normal subjects.

19

Reproducibility of the quantitative determination of the standards and of samples of plasma and/or serum was good with either method in the intra-kit tests, using highly standardized technical conditions. The statistical variations are of the same order as the 10 - 20% statistical error (1 SD) observed by Martin et al. (1-2) Another possible cause of lack of inter-test reproducibility might be instability of the label-ling or of the marker protein. In this regard, the fact that the differences in Bo/T values are greater for the CIS batches than for the Roche batches con-stitutes an argument in favor of the latter.

The calculated limiting sensitivity is clearly less for the CIS than for the Roche method, but since the value scales of the two methods differ at a ratio of 4:1, the inferiority of the former method in this respect is less than it seems.

Whether standard samples of one method are determined quantitatively with the reagents of the other, or the results of normal and pathological serum or plasma determined by the two methods are compared, we always find markedly higher values with the CIS than with the Roche method. The causes of this phenomenon were briefly considered during the international meeting held in Paris (3).

Possible technical reasons have been suggested by B. Meriadec and D.J.R. Laurence: loss of material in the course of dialysis, extraction of potential inhibitors during the perchloric extraction, effect of the medium used for the reaction (pH, temperature, etc.). In fact, however, the essential cause is the standard used for the calibration curve: quantitative determination of the same documented sample by the same method gives highly different results with use of different standards to trace the calibration curve (Table 1). The value that is calculated is essentially a function of the origin of the standard with which the calibration curve is esta-blished. Accordingly, one may be led astray by 'quan-titative' expression in nanograms, while expression in 'biological units', although vaguer, is more exact. Calibration of the standards of the two methods in relation to an international standard (4) might eliminate this problem.

With both methods, attempts have been made to avoid false-positive readings due either to the presence of factors that give a cross-reaction with CEA, particularly the glycoproteins of the blood groups, or to a small amount of CEA being present physiologically. With either method, the antibodies are adsorbed (against group antigens, various tissue extracts, etc). In the CIS method a small amount of a normal human plasma pool is added

to the standard used for the calibration curve so as
to reduce the values in serum or plasma from normal
subjects to an average of zero. This is only a minimal
theoretical source of error since a normal subject may
have a little more or a little less of cross-reacting
factors than the average of the population as a whole.
Furthermore, it has been shown that this correction
reduces the calculated value to different extents,
depending on the concentration of the test sample to
which an identical amount of the plasma in question
has been added. With the Roche method, this positive
reading in normal subjects is eliminated by using a
different medium to establish the reference curve than
is used to carry out the quantitative determinations,
as the result of which the figures are reduced by 6 ng
at point zero in the case of normal subjects and by over
10 ng in cases in which the CEA is markedly increased.

The many methodological factors:heterogeneity of
the CEA and of the antibodies obtained, technical
difficulties and labelling and preservation problems
that may impair the reproducibility, the need to take
into account cross-reactions in normal subjects_explain
why for either method it is difficult to define the
threshold beyond which the reading obtained should be
regarded as pathological.

From data obtained with both methods it is concluded that the threshold for positive values is low:
2-5 ng/ml for the Roche method and 10 ng/ml for the
CIS method. However, the literature contains numerous
cases of patients free from cancer in whom levels
beyond these limits were encountered: this occurs
especially in smokers, after consumption of alcohol, and
in patients with non-malignant pulmonary or digestive
diseases, and applies to both the Roch and the CIS
method. The results obtained in the few normal subjects
(hospital staff) included in the present investigation
confirm the earlier findings.

As regards the pathological cases, statistical
dispersion in itself explains 7 of the 10 cases that
are abnormal with the CIS method and normal with the
Roche method. However, even when we raise the threshold
of the Roche method to 6 ng, there are still 57 cases
in which this method gives an abnormal reading, whereas
the outcome obtained with the CIS method is either normal
(53 cases) or at the upper limit of normal (4 cases).

More clinical and developmental investigations will
be necessary to determine the significance of the
'false-positive' results obtained with the former and
the 'false-negative' results obtained with the latter
method.

Finally, it should be noted that, in the cases that are
distinctly pathological with either method, there is
considerable dispersion around the regression line even
though on the whole the findings obtained with one
method (CIS) are 2 to 3 times as high as those obtained
with the other; there are many cases in which one method
indicates a strong, and the other a slight, increase.
Here, also, clinical analyses will be necessary to
determine whether this disagreement is linked to certain
pathological phenomena (nature of the tumor, development,
treatment) and whether it will repeat itself in the
course of an individual patient's development.

CONCLUSION

The two methods differ only slightly as regards
reproducibility and sensitivity. At present, the Roche
is technically more difficult. Both methods use an
antigen that has not been proven to be specific, and the
difference between the antigens used may explain the
imperfect correlation in pathology. Certain 'tricks'
are required to eliminate the cross-reactions, and this
may explain the quite pronounced variability of the
readings obtained in normal subjects. Accordingly, the
threshold for pathological values should probably be
raised above that indicated in the literature, and the
same applics to the variations of the levels obtained
during the patients' follow-up.

These limitations will have to be kept in mind in
analysing the significance of the findings obtained in
pathological conditions.

ACKNOWLEDGEMENT

We gratefully acknowledge the support and help
rendered throughout this study by the Roche Diagnostica
Laboratories, by the Department of Radio-Elements of
the Atomic Energy Commission and by the staff of our own
department.

REFERENCES
1) MARTIN, E.W., JAMES, K.K., HURTUBISE, P.E., CATALANO, P., MINTON,
   J.P.: The use of CEA as an early indicator for gastrointestinal
   tumor recurrence and second look procedures. Cancer, 39, 440-
   446, 1977.
2) NEVILLE, A.M., LAURENCE, D.J.R.: Report of the workshop on the
   carcinoembryonic antigen (CEA): the present position and propos-
   als for future investigation. Int. J. Cancer, 14, 1-18, 1974.

3) Discussion générale (Symposium sur le CEA). <u>Bull. Cancer, 63</u>, 705-710, 1976.

4) LAURENCE, D.J.R., TUBERVILLE, C., ANDERSON, S.G., NEVILLE, M.: First British Standard for carcinoembryonic antigen (CEA). <u>Brit. J. Cancer, 32, 295-299, 1975</u>.

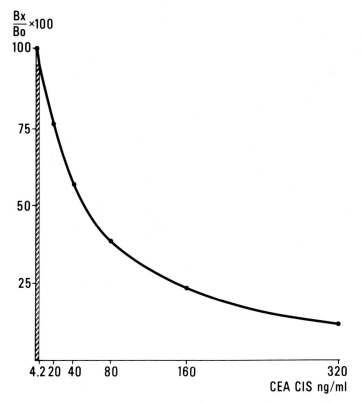

Fig. 1. CIS CEA curve in plasma medium (mean based on 10 points) using the same batch. Calculation of sensitivity at point 0.

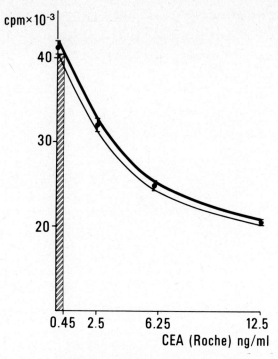

Fig. 2. Roche CEA curve in EDTA + BSA medium (mean based
on 10 points) using the same batch. Calculation
of the sensitivity at point 0.

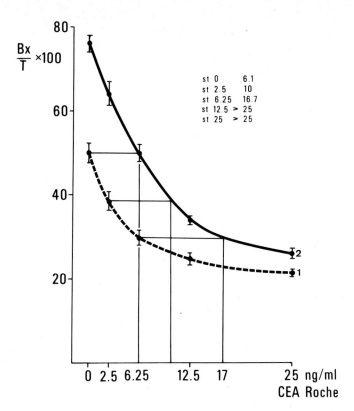

Fig. 3. Comparison of the Roche standard curve:
(1) EDTA buffer medium pH 6.5 ± 0.1 with BSA;
(2) ammonium acetate buffer medium 0.01 M
     pH 6.1 ± 0.1

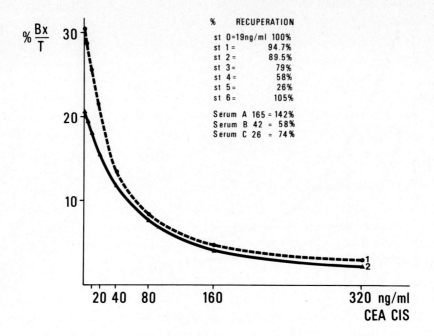

Fig. 4. Comparison of the CIS standard curve:
(1) veronal buffer medium pH 8.4 ± 0.2 + BSA
0.25%;
(2) normal human plasma

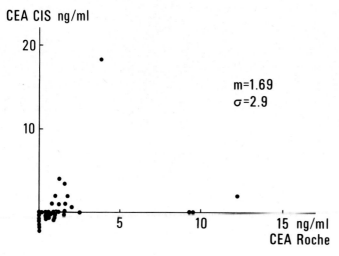

Fig. 5. 36 controls determined by the CIS and by the
Roche method.

CIS < 15 NG/ML
R < 2,5 NG/ML

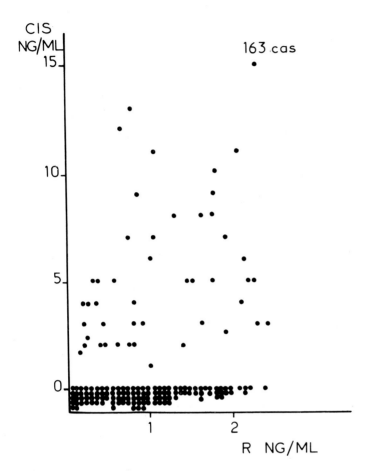

Fig. 6. 163 quantitative determinations of patient
samples, below 15 ng/ml with the CIS method and
below 2.5 ng/ml with the Roche method.

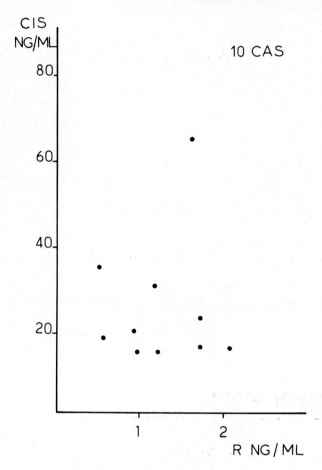

Fig. 7. 10 quantitative determinations of patient samples giving values above 15 ng/ml with the CIS method and below 2.5 ng/ml with the Roche method.

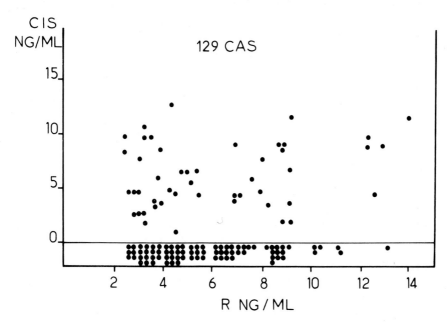

Fig. 8. 129 quantitative determinations of patient samples giving values below 15 ng/ml with the CIS method and above 2.5 ng/ml with the Roche method.

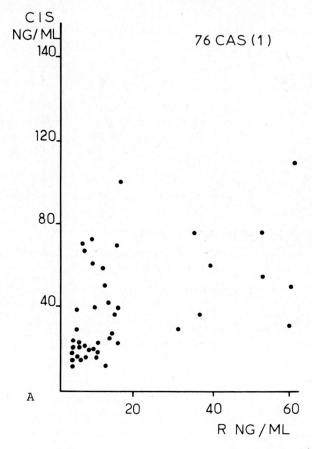

CIS > 15 NG / ML
R > 2,5NG / ML

Fig. 9. (A and B). 76 quantitative determinations of
patient samples giving values above 15 ng/ml
with the CIS method and above 2.5 ng/ml with the
Roche method.

30

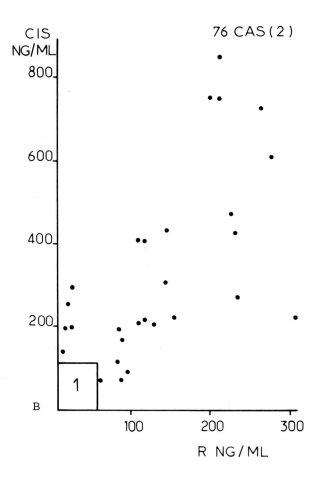

CIS > 15 NG / ML
R > 2,5 NG / ML

Fig. 9B

COMPARISON OF TWO METHODS FOR CEA DETERMINATION

G.Milano, C.Bonet, B.P.Krebs

Laboratoire de Radio-immunologie, Centre Antoine Lacassagne,
36 Voie Romaine, 06054 Nice, Cedex, France

INTRODUCTION

With the increasing interest of CEA several commercial radio-immunoassays are now available for the determination of this molecule in biological fluids.

In our Laboratory, we have been using for two years the CIS kit for blood measurement of CEA. Recently we decided to introduce the Roche Assay with the view of measuring CEA biological fluids other than plasma.

MATERIAL

CEA-CIS assay from Commissariat à l'Energie Atomique Saclay France . CEA-Roche assay from Roche France modified by ultrafiltration (system delivered by AMICON) in place of dialysis.

·RESULTS

Table 1 summarizes the respective properties of the two assays:

	CIS	ROCHE	
Perchloric acid extraction	No	Yes if CEA $<$ 25ng/ml	No if CEA $>$ 25ng/ml
Incubation			
volume (μl)	50	500	50
temperature	Room	45°	
time	28h(modif.)	1h	
Separation procedure	Double antibody	Z gel	
Range of Assay	5-640	2.5-25.0	

Figure 1 relates a study of reproductibility for the Roche Assay We measured several times the Roche quantity controls (2.5-5;5-10); more than 10). It appears that there is a small dispersion in each assay except in one case. Consequently, intra assay reproductibility is acceptable. But inter assay reproductibility is deficient and it is suggested to take into consideration the findings in quality controls to correct each assay. A series of samples (bronchial washing aspirates) have been evaluated by the two methods (fig.2). A correlation of r = 0.65 has been determined and with these two direct methods it seems that one ng of Roche is equivalent to a value between one and two ng of CIS. However, we compared simultaneous determinations obtained by indirect Roche assay and CIS. Without any doubt there is a constant difference between the results, i.e. the levels are always lower in the Roche indirect assay than with the CIS method (40 to 90 per cent of loss). We confirm this observation in the figure 3 where the recovery (40%) of the Roche indirect assay has been evaluated. We tried to give an answer to this problem in extracting a series of samples containing the same quantity of CEA (25 ng) with an increasing molarity of perchloric acid (fig.4). It appears the more perchloric acid is concentrated the more we are losing CEA. The same observation has been done before by J.J.WU et al (1).

DISCUSSION

One difference we found between the Roche and CIS methods is the problem of CEA loss with the Roche indirect assay. It seems the perchloric acid concentration used may have an influence on this phenomenon . However, this latter method is somewhat useful in the case of other biological fluids than plasma as described elsewhere by J.M.Aubanel et al. (2) . On the other hand, many serious papers have been published whose results were obtained by Roche method. In conclusion we think it is important to follow the same method all through investigations for the determination of a cut-off value between normal and pathological populations, and to take into consideration the evolutive slope of serial determinations rather than any single value.

REFERENCES

(1) Wu, J.T., et al. (1975) : Biochem.Med. 14, 305.

(2) Aubanel,J.M., Milano,G., Schneider,M., Blaive,B., Namer,M., Bonet,C., Krebs,B.P., MacDonald,E.A., Lalanne,C.M. (1978) : Proceedings, CEA Symposium, A paraître.

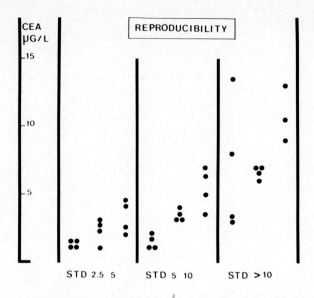

Fig.1: Intra and inter assay reproducibility for the Roche indirect CEA assay.

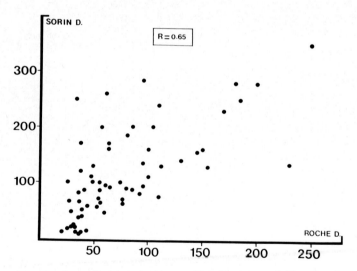

Fig.2: Correlation between the Roche and the Sorin direct methods for CEA measurements.

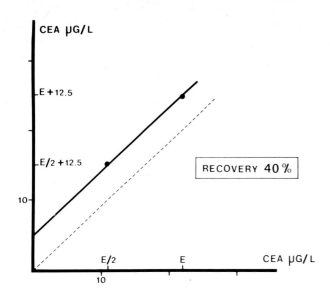

Fig.3: Study of recovery for the Roche CEA indirect assay.

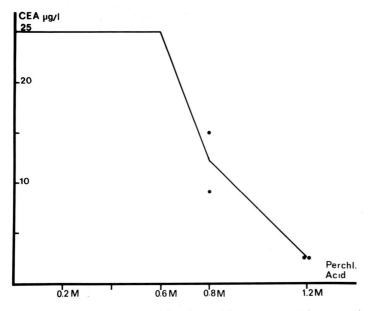

Fig.4: Effect of perchloric acid concentration on the measurement of CEA by indirect Roche assay.

DISCUSSION

MILANO G. (Nice) : You speak about reproducibility during dialysis
step. In our hand, the amicon system does not give better interassay
reproducibility.

KADOUCHE J. (Paris) : I agree with this but dialysis results in a
non negligeable immunoreactivity loss.

BOUNAMEAUX Y.(Bâle) : Concerning positive blood samples in Roche
methods and negative in CIS or reciprocally, have you data about
clinical status.

DEPIERRE A.(Paris) : We observed three groups in 19 epidermoid
bronchogenic carcinoma with no variation in CIS method : in 8 cases,
Roche method in one year follow-up showsno variation, in 6 cases,
Roche shows a non clinical related variation but in 5 cases, Roche
demonstrates a 3 to 4 months predictive values.

HEGESIPPE M. (Gif Sur Yvette) : There is, as I have said yesterday
a misunderstanding about CEA values expressed in ng without referring
to its commercial origin. Our nanograms are "CIS" ng. On the other
hand, I cannot entirely agree in increasing thresholds of positivity
proposed in the CIS system (10 ng) : in fact, on 251 non smokers
only 2% of values are positive . Dr. Krebs can confirm this incidence
of positive values (see fig. 1).

KLEISBAUER J.P. (Marseille) : Our threshold with CIS method is 40ng/ml
because in pulmonary disease, we found a lot of positive values :
mean plus 2 standard deviation gives 40ng/ml.

MASSEYEFF R. (Nice) : As all cross-reacting antigens are perchloro-
luble, why does the perchloric acid extraction step seem so necessary?

KADOUCHE J.(Paris): I cannot answer : I wonder also why this step
is performed : for other glycoproteins, like TSH or FSH, the radioimmunoassay is done directly on plasma or serum.

BURTIN P. (Villejuif) : Proteins without sugar fraction are precipi-
taded by perchloric acid, thus, this step reduces non specific inter-
ference.

SHUSTER J.(Montreal) : I was in the laboratory when the first CEA
assay was done and it was a question of choice. For particular reasons
we assumed the assay would be more sensitive and specific if the
glycoproteins were extracted from serum. In theory , if one had a
sensitive assay and wanted to do it directly without perchloric acid,
one could do so. There is no other reason for using perchloric acid.
Everyone then followed in this particular fashion.

BUFFE D. (Villejuif) : CEA and NCA are in the perchloric acid supernatant. Therefore, in CIS'method, the normal human plasma added in
the calibration curve counteracts the NCA normal present and also
a little quantity of CEA. This could explain differences between
Roche and CIS methods.

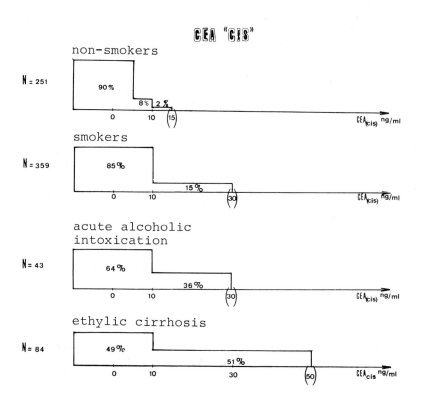

Fig. 1. CIS-CEA. Variations in threshold in non-cancerous
   populations.

IMMUNOSEROLOGIC REACTIVITY OF CEA RADIOLABELED BY TWO DIFFERENT METHODS

A. Quentmeier, B. Heymer, G. Horn and O. Haferkamp

Department of Pathology, University of Ulm, Ulm, F.R.G.

All CEA-preparations currently available exhibit heterogeneity in chemical composition, molecular size and immunologic reactivity (1,2). In addition, the CEA-molecule itself appears to possess several different antigenic groups (1,2,3), some of which cross-react with normal tissue components (3). Nevertheless, the existence of a unique CEA-specific antigenic determinant has been established (2,3,4). Therefore, it seems worthwhile to investigate all factors that potentially increase the tumor-specificity of labeled CEA-preparations used in the radio-immunoassay.

In the present studies, the hypothesis was tested that different techniques for radiolabeling might label different molecular fractions present in CEA-preparations, some of which possibly react more specifically than others.

METHODS

CEA was extracted with 1 M PCA (5) from liver metastases of patients with colon-carcinomata and purified by Sepharose 4B- and Sephadex G 200-gel filtration (5). Identically prepared CEA was kindly provided by Dr. C.W. Todd (City of Hope National Medical Center, Duarte, California, U.S.A.). Some of these preparations were further purified by concanavalin A (Con A)-chromatography (6). Equal amounts of each preparation were radiolabeled with 125-I according to the chloramine-T-method of HUNTER-GREENWOOD (7), as well as the conjugation (active ester)-procedure of BOLTON-HUNTER (8). In the former technique, tyrosine residues of CEA are directly labeled with 125-I; in the latter method an active ester is first radioiodinated and then conjugated to free amino groups of CEA (8). The immunoserologic reactivity of CEA-preparations radiolabeled according to these two different techniques (Hunter-Greenwood = HG 125-I·CEA; Bolton-Hunter = BH 125-I·CEA) was compared employing a Farr-type antigen binding assay (9), as previously described (10,11). Goat and rabbit CEA-antisera (12) were used, either non-absorbed or absorbed with human blood group A or B erythrocytes or with PCA-extracted normal liver tissue, obtained from those patients from whom the CEA was derived. In addition, normal sera and various heterologous antisera were tested: antisera to beta-hemolytic streptococci of group A (containing antibodies specific for N-acetyl-glucosamine), A variant, B, C (containing antibodies specific for N-acetyl-galactosamine), F or G, to Micrococcus luteus, to E. coli or to Candida albicans. Furthermore, the binding of the radiolabeled CEA's to the lectin concanavalin A was also studied (13).

RESULTS

CEA-preparations radiolabeled by two different methods constantly revealed distinct differences which are summarized in Figure 1. Employing identical amounts of CEA and 125-I for labeling, the specific activity of preparations radioiodinated by the HUNTER-GREENWOOD-method ranged from 12.0 to 15.7 μCi/μg, whereas that of preparations radioiodinated by the BOLTON-HUNTER procedure ranged only from 0.46 to 0.69 μCi/μg. The latter indicates the presence or availability of only a few free amino groups in CEA. In contrast to the 125-I-incorporation and the specific activity, the maximum binding of BH 125-I·CEA to CEA-antiserum as well as to Con A was considerably higher than that of HG 125-I·CEA, while the "background-binding" to normal serum did not differ significantly (Fig.1).

In Figure 2, the binding of HG and BH 125-I·CEA to serial dilutions of the same CEA-antiserum is compared. It is evident that the maximum binding of BH 125-I·CEA is higher, the slope of the binding curve steeper and the linear portion of the binding curve longer. These findings in connection with an increased sensitivity to inhibition by cold CEA indicate a greater specificity of the BH-labeled antigen.

In contrast, the slopes of the inhibition curve, which can be used as a parameter for the precision of the radioimmunoassay (8), do not differ significantly (Fig.3). It should be noted – when interpreting the latter results- that the concentration of BH 125-I·CEA employed in the inhibition assay was almost twice that of HG 125-I·CEA. Another difference between the two kinds of radiolabeled CEA's was the remarkable stability of BH 125-I·CEA. Both preparations, as revealed by Sephadex G 25-gel filtration, lost approximately 18 % of their label within two months; however, the binding capacity of BH 125-I·CEA, within the same time interval, decreased by only 1.6 % in contrast to the 35 % decrease of HG 125-I·CEA (Fig.1).

In Figure 4 data illustrating the specificity of the 125-I·CEA-preparations are summarized. Some of the differences between HG 125-I·CEA and BH 125-I·CEA previously demonstrated are also evident here. While the "background-binding" to normal rabbit serum, diluted 1:10, ranged from 10 to 14 %, the specific binding to CEA-antiserum, diluted 1:100, ranged from 70 to 80 %. Extensive absorption of CEA-antiserum with human blood group A or B erythrocytes or with PCA-extracted normal human liver did not appreciably reduce the binding. None of the heterologous antisera, including those with specificity for N-acetyl-glucosamine or N-acetyl-galactosamine, reacted markedly with either of the radioiodinated preparations. This is a good indication for the absence of measurable contamination of the CEA preparations employed with blood group A substances, since group C-streptococcal antisera are well-known to agglutinate blood group A erythrocytes (14).

In summary, data obtained in the present studies provide evidence that different molecular fractions present in commonly used CEA-preparations are labeled by the chloramine-T- and the conjugation-method. Although the specific activity of CEA radioiodinated by the latter technique is relatively low, its immunoserologic reactivity and specificity appear to exceed considerably that of CEA iodinated by the conventional Hunter-Greenwood procedure.

REFERENCES

(1) Rogers,G.T. (1976): Biochim. Biophys. Acta 458, 355.
(2) Banjo,C., Shuster,J. and Gold, P. (1974): Cancer Res. 34, 2114.
(3) Tomita,J.T., Safford,J.W. and Hirata,A.A. (1974): Immunology 26, 291.
(4) Plow,E.G. and Edgington,T.S. (1975): Int. J. Cancer 15, 748.
(5) Coligan,J.E., Lautenschleger,J.T., Egan,M.E. and Todd,C.W. (1972): Immunochemistry 9, 377.
(6) Pritchard,D.G. and Todd,C.W. (1976): Cancer Res. 36, 4699.
(7) Hunter,W.M. and Greenwood,F.C. (1962): Nature (London) 194, 495.
(8) Bolton,A.E. and Hunter,W.M. (1973): Biochem.J.133,529.
(9) Farr,R.S. (1958): J. Infect. Dis. 103, 239.
(10) Heymer,B., Bernstein,D., Schleifer,K.-H. and Krause, R.M. (1975): J. Immunol. 114, 1191.
(11) Heymer,B., Bernstein,D., Schleifer,K.-H. and Krause, R.M. (1975): Z. Immun. Forsch . 149, 168.
(12) Egan,M.L., Lautenschleger,J.T., Coligan,J.T. and Todd,C.W. (1972): Immunochemistry 9, 289.
(13) Rogers,G.T., Searle,F. and Bagshawe,K.D. (1976):

Br. J. Cancer 33, 357.
(14) Krause,R.M. (1972): Streptococci and Streptococcal
     Diseases, Academic Press, New York and London,
     1972 pp 7 - 12.

Parameters studied	Hunter – Greenwood	Bolton – Hunter
^{125}I incorporation	58.9 – 67.0 %	1.4 – 3.1 %
Specific activity	12.0 – 15.7 μCi/μg	0.46–0.69 μCi/μg
Max. binding to CEA–antiserum*	76.6 ± 5.0 %	85.0 ± 5.8 %
Max. binding to normal serum*	6.7 ± 1.1 %	5.0 ± 3.3 %
Max. binding to Con. A (10 mg/ml)*	59.3 ± 1.9 %	79.1 ± 9.1 %
Slope of inhibition curve*	24.0 %	20.5 %
Sensitivity to inhibition by CEA*	0.19 μg/ml	0.05 μg/ml
^{125}I release within 2 months	18.6 %	18.1 %
Decrease in binding capacity within 2 months	36.3 %	1.6 %

* Assay concentration: HG 0.13 μg/ml , BH 0.22 μg/ml

Fig. 1 Characteristics of CEA-preparations radiolabeled
by the Hunter-Greenwood and the Bolton-Hunter method.

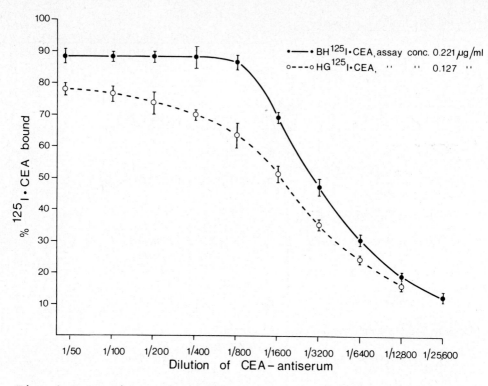

Fig. 2 Comparison of HG 125-I·CEA and BH 125-I·CEA
binding curves established with serial dilutions of the
same CEA-antiserum.

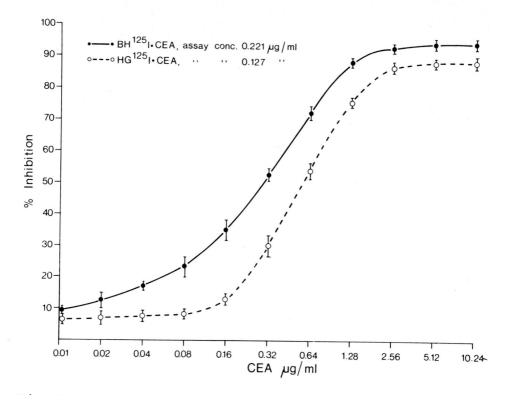

Fig. 3 Comparison of HG 125-I·CEA and BH 125-I·CEA
inhibition curves obtained by addition of cold CEA.

Sera tested	Serumdilution	HG^{125}I·CEA	BH^{125}I·CEA
Normal serum (rabbit)	1 : 1o	10.9 %	14.8 %
CEA – antiserum (rabbit):			
non – absorbed	1 : 1oo	70.1 %	80.9 %
absorbed with human erythr. (blood group A)	1 : 1oo	66.9 %	76.1 %
" " " " (" " B)	1 : 1oo	66.8 %	77.9 %
" " normal human liver (PCA extract.)	1 : 1oo	67.7 %	79.5 %
CEA – antiserum (goat)	1 : 1oo	70.7 %	80.6 %
Streptococcus – antiserum (rabbit):			
anti group A (N-ac-glucosamine-specific)	1 : 1o	8.7 %	9.7 %
" " A variant	1 : 1o	10.2 %	< 14.9 %
" " B	1 : 1o	8.7 %	n.d.
" " C (N-ac-galactosamine-specific)	1 : 1o	8.5 %	< 13.2 %
" " F	1 : 1o	7.5 %	n.d.
" " G	1 : 1o	9.5 %	n.d.
Micrococcus – antiserum (rabbit)	1 : 1o	< 11.2 %	< 11.6 %
E. coli – " "	1 : 1o	9.2 %	n.d.
Candida – albicans – " "	1 : 1o	< 9.8 %	n.d.

n.d. = not done

Fig. 4 Binding of HG 125-I·CEA and BH 125-I·CEA to non-absorbed or absorbed CEA-antisera and various bacterial antisera.

DISCUSSION

BJORKLUND B. (Stockholm) : Have you studied the role of tyrosin in the antigenicity of CEA? For example inactivation or modification of tyrosin.

QUENTMEIER A. (Ulm) : We have not done further studies, but it is likely that a modification of tyrosin will change the antigenicity of CEA.

MACH J.P. (Lausanne) : You increase the binding with excess of antibody, but at the same time, you increase your background. So you are bothered by 15% background.

QUENTMEIER A. (Ulm) : The high background comes from the normal rabbit sera and not from antibody excess. Employing other normal sera we have a background below 10%.

ISOLATION AND CHARACTERIZATION OF LOW MOLECULAR WEIGHT CEA

A. Hedin, S. Hammarström, T. Svenberg and G. Sundblad

Department of Immunology, University of Stockholm,
S-106 91 Stockholm, Sweden

ABSTRACT

A low molecular weight CEA-fraction (CEA_{low}) was purified from liver metastases of colo-rectal cancer. The purification procedure involved the following steps: PCA-extraction-ion exchange chromatography-Con A affinity chromatography-gelfiltration on Sephadex G-200 (x2)-affinity chromatography on specific anti-CEA immunoadsorbent-gelfiltration on Sephadex G-200.

Purified CEA_{low} was homogeneous on gelfiltration in 6M guanidine HCl and gave a single band on SDS-PAGE. It consisted of a single polypeptide chain and had a lower molecular weight than CEA (125,000 and 175,000 respectively, SDS-PAGE). CEA_{low} contained the same sugars and amino acids as CEA in approximately the same molar proportions. However, the carbohydrate content of CEA_{low} was lower. Polypeptide relatedness (expressed in $S\Delta Q$ units) showed that CEA_{low} was most closely related to CEA followed by NCA and BGP-I.

CEA_{low} and CEA gave a reaction of identity with 7/9 monkey anti-CEA sera. 2/9 monkey anti-CEA sera showed a weak spur, with CEA spurring over CEA_{low}. CEA_{low} spurred over NCA and BGP-I with unabsorbed rabbit and sheep anti-CEA sera. CEA_{low} and CEA gave a reaction of identity with a rabbit anti-CEA_{low} serum. This antiserum did not precipitate with NCA or BGP-I.

INTRODUCTION

Carcinoembryonic antigen (CEA) from liver metastases of colo-rectal cancer was found to be heterogeneous on gelfiltration showing a major peak (CEA) with a more or less pronounced shoulder at the descending limb (CEA_{low}). With some anti-CEA sera the low molecular weight material showed only partial immunological identity with the high molecular weight material.

In this paper we present the isolation and characterization of CEA_{low} and describe its chemical and immunochemical relationship to CEA, NCA (nonspecific crossreactive antigen) (1,2,3) and BGP-I (biliary glycoprotein I) (3,4).

chain since reduced and alkylated CEA_{low} eluted at the same volume on gelfiltration as the untreated sample.

The amino acid and carbohydrate composition of CEA_{low} was closely similar to that of CEA. The carbohydrate content of CEA_{low} was, however, lower than that of CEA (30–45% and 45–55%, respectively), Table 1. CEA_{low} and CEA lacked N-acetyl-galactosamine and methionine. CEA_{low} was precipitated by the same lectins as CEA i.e. wheat germ agglutinin (WGA), Ricinus communis agglutinin I (RCA_I) and leucoagglutinin from Phaseolus vulgaris (La) but not with Helix pomatia A hemagglutinin (HP) (3,6).

The polypeptides of CEA, CEA_{low}, NCA and BGP-I were closely related as determined from their amino acid compositions, Table 1. When compared to CEA, CEA_{low} was most closely related (S$\triangle$Q values of 5–7) followed by NCA (S$\triangle$Q values of 12–17) and BGP-I (S$\triangle$Q values of 35–40). Unrelated proteins do not give S$\triangle$Q values less than 50.

In immunodiffusion with spleen absorbed rabbit and sheep anti-CEA sera and with most monkey anti-CEA sera CEA_{low} gave a reaction of identity with CEA. However, with 2/9 monkey anti--CEA sera CEA spurred over CEA_{low} (Fig. 3). None of the nine monkey anti-CEA sera precipitated with NCA or BGP-I. With unabsorbed rabbit and sheep anti-CEA sera CEA_{low} gave a reaction of partial identity with NCA and BGP-I (CEA_{low} spurring over NCA and BGP-I). Rabbit anti-NCA serum precipitated weakly with CEA_{low} but not at all after absorption of this antiserum with CEA_{low} (Fig. 3). One rabbit anti-CEA_{low} serum was prepared. This antiserum gave a reaction of identity between CEA_{low} and CEA. Most interestingly, however, the antiserum did not precipitate with NCA (Fig. 3).

When compared in an enzyme linked immunoadsorbent assay (ELISA) with immunoadsorbent purified monkey anti-CEA antibodies CEA_{low} showed about half the activity of CEA when compared on a weight basis. It was, furthermore, noted that the inhibition curves were not parallel. NCA did not inhibit at a 500 times higher concentration.

No difference between the two CEA_{low} preparations has been noted in the different immunological and physico-chemical tests applied so far.

DISCUSSION

The chemical and immunochemical analysis show that CEA_{low} is not contaminated with CEA, NCA or BGP-I to any significant degree. CEA_{low} is closer related to CEA than to NCA and BGP-I. However, molecular weight determinations show that CEA_{low} is distinct from CEA. Both CEA_{low} and CEA lacked methionine in contrast to NCA. CEA_{low} gave a reaction of identity with CEA

MATERIALS AND METHODS

CEA_{low} was purified from two individual liver metastases of colo-rectal cancer using the procedure shown in Fig. 1. CEA was purified from these tumors and from additional tumors of the same origin. NCA was purified from pooled adult spleens (S-NCA) and lungs (L-NCA) and BGP-I from normal human bile (3).

Antisera were raised in rabbits (CEA_{low}, CEA, NCA, BGP-I) sheep (CEA) and monkeys (CEA) by 3-5 intramuscular injections of 50-200 µg of purified antigen in Freund's complete adjuvant. The IgG fraction from rabbit and monkey antisera was prepared by protein A-Sepharose affinity chromatography. Sheep IgG was prepared by $(NH_4)_2SO_4$ precipitation followed by DEAE-cellulose chromatography. Monkey anti-CEA antibodies was purified on an immunoadsorbent column, containing CEA covalently bound to Sepharose 4B. Sheep and rabbit anti-CEA sera were used unabsorbed or after absorbtion with 1M perchloric extract of human spleen (3-5x10 mg/ml antiserum). One anti-NCA serum was absorbed with PCA extract of tumor with low CEA and NCA content until specific for NCA as tested by immunodiffusion.

Molecular weights were determined by gradient polyacrylamide gel electrophoresis (7,5-15%) in sodium dodecylsulphate using a discontinous buffer system and by gelfiltration on Sepharose 4B in 6M guanidine HCl. In both analysis reduced and alkylated 125I-labelled samples were studied. Molecular weights were determined from mobility (PAGE) and K_{av}-value (gelfiltration) by comparison to a series of 7 standard proteins. Hexoses and methylpentoses were determined by gas/liquid chromatography as their alditol acetates. Amino acids and hexosamines were quantified on an amino acid analyser after hydrolysis of samples at 110°C for 24 hr. Half-cystine and methionine were determined after performic acid oxidation. Polypeptide relatedness between CEA_{low}, CEA, NCA and BGP-I was calculated from their amino acid compositions by the statistical method of Marchalonis and Weltman (5).

RESULTS

Purified CEA_{low} gave a single band on SDS-PAGE (Fig. 2) and a single homogeneous peak on gelfiltration in 6M guanidine HCl and in phosphate buffered saline, pH 7.3.

Molecular weights of CEA_{low}, CEA, NCA and BGP-I are presented in Table 1. Molecular weights were determined by SDS-PAGE and gelfiltration on Sepharose 4B in 6M guanidine HCl. The two methods gave similar values for CEA (170-180,000) and BGP-I (80-90,000) but not for CEA_{low} and NCA. The values for CEA_{low} was 125,000 and 90,000 (SDS-PAGE and gelfiltration, respectively). For NCA the values were 115,000 and 60,000, respectively. The lower NCA-value (60,000) is in accordance with data presented by others (2). CEA_{low} appears to consist of a single polypeptide

47

with most anti-CEA sera tested. However, with 2/9 monkey anti-
-CEA sera CEA showed a weak spur over CEA_{low} indicating that
CEA_{low} may lack antigenic determinants present in CEA. Anti-
-CEA_{low} serum did not detect unique CEA_{low} determinants indicating that CEA_{low} may be derived from CEA.

CEA_{low} has a lower molecular weight and appears less glycosylated than CEA. It may also have a shorter polypeptide chain,
however, direct evidence for this is lacking.

CEA_{low} may originate from cleavage of CEA in vivo or be a
less glycosylated form of CEA. It appears unlikely that CEA_{low}
is formed during PCA extraction since we have shown that purified CEA is resistant to 1M PCA for up to 3 hr at 40°C. Our
purification procedure includes PCA extraction at 4°C. The presence of CEA_{low} was studied in four individual tumors. It was
found in significant amounts in two tumors, in small amounts in
the third and in trace amounts in the fourth tumor. These data
may indicate that in vivo degradation determines the presence of
CEA_{low}.

The isolation of a large natural fragment of CEA may be
helpful in the analysis of the covalent structure of CEA. It may
also be of use in the identification and localization of different antigenic determinants.

ACKNOWLEDGEMENTS

We thank Ms. Sari Feld for skillful technical assistance.
This work was supported by a grant from the Swedish Cancer
Society (no. 706-B76-04XA).

REFERENCES

(1) Von Kleist, S., Chavanel, G. and Burtin, P. Proc. Nat. Acad.
    Sci. USA 69, 2492, 1972.
(2) Mach, J.-P. and Pusztaszeri, G. Immunochem. 9, 1031, 1972.
(3) Hammarström, S., Svenberg, T., Hedin, A. and Sundblad, G.
    Scand. J. Immunol., suppl. 6. 1977 (in press).
(4) Svenberg, T. Int. J. Cancer 17, 588, 1976.
(5) Marchalonis, J. and Weltman, J. Comp. Biochem. Physiol. 38,
    (B), 609, 1971.
(6) Hammarström, S., Engvall, E., Johansson, B., Svensson, S.,
    Sundblad, G. and Goldstein, I. J. Proc. Nat. Acad. Sci.
    USA 72, 1528, 1975.

TABLE 1 Chemical and physicochemical properties of CEA_{low}, CEA, NCA and BGP-I

	CEA_{low}	CEA	NCA	BGP-I
Mol.wt.x10^{-3} (SDS–PAGE)	125$\pm$6	175$\pm$8	115$\pm$7	83$\pm$4
Mol.wt.x10^{-3} (Seph.4B, 6M GuaHCl)	90	170	60	94
Carbohydrate (%)[*]	29–38	46–54	22–33	38–43
Polypeptide relatedness as compared to CEA, sample 1. (SΔQ units)	5,0–7,1	1,0–2,5	12,0–17,2	34,9–39,6

[*]Carbohydrate % = $\dfrac{\text{residue weight CHO}}{\text{residue weight CHO + aa}}$ x 100. Tryptophane and sialic acid not included. The following monosaccharides were found in all samples: fucose, mannose, galactose and N–acetyl-glucosamine. CEA_{low} 2 samples; CEA 7 samples; NCA 3 samples and BGP-I 2 samples.

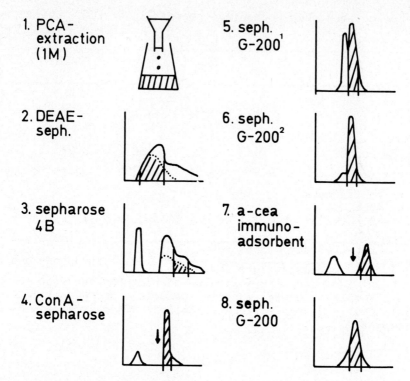

1. PCA-
   extraction
   (1M)

2. DEAE-
   seph.

3. sepharose
   4B

4. ConA-
   sepharose

5. seph.
   G-200^1

6. seph.
   G-200^2

7. a-cea
   immuno-
   adsorbent

8. seph.
   G-200

Fig. 1 Purification of CEA_{low} from liver metastases of colo-rectal cancer. The shaded areas indicate CEA_{low}-active material as
determined by fused rocket immunoelectrophoresis and ELISA
(dotted line in steps 2 and 3). The solid line shows optical density at 280 nm. Material was pooled as indicated by lines through
the abscissa.

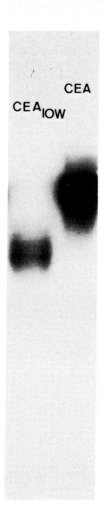

Fig. 2 Sodium dodecylsulphate-polyacrylamide gel electrophoresis
(7,5-15%) of purified CEA_{low} (left) and CEA (right) after complete reduction.

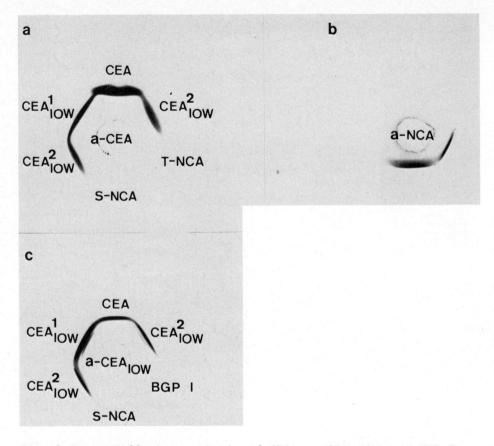

Fig. 3 Immunodiffusion analysis of CEA_{low}, CEA, NCA and BGP-I with monkey anti-CEA serum (a), rabbit anti-NCA serum (b) and rabbit anti-CEA_{low} serum (c) in central wells. Antigens added as indicated in figure.

DISCUSSION

VON KLEIST S. (Villejuif) : I was struck by the fact that your NCA has about twice the molecular weight usually given by the authors (Did you have any explanation for that, i.e. bimer formation?).

HEDIN A. (Stockholm) : We have determined the molecular weight of NCA by SDS-PAGE and by gel filtration in 6 M guanidine hydrochloride and we get 115.000 and 60.000 respectively. We have as yet no explanation for this discrepancy. CEA gives 175.000 with both methods. The higher M.W. for NCA is in accordance with that found by Engvall et al.: Normal crossreacting antigen, NCA. Chemical basis for its immunological crossreaction with CEA. 5th IRGCP meeting Copenhagen ,Aug.1977.

RAPP W. (Heidelberg) : Ruoslahti showed that monkey do not react with NCA. Could this be the explanation for your non-reactivity with NCA like substances?

HEDIN A. (Stockholm) : Well, what I was trying to show with my monkey antiCEA antiserum was that CEA-low really precipitates with this antiserum and NCA does not precipitate.

CLINICAL INTEREST OF NCA (NON SPECIFIC CROSS REACTING ANTIGEN)

S. von Kleist, and M. King

Institut de Recherches Scientifiques sur le Cancer, 94800 Villejuif, France.

In human colonic tumors three main antigens have been characterized, the most famous of which is the CEA (carcinoembryonic antigen), discovered more than ten years ago by Gold and Freedman (1). Since then many antigens have been described in literature which were said to crossreact with CEA, but only few of them have been sufficiently purified as to allow further studies of their physico-chemical nature and eventual medical interest. NCA is a substance which has been published independantly under six different names : We named it according to its relationship with the CEA nonspecific crossreacting antigen (NCA) (2) ; the other abbreviations are NGP (Normal Glycoprotein) given by Mach and Pusztaszeri (3), CCAIII (Newman et al., 4) and CE-X, alias CCEA-2 used by Darcy et al. (5) and Turberville et al. (6) and Beta E by Ørjasaeter (7). These six antigens are immunochemically identical. The NCA is regularely present in PCA extracts of human tumors and it is a tenacious contaminant of CEA preparations in which it is difficult to detect, because of the strikingly similar properties and shared immunoreactive sites on the two molecules. Both antigens, however, are distinguishable by their molecular weight and by their individual antigenic determinants which permit their specific detection in tissues and fluids, in which CEA and NCA are distributed in a ubiquitous fashion.

Since we showed that NCA (like CEA) circulated in the blood of healthy individuals, and subsequently also in benignly or malignantly diseased patients, we asked the question, wether this antigen might bear any clinical importance comparable to that of CEA, specially in respect to oncology. So we assayed 300 patients' sera by the RIA, using a micromethod on whole serum and the double antibody technique adapted from Laurence et al. (8) to measure both antigens in parallel. The sera were divided into three groups : 1. controls, 2. non cancerous diseases, 3. cancers. All results have been statistically evaluated, in order to precise the following questions :

- Is there any relationship (or dependancy) between the serum levels of the two antigens, as observed on a single trial basis and/or during the evolution of a neoplastic affection ?
- Are there statistically significant differences between antigen values in blood donors' sera and patients having cancerous or non cancerous diseases, and finally,
- Is there a relationship between factors like blood group, sex, or age and the NCA and CEA serum levels ?

As far as the first question is concerned it has been proved statistically, that the serum values of the two antigens in all three groups, are not significantly linked. The coefficient of correlation is 0.77 for the blood donors, (Fig. 1) of whom we studied 51, and for the two other groups 0.51 and 0.56 respectively (Fig. 2). Yet it was in this group where at first view a rather satisfactory correlation has been stated. Having obtained quite dispersed values ranging from 30-510 ng/ml in the donors of whom we knew only that they were hepatitis free, we chose 150 ng/ml as cut off point for "normal" for our clinical studies, though the average value obtained was 130 ng/ml. Then 35% of our donors had elevated NCA serum levels which is quite comparable to the 31 % observed for CEA, for which we chose 4 ng/ml as upper normal limit.

In order to answer the second question, we compared average values obtained in the two groups of patients (non malignant diseases: 90 cases, cancers : 95 cases) with the controls. The difference is highly significant between the controls and the two groups of patients. However, between cancerous and non cancerous diseases no significant difference had been observed.

If it is now widely accepted that there is a critical upper CEA serum value above which the presence of neoplasia in the patient is more than likely ; there is nothing the like with NCA : this antigen is generally little augmented in malignancy and 2/3 of the tumors fall into a zone of moderate elevation of 150-260 ng/ml. Apparently this is a typical phenomenon, because carcinomas, analyzed organ by organ, also follow this pattern. T. Edgington (personal communication) has made similar observations. So we wanted to know whether malignancy would diminish-rather than augment-NCA. We chose pulmonary affections for this study, because lung tissue is particularely rich in NCA. We looked also at liver diseases known to be frequently accompanied by serum glycoprotein disturbances. Results can be summarized as follows: NCA was augmented in all (31) cases of benign lung carcinomas, in whom augmentation is not the rule. Hence NCA measurements are not a means for detecting a cancer developing in a chronic pulmonary affection. In contrast, in hepatic illnesses NCA is rarely elevated, i.e. in about 30 % , which is the same percentage observed in our controls.

Digestive tract diseases form an intermediate group : again half of the intestinal and gastric carcinomas are only moderately augmented. Here we had the possibility to verify the "behaviour" in cancer of NCA in a horizontal study thanks to Prof. E. Cooper, Univ. of Leeds, who graciouly furnished us 55 serum samples representing 12 cases of colonic cancer cases. We could thus prove that NCA, indeed, augments very little as compared to CEA and that it levels off at around 130-150 ng/ml. As to the last question : we could not find any liaison between the age or blood groups and the two tested antigens in any of the three groups. As far as sex is concerned, there were significantly higher NCA serum values in men than in women (p = 0.002) in non cancerous diseases, while for CEA there was no difference noted. In the cancer group the CEA had significantly higher avarage values in men than in women. Wether this holdstrue in larger series leaves to be seen.

So in conclusion we can say that, since it is above all the existence of a significant difference in the antigen serum levels in cancerous and non cancerous diseases that bestow clinical importance on an antigen in oncology, it is evident that NCA has little if any. NCA measurements cannot -not more than CEA- distinguish between a malignant and benign affection. Nevertheless : perhaps NCA will be of some use in the handling of pulmonary diseases one day.

REFERENCES

(1) Gold, Ph, and Freedman, S.(1965) : J. Exp. Med. 122, 467
(2) von Kleist, S., Chavanel, G. and Burtin, P. (1972) : Proc. Natl Acad. Sci. (USA) 69, 2492
(3) Mach, J.P., and Pusztaszeri, G. (1972) : Immunochem. 9, 1031
(4) Newman, S.E., Petras, J.G., Hamilton, H.J. et al. (1972) : Fed. Proc. 31, 639
(5) Darcy, D.A.,Turberville, D., and James, R. (1973) : Brit. J. Cancer 28, 147
(6) Turberville, C., Darcy, D.A., Laurence, D.J., et al. (1973) : Immunochemistry, 10, 841
(7) Ørjasaeter, H., Frederiksen, G. and Liavag, J. (1974) : Acta Path. Microbiol. Scand. (B) 82, 387
(8) Laurence, D., Stevens, D., Bettelheim, U. et al. (1972) : Brit. Med. J. 3, 405

CEA & NCA values in(N)donors' sera

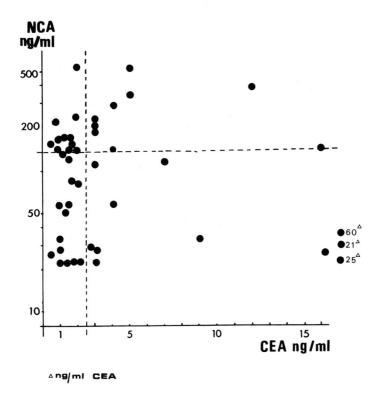

Fig. 1 Relationship of CEA and NCA serum values in blood donors' sera.

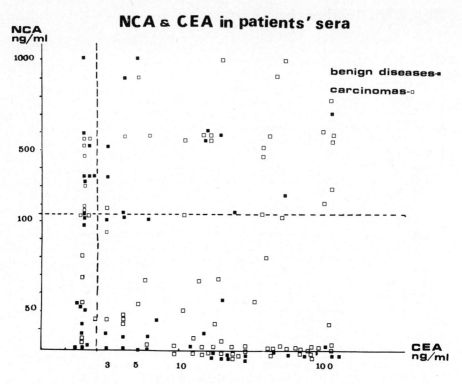

Fig. 2 Relationship of CEA and NCA serum values in the sera of patients with non cancerous diseases and carcinomas.

DISCUSSION

COOPER E.H. (Leeds) : Do you think, because the values become asymptomatic, that a feed back control mechanism stops rising after a certain level?

VON KLEIST S. (Villejuif) : I do not believe that : I think the mechanism might be that the NCA gets triggered off and just goes on on this certain level. If there was a feed back then there should be some fluctuations of NCA, but we have never seen that.

RAPP W. (Heidelberg) : I want to demonstrate that recent findings concerning NCA like substances, or better "commonsite antibodies" (Primus, J. et al. Immunol. 118,55,1977) seem to be much more important than hitherto assumed :
i) commonsite antibodies are excellent markers in immunohistology for leukocytes (PMN) and monocytes as demonstrated by Burtin et al.

ii)Using these marker antibodies we could demonstrate that in normal gastric mucosa there are no PMN, but only in heavy inflammatory states, especially in tumour adjacent mucosa we have observed PMN.

iii)Areas with CEA positive dysplastic and intestinalized cells show less leukocyte infiltration.

TISSUE POLYPEPTIDE ANTIGEN; REVIEW OF PHYSICAL CHEMISTRY AND CLINICAL APPLICATION

Bertil Björklund

Cancer Immunology Section, National Bacteriological Laboratory, Stockholm, Sweden

TPA is a specific single chain polypeptide isolated from a large variety of human malignant tumors and from placenta (1). TPA has a molecular weight of approx. 25 000 and possesses a number of characteristic properties such as fluorescence at 350 nm, when excited at 288 nm, absorbance at 230 nm, and solubility at low pH.

TPA is fairly well characterized chemically; the sequence of more than one hundred of its amino acids is known (2). On the basis of the extracted knowledge it has been possible to synthesize peptides with specific activity in the TPA test. An example of an active sequence is given here:

Ala Leu Leu Asn Asp Glu Leu Ala Gln Tyr Leu Asp Leu
Val Arg Ala Leu Glu Ala Ala Asn Gly Arg Leu Glu Val

The most dominating amino acids in TPA are glutamic acid, aspartic acid, and leucin. The specific immunologic activity is independent of tryptophan and cysteine but dependent on tyrosine and arginine. Modification of tyrosine with iodine leads to inactivation up to 85 % with regard to monospecific antibody. Modification of arginine with cyclohexandione leads to complete inactivation of the molecule. This effect can to a large extent be reversed with hydroxylamine. The lysine amino groups are insensitive, which has made it possible to use the Bolton-Hunter reagent and attach iodine to TPA without disturbing the sensitive tyrosine site. It has also been possible to label TPA with fluorescein isothiocyanate without loss of activity.

CD-studies in conjunction with studies of the effect of various denaturating compounds and also the specific activity of short synthetic peptides indicate that the specific determinant of TPA is of a sequential nature and not a conformational one (3).

TPA is determined routinely by means of a modified, standardized hemagglutination inhibition technique (1). Microquantities are used (25 and 50 µl). In brief, TPA in sample inhibits the ability of the antiserum (anti-TPA) to agglutinate sheep red blood cells (SRBC) that are labelled with TPA. The specimen is titrated by serial dilution in five steps and 25 µl anti-TPA serum is added to each dilution. Then SRBC labelled with TPA are added and will form a thin, agglutinated film on the bottom of the reaction well unless the anti-TPA serum is neutralized by TPA in the specimen.

The reproducibility of the technique has been studied within and between laboratories and within and between different individuals who

performed and read the test. A total of 500 human sera were each
divided in aliquots of 200 µl and stored at -90°C. The TPA value of
the sera varied from negative to strongly positive. The sera were
derived from blood donors, patients with cancer and patients with
other diseases than cancer. In 59 cases pools of serum were tested.
As a measure of the reproducibility the correlation coefficient (r)
was used. The correlation was 0.99 when duplicate tests were
performed on absorbed sera. Within and between laboratories the
correlation was 0.9. Within and between different individuals a
higher figure was obtained. Thus, the reproducibility of the
hemagglutination inhibition test for TPA is satisfactory.

Conversion tables for convenient reading of the TPA values have
been constructed from inhibition curves illustrating how various
amounts of TPA inhibit different concentrations of anti-TPA. New
instruments, which have been developed, in conjunction with
standardization of the procedures have made the hemagglutination
inhibition quantitative and opened up new possibilities for further
studies.

So far free TPA has been determined. For some time, however, it
has been hypothesized that TPA reacts with anti-TPA antibody in the
blood stream and that immune complexes are being formed. Recently a
procedure was worked out to release TPA from such complexed antibody,
thus making it possible to determine the total amount of TPA in serum.
Preliminary results indicate that the ratio between free and total
TPA is different for different groups of patients and that a maximum
is reached beyond which the ratio decreases. Healthy blood donors
exhibit a fairly constant ratio, while changes can be seen in cancer.
These findings together with analyses of free anti-TPA antibody will
continue. They may throw additional light on the formation and
breakdown of TPA and anti-TPA.

TPA is present in the membrane structures of human cancer cells.
It can be detected there by the effect of cytotoxic antibodies, or by
the localization of fluorescent or peroxidase-labelled monospecific
anti-TPA antibodies. Tumor cells like HeLa-cells in culture exhibit
typical membrane fluorescence.

TPA is released from growing and multiplying human cancer cells
in vitro and can be specifically demonstrated in the culture medium.
Human cancer tumors in general, regardless of type and origin have
been found to contain large amounts of TPA. Several hundred
individual tumors have been analyzed and no significant exceptions
have been found. These observations are corroborated by clinical
studies, which have revealed that TPA is present in serum in most
cancer patients, regardless of type and site of the cancer. Thus, TPA
is released from a wide spectrum of cancerous tumors. Healthy persons,
on the other hand, rarely exhibit positive levels of TPA in serum (1).

High levels of TPA were found in each of more than a hundred
individual placentae. TPA has also been found in high concentrations
in various fetal organs such as liver, the intestinal tract and in
the urine. TPA has also been found in mother's milk, ascitic fluid
and other body fluids.

TPA is present also in a wide variety of different animal species
ranging from apes through hoofed animals and rodents, down to
different fishes but not in a number of bacterial strains (4).

A number of clinical studies have been performed in various

hospitals and countries in order to test the possibility that TPA may
be of use as a monitor of cancerous diseases and various other
diseases as well (5).

Initially, more than 3,000 patients were studied clinically and
in the laboratory by blind and double-blind techniques (1). The
patients were classified in groups. The percentage of individuals
or samples with elevated TPA in serum within the different groups
was established. Values higher than or equal to 0.09 U TPA/ml of
serum were considered to represent antigenemia, while all lower
values were considered negative. This arbitrary borderline was used
throughout. The highest percentage of antigenemia was obtained for
the group "cancer with metastases" (73 ± 10%) and the lowest
percentage for the group "healthy persons" and "blood donors"
(2 ± 1%). For the 760 blood donors the percentage of antigenemia was
1 ± 1 %. Similar findings were made by Menendez-Botet and Schwartz
(6) who reported 378 of 513 cancer patients as TPA-positive, which
corresponds to 74 %. They too found a high percentage of positivity
in a multitude of different types of cancers.

Consecutive studies of human cancer cases have demonstrated that
a persistent elevation or a steady increase of TPA reflects the
progressive nature of the disease (7, 8). In benign diseases clinical
investigations have shown that elevated TPA values are temporary and
that TPA returns to normal: Lundström et al studied 2,632 patients in
Eskilstuna, Sweden during the period 1971-1975 with regard to
clinical conditions and TPA (9). The patients were grouped in
infectious diseases, other non-malignant diseases, cancer mixed
group and healthy individuals. The patients in the two first groups
represented 101 different diseases. During illness 22-25 % were
positive. Repeated testing showed that there was a significant drop
of TPA-positives among the benign cases. This was in contrast to the
cancer group.

Mattsson and Borgström performed a blind study of consecutive
patients with metastatic mammary carcinomas (10). TPA was analyzed
prior to every course of chemotherapy and monthly during hormonal
treatment. They found that TPA decreased in patients who responded
well to cytostatic therapy. By contrast TPA increased in patients with
a poor response to treatment.

The prognostic value of TPA has been studied by Eklund et al
(11, 12). Among 372 cases of cancer of various types, stages,
localizations, and different types of therapy, 190 died. The others
were followed for up to 4 years, with a median follow-up period of
12 months. All patients were grouped in four classes with respect
to their serum TPA values. A considerably lower mortality was
observed in the negative class as compared to each one of the other
classes. Within the class with the highest values of TPA 80 %
mortality was seen in 5 months. The analyses demonstrated that high
values of TPA in patients with a diagnosis of cancer preceded a high
rate of mortality and that low values of TPA were indicative of a
low mortality rate. The correlation between mortality and TPA was
statistically very highly significant and neither related to type
and site of the cancers nor to therapy.

61

SUMMARY

Determination of TPA in serum may be of value in the management of the patient when cancer is suspected or diagnosed. Measurements of the level of TPA can be used to monitor the effect of carcinostatic and/or other treatment of cancer; it may also be possible to obtain an early indication of tumor recurrence or the presence of undetected metastases. There is a highly significant correlation between the TPA level in serum and survival in cancer; a therapeutically induced decrease of TPA may be a favourable sign with regard to prognosis.

A single TPA determination is not a test for malignancy; it is rather an indication of the degree of proliferation of cells in the organism. Since termporary elevations of TPA are seen in certain benign diseases and steadily increasing levels are observed only in progressive cancer, repeated testing for TPA may establish the nature of observed elevations.

ACKNOWLEDGEMENT

This work was supported by the Swedish State, The Bonnier Group, the Folksam, and the County of Södermanland, Sweden.

REFERENCES

(1) Björklund, B., Björklund, V., Wiklund, B., Lundström, R., Ekdahl, P.H., Hagbard, L., Kaijser, K., Eklund, G. and Lüning, B. (1973): Immunological Techniques for Detection of Cancer, 1973. pp. 133-187, Bonniers, Stockholm.
(2) Lüning, B., Redelius, P., Wiklund, B. and Björklund, B. (1976): Onco-Developmental Gene Expression, 1976. pp. 773-777, Academic Press, New York.
(3) Lüning, et al (1977): The Annual Meeting of the Swedish Medical Association 1977.
(4) Björklund, B., Björklund, V., Lundström, R. and Eklund, G. (1976): Advances in Experimental Medicine and Biology, Vol. 73B: The Reticuloendothelial System in Health and Disease: Immunologic and Pathologic Aspects, 1976. pp. 357-370, Plenum Press, New York.
(5) Björklund, B. (1977): Antibiotics and Chemotherapy, 1977. pp. 97-112, Vol. 22, S. Karger, Basel.
(6) Schwartz, M.K. (1976): Report from Sloan-Kettering Institute, Clinical Bulletin, 6, pp. 62-68, No. 2.
(7) Björklund, B., Lundström, R., Eklund, G. and Lüning, B. (1973): Immunological Techniques for Detection of Cancer, 1973. pp. 237-242, Bonniers, Stockholm.
(8) Lundström, R., Björklund, B., and Eklund, G. (1973): Immunological Techniques for Detection of Cancer, 1973. pp. 243-247, Bonniers, Stockholm.
(9) Björklund, B. (1976): Onco-Developmental Gene Expression, 1976. pp. 501-508, Academic Press, New York.
(10) Mattsson, W. and Borgström, S. (1976): 3rd International Symposium on Detection and Prevention of Cancer, April 26 - May 1, 1976, New York.

(11) Eklund, G., Björklund, B. and Lundström, R. (1975): The Folksam
     Symposium on TPA, November 13-14, 1975, Stockholm.
(12) Björklund, B. (1976): Protides of the Biological Fluids, 1976.
     pp. 505-512, Pergamon Press, Oxford.

DISCUSSION

VON KLEIST S. (Villejuif): Do you have any idea about tumour staging
and the positivity of TPA. Do you know if a T1 NO MO would give
a positive test.

BJORKLUND B. (Stockholm): Some authors found correlation between
the differentiation of the tumours and the level of TPA. The size
of the tumour is probably reflected by TPA. A big tumour produces
higher values.

CEA IN DIAGNOSIS, PROGNOSIS, DETECTION OF RECURRENCE, AND
EVALUATION OF THERAPY OF COLO-RECTAL CANCER*

Norman Zamcheck, M.D.

Chief, Mallory Gastrointestinal Research Laboratory, Boston City
Hospital and Associate Clinical Professor of Medicine, Harvard
Medical School, Boston, Massachusetts

INTRODUCTION

In his introductory remarks, Dr. Lalanne stated that the aim of
this Symposium was to define the practical clinical applications of
the CEA assay. It is impossible to review the present status of CEA
in all digestive tract cancers. Hence, I shall concentrate on a few
aspects which appear to me to have practical clinical potential.

The initial studies of Gold and co-workers were performed on
colo-rectal cancer (1) and by far the greatest amount of subsequent
work has also been done on this malignancy. Contrary to the initial
hopes for a specific test for the detection of early cancer, the
studies from many laboratories have established the fact that the
CEA assay is a good indicator of invasive colonic cancer, and particularly of metastases to the liver (2,3). CEA elevation in
patients with localized disease (Dukes Stage A) occurs in less than
50% of patients.

The circulating CEA level depends upon several factors, including the pathological stage and the degree of differentiation of the
primary tumor, the presence of invasion of lymphatics, blood vessels
or perineural spaces, the extent of distant spread of tumor, and the
total mass of CEA-producing tumor (4). We believe the involvement of
the liver and its functional status is of especial importance (5).

PROGNOSIS AND DETECTION OF RECURRENCE

The CEA assay has proved to be a useful index of prognosis. The
higher the pre-operative level the poorer the prognosis. While a low
or normal pre-operative determination does not guarantee a localized
tumor, a markedly elevated level is consistent with widespread metastases especially to the liver (2,3).

Herrera, Chu and Holyoke showed that only 1 of 20 patients with
a pre-operative CEA level less than 2.5 ng/ml recurred in 18 months
compared with 7 of 9 patients with levels above 7 ng/ml who had recurrences within 2 to 4 months. Six of 11 patients with CEA levels
between 2.6 and 7.0 had a mean recurrence time of 11 months (6).

*Supported in part by Grant CA-04486 from the National Cancer Insti-
tute and IM-18 from the American Cancer Society.

These workers compared the prognostic and post-operative monitoring capabilities of CEA assay with (a) pathological staging of the
tissue specimens and (b) with clinical and laboratory follow up, including DNCB testing and alkaline phosphatase and transaminase measurements. CEA was considered superior to Dukes staging and TNM
staging. In addition it was easier to do, faster and more economi-
cal. It was also superior in prompt recognition of recurrence.
A pre-operative CEA greater than 4.5 predicted a greater than 80%
chance of recurrence within 18 months of resection. Alkaline phosphatase and SGOT levels correlated poorly with presence or absence of
recurrence. CEA detected 20 of 23 recurrences at the time of clinical evidence and in 14 patients preceded clinical diagnosis by any
other test by more than 3 months.

Studies with Dr. Sugarbaker and Dr. Moore at the Peter Bent
Brigham Hospital disclosed nine patients with completely resected
colo-rectal cancers whose CEAs remained low for more than 2 years
after surgery; none has shown evidence of metastasis (7); CEA levels
were drawn monthly and the patients were examined physically at 3
month intervals (Fig. 1). Note that all but three of these patients
had normal CEA levels pre-operatively.

In contrast, the monthly serial CEA titers in 12 patients who
developed recurrent or metastatic colo-rectal cancer are seen in Fig.
2. The arrows indicate the point in time when the first objective
clinical evidence of recurrence was detected. In 7 patients rising
CEAs preceded this clinical evidence. The circles indicate the point
in time when it was considered clinically that the CEA levels had indeed risen significantly. Four of our patients did not show rising
CEA levels preceding objective evidence of recurrence. Note that
these patients had minimal or no elevations of CEA pre-operatively,
thus differing from the others.

In 7 patients rising CEA trends gave the first objective evidence of recurrence (excluding non-specific symptoms). Physical
findings and symptoms were noted first in 3, both were observed at
the same clinic visit in 1 patient. One patient was re-explored for
a surgical complication.

TABLE 1   Use of CEA in colo-rectal cancer as the first indicator of
recurrence

		No. of Pts.	
		A*	B*
I.	Rising CEA	4	7
II.	Physical findings or symptoms	5	3
III.	I and II simultaneously	2	1
IV.	Surgical re-exploration	1	1
V.	Battery of laboratory and x-ray tests	0	0

*A - Includes non-specific symptoms.
*B - Includes only objective signs and tests.

None of the numerous other laboratory and roentgen tests which were done at six monthly intervals, including hematocrit, alkaline phosphatase, chest x-ray, liver scan, barium enema, or sigmoidoscopy provided early objective evidence of recurrence, although they helped to confirm the CEA observations.

The onset and mean time of occurrence of the first indication of recurrence is noted in Table 2 below. The first CEA rise was observed at 3 - 16 months post-resection in 8 patients with a mean of 7.8 months. Four had no rise in CEA. Three monthly review of symptoms and physical examination gave evidence of recurrence at 8.9 months (mean) in 10 patients.

TABLE 2   Onset and mean of first evidence of recurrence of colon cancer

I.	Monthly CEA	8 Pts.	3-16 Mo.*	Mean, 7.8 mos.
		4 Pts.		No rise
II.	3-Month physical examination and history	10 Pts.	3-13 Mo.#	Mean, 8.9 mos.
		2 Pts.		No signs or symptoms
III.	6-Monthly laboratory and radiologic tests	6 Pts.	6-20 Mo.	Mean, 11.2 mos.
		6 Pts.		No tests pos.

* Rise first Noted.   #Symptoms or signs first noted.

In this study CEA was found not to be a substitute for careful clinical follow-up, but it was a useful adjunct for the detection of early recurrent cancer, especially intra-hepatic or retroperitoneal disease recurring in patients with elevated pretreatment CEA levels.

An example of one of our patients who had a modest elevation of CEA prior to resection of a Dukes C rectal cancer, but had no increase in CEA titer despite evidence of recurrence proven by biopsy is seen in Fig. 3.

"SECOND LOOK" SURGERY

When it became apparent that rising serial CEA levels could yield evidence of recurrence in otherwise asymptomatic patients it was logical that this be considered for use as an indicator for "second-look" surgery, and several groups, including Dr. Mach's (Lausanne), Martin, Minton and their associates (Ohio State Medical School), and Staab, Anderer and associates (Tubingen) are presently assessing the potential usefulness of this approach. Since reports from these groups are presented elsewhere in this Symposium, I shall not review their findings.

It is fair to state, however, that insufficient experience has accumulated to date to draw firm conclusions on the usefulness of CEA for "second-look" surgery.

TRANSIENT RISES IN CEA: A LIMITATION IN THE USE OF SERIAL CEA
LEVELS AS AN INDICATOR FOR SECOND-LOOK SURGERY?

My surgical colleagues in Boston have performed relatively few
second-look procedures on the basis of rising CEA alone. In review-
ing our experience with 69 prospectively followed patients with
colo-rectal cancer we found 24 who demonstrated significant rises
greater than the 95% confidence limits (3.0 - 9.8 ng/ml) (8). Ten
of them subsequently showed unexplained falls in CEA levels approaching the baseline. These patients had an average of 18 post-operative
determinations. Only one, fourteen months after surgery, developed
a recurrence (anastomotic site). The other nine, followed for a
mean of 27 months post-operatively, showed no evidence of recurrence. One patient had hepatitis demonstrated by biopsy at surgery.
Another patient had an unexplained rise and fall of alkaline phosphatase paralleling the CEA and attributed to hepatitis. A third
patient had congestive heart failure.

Fourteen of the 24 patients showed continued CEA rises, 11 of
whom have already had documented recurrences. Others continue to be
followed. Other possible explanations for the reversible CEA rises
include heavy smoking, liver malfunction, transfusion of CEA-
positive blood: (Four of our patients had received transfusions.)

Thus, even when laboratory variation as a cause of the CEA
rises is eliminated, biologic causes other than cancer, especially
non-malignant liver disease, are not ruled out. It must be emphasized that although rising serial CEA levels are undoubtedly helpful
in making the decision for reexploration they do not substitute for
complete clinical assessment. Because of the importance of the
liver status, we recommend that complete liver assessment, including needle biopsy, be done routinely as part of the pre-operative
work-up when a rising CEA is the sole indication of tumor recurrence. We shall refer again (below) to the liver.

CEA AS A MONITOR OF CHEMOTHERAPY

Numerous collaborative studies, underway in many countries, are
testing the effectiveness of combinations of surgery, chemotherapy,
radiation therapy and immunotherapy on metastatic digestive tract
cancer. There is urgent need for objective monitors of the
patient's response to treatment to supplement clinical, laboratory
and roentgenographic examinations. Serial CEA determinations appear
to provide such objective evidence of changing status and in some
clinics changing trends of CEA are being used as one indicator for
making therapeutic decisions.

We have studied several series of patients at the Sidney Farber
Cancer Institute (9,10,11). Most recently Dr. Robert Mayer and
associates studied 47 patients with documented metastatic colo-rectal
cancer (11). Thirty patients received chemotherapy and had serial

CEAs. Four (13.3%) demonstrated "probable tumor regression" and seven (23.3%) had "stable disease". Of nineteen (63.3%) who showed "disease progression," eleven have already died and in 14 (74%) the CEA value doubled.

CEA titers declined in all four responders (Fig. 4), but in only one instance did the level fall to below 4.0 ng/ml and provide evidence of a tumor response not appreciated clinically. The only cytotoxic drugs effecting tumor regression were 5-FU and FUDR. CEA levels usually rose as disease progressed, but once elevated, absolute values did not correlate directly with tumor burden. The further usefulness of CEA assays in monitoring disseminated colo-rectal cancer must await the development of improved chemotherapeutic agents.

A 52 year old man with metastatic rectal cancer had an apparent response to hydroxyurea and 5-FU with disappearance of adenopathy, but this response did not persist as was indicated by the rising CEA trend (Fig. 5).

A 73 year old woman who underwent sigmoid resection for a Dukes C adenocarcinoma, showed a progressive rise in CEA titer eight months before any other sign of tumor recurrence could be detected (Fig. 6). Note that the elevated pre-operative CEA never fell to normal. This is a poor prognostic finding.

In another patient, a 63 year old woman, falling CEA levels correlated well with objective regression of disease. Figure 7 shows the advantage of the use of the diluted CEA assay (in this instance the direct Roche assay) which permits measurement of levels of 10,000 ng/ml or higher. In this patient alkaline phosphatase values reached normal levels, while CEA levels were still markedly elevated.

Dr. Mayer summarized the role of CEA as a monitor of chemotherapy in metastatic colo-rectal cancer as follows:

1. If elevated, serial CEA levels provide a measurable index of residual disease otherwise clinically undetectable.

2. Rising CEA levels may pre-date clinical evidence of tumor resistance to previously effective chemotherapy, indicating the need for a change in therapy.

3. A rising CEA level is incompatible with disease regression.

CEA MONITORING OF RADIATION THERAPY

Preliminary findings by Sugarbaker and associates at the Peter Bent Brigham Hospital suggest that serial plasma CEA levels are useful for monitoring radiation therapy for rectal cancer (12). Serial CEA assays were performed on 16 patients receiving pre-operative radiation therapy of rectal cancer or radiation of recurrent or metastatic colo-rectal cancer. Radiation therapy of localized colo-rectal cancer reliably reduced previously elevated circulating titers. Significant decrease of elevated CEA titers with accumulating doses of radiation indicated that the bulk of CEA-producing tumor was within the radiation treatment portal. When disseminated disease was extensive compared to the treated lesion, radiation therapy failed to lower CEA values. A rebound in CEA levels strongly suggested that the initial decline did not presage long term control. Thus the serial trends assisted in management decisions -- including the timing, nature and extent of surgery. Sugarbaker was careful to point out, however, that such decisions must be made cautiously with full understanding of the entire clinical and laboratory status of the patient, as well as of the limitation of the assay.

A 43 year old man received 4500 rads of pre-operative radiation therapy for a large posteriorly fixed rectal cancer (Fig. 8). The CEA level fell to undetectable levels and abdominal-perineal-sacral resection was then carried out. The patient has remained apparently disease-free for three years after therapy, confirmed by the serial CEA levels.

Another patient was a 44 year old woman who, 1 and 1/2 years after resection of a Dukes B2 sigmoid colon cancer, developed, concurrent with an expanding left hilar mass, a CEA rising from normal to 20 ng/ml (Fig. 9). The left lung was totally atelectatic. Treatment with 4500 rads caused the CEA to fall to 3 ng. Within 2 months, however, along with reexpansion of the hilar mass the level rose, reaching a height of 100. Following left pneumonectomy it fell rapidly to normal levels. The serial levels in this patient correlated closely with tumor status and apparent effect of therapy.

THE ROLE OF THE LIVER

The liver status is relevant to the clinical use of CEA in patients with digestive tract cancer (5,11). Using the original Thomson radioimmunoassay for CEA, Moore et al (1972) (13) showed that CEA elevations were obtained in 45 percent of patients with severe alcoholic liver disease, none of whom had evidence of gastrointestinal malignancy. Circulating CEA levels were usually lower in patients with alcoholic liver disease than in patients with colonic or pancreatic cancer.

Khoo and Mackay (14) found elevated serum CEA levels using MacSween's method in primary biliary, cryptogenic and alcoholic cirrhosis and noted that the levels correlated with degrees of impairment of liver function as indicated by BSP retention and alkaline phosphatase and transaminase levels.

Early clinical evidence suggested a role of the hepatobiliary system in the regulation of circulating CEA levels. In patients with digestive tract cancer a rapid rise of CEA was often associated with the onset of jaundice (9). Whether this was due to increased production of CEA by tumor, to impaired metabolism due to liver cell failure, or to biliary obstruction was uncertain. Accordingly, Lurie,

Loewenstein and Zamcheck studied 29 jaundiced patients with benign extra-hepatic biliary tract obstruction and inflammation (15). During the obstructive and inflammatory phase, 52 percent of the patients had CEA levels greater than 2.5 ng/ml. Elevated levels were associated more frequently with common duct stones (and cholangitis) than with gall bladder stones (and cholecystitis) alone. Some with common duct stones had levels greater than 5.0 ng/ml, which returned to normal following surgical relief of obstruction in seven of ten patients. The levels increased, however, in three patients with progressive inflammation. The highest values were seen in two patients with liver abscesses (Fig. 10).

Highest CEA levels are repeatedly found in metastatic disease of the liver. Terminal failure of the liver to metabolize and/or excrete CEA in the face of an increasing CEA load probably contributes to the rapid rises so often observed. It would seem unlikely that such elevations are caused solely by a rapid increase in production of CEA by the tumor masses. Whether liver toxicity by chemotherapeutic agents contributes to elevated CEA levels in some patients also needs study. Thus concomitant monitoring of the liver function is essential for the correct interpretation of CEA levels. Cooper, et. al. (16) showed liver involvement by metastatic colorectal cancer could be reliably predicted many weeks in advance by combined measurement of CEA and gamma-glutamyl transpeptidase. Similarly, Munjal, et. al. (17) found that elevations of phosphohexose isomerase occurred commonly in the presence of liver metastases from colo-rectal, breast and lung cancer, whereas non-hepatic metastases less frequently gave rises.

METHODOLOGY

Several methods are now widely used for assay of CEA. Effective use of the CEA assay, as with any laboratory test, requires understanding of the limitations of the method used. With the Hansen method (CEA-Roche), widely used in the United States plasma specimens are first tested by an "indirect" method in which perchloric acid extraction precedes the actual radioimmunoassay; this indirect assay measures CEA concentrations reliably up to approximately 20 ng/ml. Specimens shown to have CEA concentrations greater than 20 ng/ml by the initial assay are reassayed by a "direct" method (without perchloric acid extraction) and the latter values are reported. Values obtained by the direct method are higher than those obtained by the indirect method on the same specimen. This is relevant to the use of serial levels (18). An apparent sudden increase in a patient's serial values at 20 ng/ml (Fig. 11) may be caused by the shift in method rather than by a worsening in the patient's status (due to tumor growth or spread). Similarly, a sudden decline in reported results from, say 52 to 19 ng/ml (Fig. 12) may largely reflect the change in method rather than tumor regression. The existence of the discrepancy need not impair the clinical usefulness of the assay; but clinicians who are unaware of the disparity of assay values may misinterpret serial levels traversing 20 ng/ml.

CONCLUSIONS

When used with full awareness of its limitations, the CEA assay is useful in the management of the cancer patient by helping (a) to assess prognosis, (b) to determine incompleteness of surgical resection, (c) to detect recurrence of cancer, and (d) to monitor chemotherapy and radiation therapy.

No CEA assay value or series of values can substitute for complete clinical and laboratory evaluation, including assessment of liver function, histopathology and staging of malignancy. The assay supplements the use of tumor histopathology in assessing prognosis.

It remains to be shown whether changes in serial CEA levels occur early enough to permit curative therapy such as "second look" surgery or beneficial change of chemotherapy or radiation therapy.

REFERENCES

(1)   Thomson, D. M. P., Krupey, J., Freedman, S. O., and Gold, P. (1969): Proceedings of the National Academy of Sciences of the U.S.A., 64, 161.

(2)   Zamcheck, N. (1975): Cancer, 36, 2460-2486.

(3)   Zamcheck, N., Moore, T. L., Dhar, P., and Kupchik, H. Z. (1972): New England Journal of Medicine, 286, 83-86.

(4)   Zamcheck, N., Doos, W. G., Prudente, R., Lurie, B. B., and Gottlieb, L. S. (1975): Human Pathology, 6, 31-45.

(5)   Loewenstein, M. S. and Zamcheck, N. (1977): Gastroenterology, 72, 161-166.

(6)   Herrera, M. S., Chu, T. M., and Holyoke, E. D. (1976): Annals of Surgery, 183, 5.

(7)   Sugarbaker, P. H., Zamcheck, N., and Moore, F. D. (1976): Cancer, 38, 2310-2315.

(8)   Rittgers, R. A., Steele, G., Zamcheck, N., Loewenstein, M.S., Sugarbaker, P. H., Mayer, R. J., Lokich, J. J., Maltz, J., and Wilson, R. E. (1977): Clinical Research, Abstract, in press.

(9)   Skarin, A. T., Delwiche, R., Zamcheck, N., Lokich, J. J., and Frei, III, E. (1974): Cancer, 33, 1239-1245.

(10) Sugarbaker, P. H., Skarin, A. T., and Zamcheck, N. (1976): Journal of Surgical Oncology, 8, 523-537.

(11) Mayer, R. J., Garnick, M. B., Steele, G. D., and Zamcheck, N. (1977): Cancer, in press.

(12) Sugarbaker, P. H., Bloomer, W. D., Corbett, E. D., and Chaffey, J. T. (1976): American Journal of Roentgenology, 127, 641-644.

(13) Moore, T. L., Dhar, P., Zamcheck, N., Keeley, A., Gottlieb, L., and Kupchik, H. Z. (1972): Gastroenterology, 63, 88-94.

(14) Khoo, S. K., and Mackay, I. R. (1973): <u>Journal of Clinical</u>
<u>Pathology</u>, 26, 470-475.

(15) Lurie, B. B., Loewenstein, M. S., and Zamcheck, N. (1975):
<u>Journal of the American Medical Association</u>, 233, 326-330.

(16) Cooper, E. H., Turner, R., Steele, L., Neville, A. M., and
Mackay, A. M. (1975): <u>British Journal of Cancer</u>, 31, 111-117.

(17) Munjal, D., Chawla, P. L., Lokich, J. J., and Zamcheck, N.
(1975): <u>Proceedings of the Annual Meeting of the American</u>
<u>Society for Clinical Oncology</u>, 16, 260.

(18) Loewenstein, M. S., Kupchik, H. Z., and Zamcheck, N. (1976):
<u>New England Journal of Medicine</u>, 294, 1123.

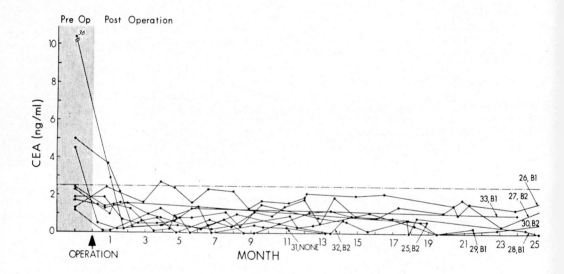

Fig. 1   Serial CEA levels in 9 patients with completely resected
colo-rectal cancers.

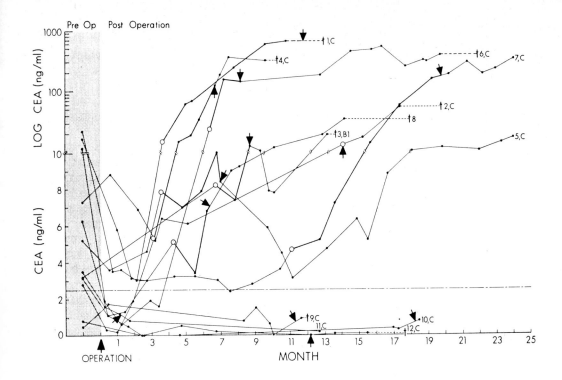

Fig. 2 Serial CEA levels in 12 patients who developed recurrent or metastatic colo-rectal cancer. (From Ref. 7)

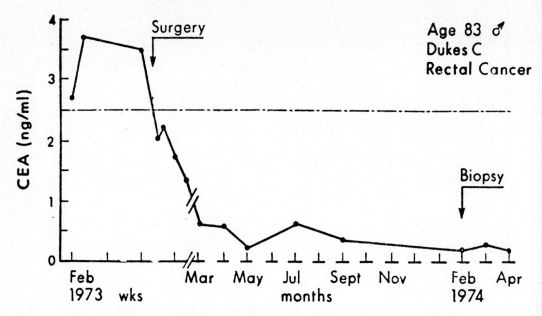

Fig. 3 This patient, despite biopsy evidence of recurrence, did not have a rise in CEA. (From Ref. 10)

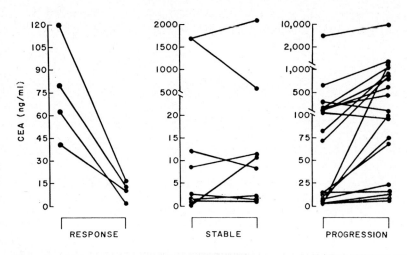

Fig. 4 Changes in serial CEA levels during chemotherapy. (Note differences in the ordinate scales of the three categories.) (From Ref. 11)

74

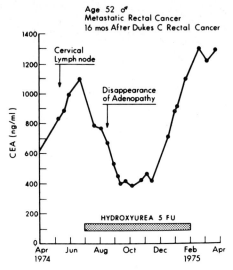

Fig. 5 A rapidly rising CEA trend signalled the need to change chemotherapy. (From Ref. 10)

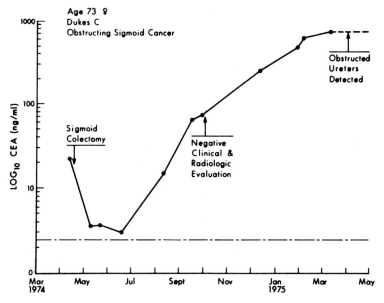

Fig. 6 A progressive rise in CEA was seen 8 months before any other sign of recurrence was detected. (From Ref. 10)

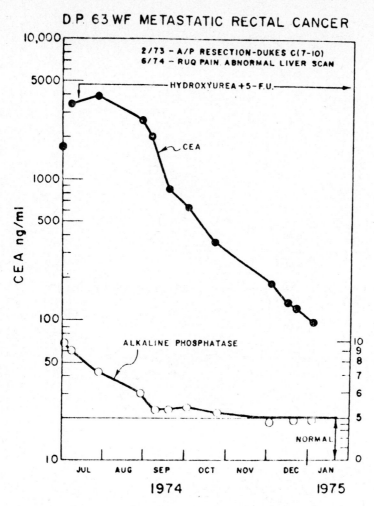

Fig. 7 In this 63 year old woman a falling CEA correlated well with objective regression of disease. (From Ref. 10)

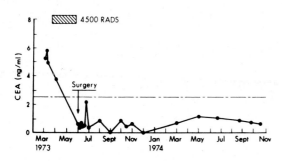

Fig. 8 Serial CEA levels in radiation treated rectal cancer followed by surgical resection. (From Ref. 12)

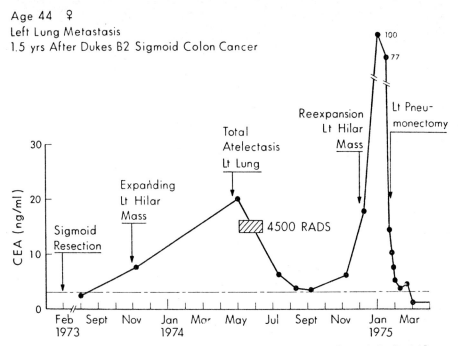

Fig. 9 Serial CEA values in a patient with an isolated left hilar metastasis treated with 4500 rads followed by pneumonectomy. (From Ref. 12)

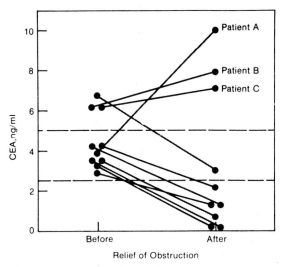

Fig. 10 CEA levels before and after relief of common bile duct obstruction by stones. Patients A and B developed cholangitis and liver abscesses and died. (From Ref. 15)

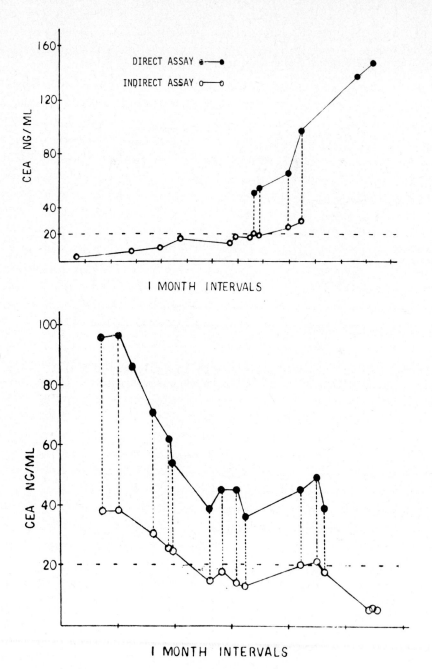

Figs. 11 and 12 Disparity between indirect and direct CEA methods.
Dotted lines join values obtained on the same plasma specimens.
Fig. 11 - Rising CEA values. Fig. 12 - Falling CEA values. (Fig. 11
from Ref. 18)

DISCUSSION

ROCHMAN H. (Chicago): You compared CEA on peritoneal fluid with cytology. Was the CEA done on peritoneal fluid or in peripheal blood.

ZAMCHECK N. (Boston): They were all done on peritoneal fluid.

NAMER M. (Nice): Can the absolute level of CEA be predictive of an event, for example efficiency of chemotherapy or death.

MACH J.P. (Lausanne): The group of Holyoke (Herrera et al., Ann.Surg. 183, 5, 1976) have requested results showing that high preoperative CEA values are correlated with a bad prognosis.
I have no response concerning chemotherapy in colo-rectal cancer, but in a recent article from Tormey et al. (Cancer 39, 2397, 1977) it is demonstrated that high levels of CEA in breast cancer correspond to low response rates to chemotherapy.

COOPER E.H. (Leeds): We examined the levels of CEA during the last year of life in patients treated with chemotherapy or left untreated. There is no evidence that the level of CEA at the beginning of the last year of life is predictive of how long the patient can survive.

BOUNAMAUX Y. (Bâle): I agree that the variation of CEA is more important than absolute level, but actual level is important, for example stomach cancer patients with more than 5 ng Roche /ml has little possibility for complete resection of tumour.

ZAMCHECK N. (Boston): There are many factors which influence the absolute circulating level of CEA. 1) The amount of CEA produced by the tumour; in tissue culture this is extremely variable. Tissue culture studies, however, do not necessary correspond to what take place in vivo .2) Invasion by the tumour. 3) The liver plays an important role in CEA excretion. The liver's ability to excrete CEA may be exceeded by CEA load. In general, the higher the CEA level the worse the prognosis. On the other hand, one cannot attribute to any single individual level a quaranteed outcome - say for, effective chemotherapy or death. Serial trends in the same patient, of course, are helpful.

CEA IN THE MONITORING OF COLO-RECTAL CARCINOMA PATIENTS;
DESCRIPTION OF A FEW SELECTED CASES.

H. Vienny, J.-P. Mach, B. Haldemann and J. Pettavel

Departments of Biochemistry and Surgery, University of Lausanne and
Unit of Human Cancer Immunology, Lausanne Branch, Ludwig Institute
for Cancer Research, 1066 Epalinges s/ Lausanne, Switzerland.

INTRODUCTION

        Since the first report of Thomson et al. in 1969 (1),
describing the radioimmunoassay (RIA) of carcinoembryonic antigen
(CEA) as a specific test for the diagnosis of colo-rectal carcinoma,
numerous articles in the literature have shown that various other
types of carcinoma can be associated with marked elevations of circulating CEA and that a moderate increase of CEA values can also be
observed in several non-malignant inflammatory diseases,for review
see Zamcheck (2), Hansen et al. (3), Neville and Cooper (4), and
Mach et al. (5).
        In spite of the lack of tumor and organ specificity of CEA,
precluding the use of the CEA assay for the screening of cancer, it
is now accepted that repeated measurements of CEA in patients operated
for a large bowel carcinoma can provide interesting information concerning tumor recurrences, earlier than other conventional tests.
The problem is now to determine the importance of the CEA results in
the management of colo-rectal carcinoma patient.
        Recently, two groups, Martin et al. (6) and Staab et al (7)
reported results suggesting that second look operations based exclusively on moderate elevation of circulating CEA levels could lead to
the discovery of resectable local tumor recurrences in a high percentage of colo-rectal carcinoma patients. These optimistic results
contrast with the conclusion of other groups having a long experience
with the CEA assay in patients with large bowel carcinoma, like
those of Zamcheck (2), Holyoke (8), Neville (4) and Mach (5) who
found that the discovery of still resectable local tumor recurrences
was rather the exception than the rule. Of course, these differences
in results might be due to more conservative or aggressive attitude
of the groups concerning second look surgery. The purpose of this
communication is to report our experience in 4 representative cases
selected from a series of 80 patients followed up by repeated CEA
assays after a complete resection of colon or rectum carcinoma. A
more complete report of these results will be published elsewhere (9).

METHODS

The radioimmunoassay of CEA was performed according to the
method of Gold (1) as modified by Mach et al. (5). The major modification was that duplicates of 1 ml of plasma (10 ml of blood was
collected in tubes containing 33 mg of dry E.D.T.A. K3) instead of
5 ml of serum, were extracted in 1 M perchloric acid. The sensitivity
of the test is 1 ng/ml. The normal value determined in 90 non smoking
blood bank donors ranges between 0 to 3.5 ng/ml (5). Our CEA assay
is similar to the Hansen method (3), however, our numerical values
are slightly higher and should be divided by a factor of 1.5 in
order to make a direct comparison.

RESULTS

A brief clinical history of 4 selected representative cases
will be presented with the evolution of their CEA levels.

Patient No 1 (Fig. 1) is a 60 year old woman who had a complete
removal of the rectum for a Dukes' C carcinoma, in October 1973.
There was no evidence of hepatic metastasis at the time of operation.
The CEA levels decreased after surgery from 6.2 ng/ml to 2.5 ng/ml
and then increased to 7.4 ng/ml 5 months later. The CEA values
remained moderately elevated around 8 ng/ml for the 12 following
months, then progressively increased up to 100 ng/ml during the next
7 months. This relatively thin patient (44 kg) had no weight loss,
no clinical evidence of tumor relapse and negative scan and arteriography of the liver. She remained subjectively perfectly well for
the next 7 months with CEA values of 100 ng/ml. Only at that time,
26 months after the first increase of CEA level, the liver scan and
ultrasonography showed evidences of multiple hepatic metastases. One
month later, she was found to have multiple small pulmonary metastases and she died 6 months later with disseminated disease.

Retrospectively, the 26 months lead time between the
first elevation of CEA level and the clinical diagnosis of tumor
metastases does not seem to have been used optimally. However, this
patient had a 2.5 year symptom free period with no clinical evidence
of local recurrences. It is not certain that a second look surgery
would have prevented the occurrence of liver and pulmonary metastases.

Patient No 2 (Fig. 2) is a 61 year old woman who was operated
in February 1973, for a Dukes' B sigmoid carcinoma. Palpation and
inspection of the liver at operation did not show any hepatic metastasis. The CEA level decreased from 5 to 0.5 ng/ml after the complete tumor resection but then increased slowly up to 11 ng/ml during
the next 15 months. The patient was subjectively well with no weight
loss, normal bowel movements, and no blood in the stool. One month
later, however, she was hospitalized with acute abdominal pain. At
operation a large local tumor recurrence infiltrating the right colon
was removed and several small hepatic metastasis in the liver were
observed. The CEA level decreased to 6.2 ng/ml after surgery, but
10 months later increased up to 20 ng/ml and the patient died with
disseminated disease 20 months after the second operation.

In this case, with the CEA giving a lead time of 10 months, we should have been able to detect earlier the local tumor recurrence by a barium enema. It is important to note, however, that liver metastases developed with a relatively slow increase of CEA levels.

Patient No 3 (Fig. 3) is a 56 year old woman who was operated on for a Dukes' C stenosing colon carcinoma of the hepatic flexure. Her first CEA values, obtained 3 and 7 months after surgery, were below 2 ng/ml. Three months later her CEA level increased to 9 ng/ml and remained around 10 ng/ml for the next 8 months. At this time the ultrasonography of the liver was within normal limits, whereas hepatic scan and arteriography suggested the presence of a liver metastasis. A second look operation was performed, no liver metastasis was detected, but a tumor in the right ovary measuring 7 cm diameter was found and removed. The histologic diagnosis indicated that the ovarian tumor was derived from the colon carcinoma and that 2 regional lymph nodes were infiltrated with tumor cells. The CEA decreased after surgery to 3.3 ng/ml and to 1.5 ng/ml one month later. In this case, the resection of tumor recurrence was made possible by the observation of elevated CEA values. This second tumor resection may increase the long-term survival of this patient.

Patient No 4 (Fig. 4) is a 69 year old woman who was operated for a relatively large Dukes' A stenosing colon carcinoma of the splenic flexure, in February 1973. A splenectomy was performed with the partial colectomy because of suspicion of tumor infiltration of the spleen which was not confirmed by histologic examination. The gall-bladder was also removed at the same time because of cholelithiasis. This patient belongs to the category of patients that we recently described who exhibited moderately elevated CEA values without clinical evidence of tumor relapse (9). Her CEA level dropped from 14 ng/ml to 0 ng after the operation. It then increased up to 6.9 ng/ml during the next 3 months. These moderately elevated CEA values were observed in 5 different CEA assays during a period of 5 months. At the same time the alkaline phosphatase was also moderately elevated but the transaminases were normal. A barium enema was found within normal limits. Two liver scans showed some degree of heterogeneity of the right upperlobe. The patient was considered for a second look laparotomy but she refused a new operation. Four months later her CEA level decreased to 3.4 ng/ml, it remained at this level for 10 months and then decreased to below 2 ng/ml. The patient is still alive and without evidence of tumor recurrence 3 years after her first elevated CEA value.

In this case, we did not find any satisfactory explanation for the elevated CEA values. In particular, it was difficult to understand these repeated CEA elevations, because they followed a definite drop of CEA to normal values after surgery.

DISCUSSION

The first case presented illustrates the use of serial CEA assays as an indicator of prognosis. It shows that CEA elevation can precede clinical diagnosis with a lead time of more than 20 months.

It also confirms the usual observation that marked elevations of CEA level (higher than 20-30 ng/ml) are associated with liver metastases or tumor dissemination. At these levels, the CEA test is definitely more specific than liver enzyme assays, and can detect metastases earlier than liver scan and arteriography.

In patients with moderate elevations of CEA level (between 3-10 ng/ml) the interpretation is more difficult. One has always to consider three possibilities, either a local tumor recurrence, or distant metastases of moderate size without local tumor recurrence, or the presence of a non-malignant disease known to increase the circulating CEA level. In a population of patients with colo-rectal carcinoma who have an average age of more than 60 years, there is a large percentage of individuals with heavy smoking habits, chronic bronchitis or liver diseases. Some of these patients may never have normal CEA values after the first tumor resection, but others can show a decrease of circulating CEA level post operatively, followed by a moderate increase mimicking a tumor relapse, because they have started to smoke or to drink again, after a temporary interruption of their habit during hospitalization and convalescence. Others may also develop post-transfusional hepatitis, which may provoke an increase of CEA levels.

For these reasons the decision to perform a second look operation based exclusively on moderate elevations of CEA levels does not appear to us to be as obvious and well defined as in the recommendation of Martin et al. (6) and Staab et al. (7).

Practically, we suggest that patients followed after resection of colo-rectal carcinoma who have a CEA level at least two times higher than the base line observed postoperatively and exceeding 4-5 ng/ml, should have two more CEA tests within the next 3 months and a complete clinical work up. If during that period of time the CEA increased at least to 50 percent of its last elevated value and no reason for a non-specific elevation of CEA is found, then a second look operation can be reasonably considered. However, these second look operations motivated by the detection of increased circulating CEA levels should not be performed routinely and should be limited to carefully controlled studies because it has not been proven yet that removal of local recurrences can modify the patient's prognosis. Only randomized studies will determine if this approach can improve the quality and length of survival of the patients.

REFERENCES

(1) Thomson, D.M.P., Krupey, J., Freedman, S.O. and Gold, P. (1969) : Proc. nat. Acad. Sci. U.S.A. 64, 161.
(2) Zamcheck, N. (1975) : Cancer 36, 2460.
(3) Hansen, H.J., Snyder, J.J., Miller, E., Vandervoorde, J.P., Miller, O.N., Hines, L.R. and Burns, J.J. (1974) : Hum. Path 5, 139.
(4) Neville, A.M. and Cooper, E.H. (1976) : Ann. Clin. Biochem 13, 282.

(5) Mach, J.-P., Jaeger, P.-H., Bertholet, M.-M., Ruegsegger, C.H., Loosli, R.M. and Pettavel, J. (1974) : <u>Lancet II</u>, 535.
(6) Martin, E.W., James, K., Hurtubise, P.E., Catalano, P. and Minton, J.P. (1977) : <u>Cancer 39</u>, 440.
(7) Staab, H.J., Anderer, F.A., Stumpf, E. and Fischer, R. (1977) : <u>Dtsch. med. Wschr. 102</u>, 1082.
(8) Herrera, M.A., Chu, T.M. and Holyoke, E.D. (1976) : <u>Ann. Surg. 183</u>, 5.
(9) Mach, J.-P., Vienny, H., Jaeger, Ph., Haldmann, B., Egely, R. and Pettavel, J. (1977) : <u>Cancer</u>, in press.

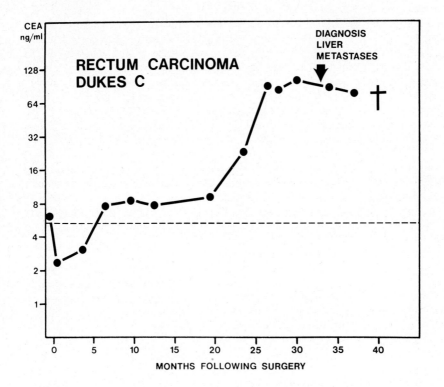

Fig. 1 Serial CEA values in a patient who had a complete removal of the rectum for a Dukes' C rectum carcinoma. The black arrow indicate the first evidence of hepatic metastases detected by liver scan and ultrasonography 26 months after the first increased CEA value.

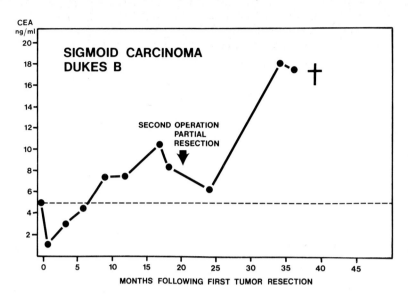

Fig. 2 Serial CEA values in a patient who had had a complete resection of a Dukes' B sigmoid carcinoma. The black arrow indicate the time of a second operation performed because of partial abdominal obstruction. At operation a large local tumor recurrence was removed but several small liver metastases were already present.

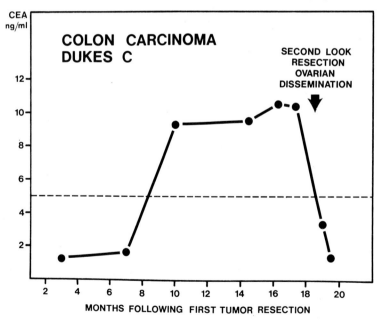

Fig. 3 Serial CEA levels in a patient who had a complete resection of a Dukes' C colon carcinoma of the hepatic flexure. The black arrow indicate the time of a second look operation motivated by the elevation of circulating CEA. At operation an unsuspected tumor recurrence in the right ovary was removed.

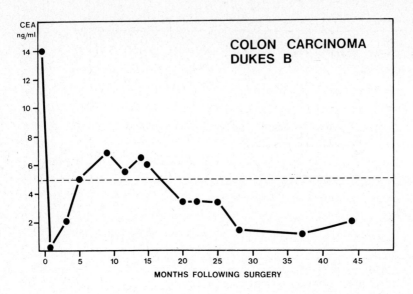

Fig. 4 Serial CEA values in a patient who had a complete resection of a Dukes' A colon carcinoma of the splenic flexure. This patient had several moderately elevated CEA values for 5 months without clinical evidences of tumor recurrence. No satisfactory explanation was found for these well documented increased CEA values.

DISCUSSION

LALANNE C.M.(Nice): Occult metastases disappearing spontaneously through immunology or other mechanism might explain the slight elevated values after surgery.

MACH J.P. (Lausanne): I agree with you,but the frequency of this phenomenon, spontaneous remission is rare .

MASSEYEFF R. (Nice): I was strucked by some of the curves you showed. I have noted that the slope of decrease varied widely. It seems that the slope of AFP in Yolk-sack tumours after surgery could be predictive for residual disease. I wonder if the same could apply to CEA. Do you know enough about the half life of CEA and have you some remarks about the slope.

MACH J.P. (Lausanne): In fact, there is no precise information concerning the half life of CEA, but one should wait at least one month after surgery before drawing any conclusion from the CEA assay concerning the evaluation of tumour resection.

86

DELMONT J.(Nice): Can we notice an overshoot of CEA when patients stop smoking or drinking, as we have observed this in alcoholic patients with AFP at entrance in hospital.

MACH J.P. (Lausanne): I cannot answer your question, because in my knowledge, there is no data in the literature.

STAAB H.J.(Tubingen): I just want to make a further comment on the alcoholic malfonction of the liver. I have never seen liver malfonction with CEA level higher than 10 ng/ml according to the Roche assay.

MACH J.P.(Lausanne): Nevertheless, I think that you have to wait about 3 months to see the trend of increase of CEA level before making a decision concerning second look surgery.

A RETROSPECTIVE AND PROSPECTIVE ANALYSIS OF THE SECOND-LOOK PROCEDURE, USING SERIAL CEA DETERMINATIONS TO DETECT RECURRENT GASTROINTESTINAL CANCER.

E. W. Martin, Jr., L. Rinker, M. Cooperman, John P. Minton, and L. C. Carey

Departments of Surgery and Pathology, The Ohio State University Hospital, Columbus, Ohio 43210, USA

The second-look procedure was first proposed in 1951 by Wangensteen et al. (6,7), and shortly thereafter fell into disrepute because of the high morbidity and mortality. The arbitrary time interval as an indication for second-look surgery was too imprecise, and a better indication was needed. The nonspecific CEA tumor marker, described in 1965 by Gold et al. (1), is now presented as a more precise indicator of recurrent tumor and early reoperation. The frequency of preoperative and serial postoperative determinations is emphasized (every 4 to 6 weeks for the first year). Our seven-year experience with the CEA radioimmunoassay has enabled us to interpret values obtained in our laboratory and to place reliable clinical significance on numerical value changes. The CEA NOMOGRAM is used as a simple scale for evaluation of the significance of the CEA value. If the follow-up determination indicates a significant change from the postresection baseline, the rise should alert the physician to the possibility of recurrent tumor, and, in the absence of other clinical or laboratory explanations for the elevation, indicate reoperation.

MATERIAL AND METHODS

Storage of Samples

All CEA samples are drawn in lavender-stoppered tubes (EDTA tubes) and cells are separated from plasma. Each plasma sample is stored at -20° C so that it can be compared with a subsequent plasma level when serial reevaluations are performed. To make the comparison, each sample is thawed and centrifuged at 3000 rpm for 5 minutes prior to retesting with the current sample (5). We propose that assays be done every month for the first year, bimonthly for the next two years, and every 3 months for the following two years.

Radioimmunoassay (Technic Modified)

Plasma samples were analyzed for CEA content by the Hansen Z-gel method (2) specified by Roche Diagnostics. (CEA Roche TM) Results were reported only if the duplicate values were within the limits of reproducibility established in the Roche procedure manual (5).

Since February 1977, we have used an AMICON filter which eliminates the dialysis step (5). Use of a neutralized perchloric acid-extracted CEA sample removes the variable time-contact of each sample by the rapid addition of TRIS buffer solution after a time-controlled separation technic. The free CEA molecules are trapped on a filter membrane, rinsed free of extraneous materials, and suspended in ammonium acetate buffer (pH 7.1 ± 0.2). The time required for this procedure is three and one-half hours per twenty paired samples, thus the total assay procedure time is decreased to approximately 18 hours, or less than one day.

CEA Nomogram

The accuracy and reproducibility of the CEA-Roche assay were determined by assessing the sources of error not only within a given assay, but also between assays (4). Intraassay error was evaluated by preparing samples of five different concentrations within the critical range of 1-12 ng/ml and assaying each sample in duplicate 25 times. Interassay error was evaluated by preparing samples of four different concentrations within the same critical range and a fifth sample above 100 ng/ml. Aliquots of these samples were frozen at -20° C and, over a three-month period, were thawed and assayed in duplicate in 25 separate assays.

Reproducibility of the duplicate samples was well within the acceptable limits stated by the kit manufacturer. Mean, standard deviation, coefficient of variation, and range were established for each set of 25 duplicates (4,5).

Data were then plotted on linear graph paper with equal axes to demonstrate the standard deviation of the assay in this laboratory, i.e., the 95% confidence limit for any given result. Use of this plot as a NOMOGRAM for interpretation of the statistical significance of serial CEA levels obtained in a laboratory has been proposed (Fig. 1) (4,5). For example, a value of 3 ng/ml, read off the vertical axis (assay reported value) can be interpreted by drawing a line parallel to the horizontal axis to determine the 95% confidence statistical range of 2.2-3.8 ng/ml. To be significant, according to the NOMOGRAM, any subsequent value must not fall within that range, i.e., must be greater than 4.7 ng/ml (Fig. 2).

Assay variance greater than that demonstrated by these data does occur. To assess further variance, assayed samples were stored at -20° C for reevaluation with subsequent samples. If the follow-up sample demonstrated an increase outside the 95% confidence limit, both samples were reanalyzed at the same time under the same conditions; thus, the patient's own sample was used as his control.

Patient Selection

All patients had histologically proved adenocarcinoma at primary operation. Postoperative serial CEA determinations were made at three-month intervals. When a significant CEA elevation occurred, the test was repeated and if the repeated CEA value remained elevated, it was considered to be an indication for further clinical evaluation and, if no other explanation was perceived, then a second-look operation was performed.

RESULTS

Between 1972 and 1975, we reoperated upon 22 patients, and found recurrence of tumor in 19 (86%)(4). Among these 19 patients, only 6 (26%) had a resectable tumor; the remaining 13 had distant disease and only confirmation of recurrent tumor could be made. Of the 3 additional patients who underwent second-look but in whom no tumor was found, 2 subsequently proved to have positive bone scans and one a positive brain scan.

During the past 19 months, an additional 16 patients have been reoperated upon, and 13 of the 16 (81%) had localized recurrent tumor (Table I). In all 13, all gross tumor was removed at second-look, and the CEA level subsequently fell to the baseline value established after the primary procedure.

The improved result (81% resectable tumors) in the recent group differs from that in the earlier group (26% resectable tumors) in the time delay between identification of a significant rise in CEA value and reoperation. In the retrospective group, the delay between the first significant CEA elevation and the actual second-look was 7 months; in the prospective group, the delay was reduced to 1.4 months. We believe that shortening the delay between detection of localized recurrent tumor and reoperation increased the proportion of resectable tumors encountered from 26% to 81%.

The magnitude of the rise in CEA level continues to be a good predictive index of the extent of recurrent tumor. In addition, when the CEA level fails to return to the baseline established after the primary operation. it probably indicates residual tumor, and we included these patients in the nonresectable group (distant metastases).

TABLE I

Patients	Number	Tumor Loc/Dist		Negative Second Look	Av CEA (ng/ml) Loc/Dist		Av Delay (months) Loc/Dist		Per cent Localized Tumor
Retrospective	22	6	13	3	7.2	20	3.5	7	27
Prospective	16	13	3	0	6.4	15.5	1.4	4.5	81
Total	38	19	16	3	6.65	20	2.2	6.5	50

Table I Retrospective group compared with prospective group, showing increase from 27% to 81% in localized tumors encountered and definite decrease in time delay before reoperation.

DISCUSSION

It is believed that 90-95% of colorectal malignant tumors produce carcinoembryonic antigen (CEA); thus, CEA assay provides a serologic monitor of the disease. Our experience points to the fact that a rising CEA value can identify tumor recurrence early enough to make complete resection possible. The use of a significant rise in CEA to indicate early second-look operation has provided one patient in this series with 61 months of tumor-free survival since her initial operation; in fact, 5 of the 6 patients in the retrospective group who had localized recurrent tumor removed continue to survive 19 to 61 months after the first operation. However, shortening of the delay between a significant rise in CEA and second-look operation is paramount; all 16 patients in the retrospective group who were found at reoperation to have distant spread of tumor have died. It is still too early to evaluate long-term results in the prospective group.

It appears that serial CEA determinations at frequent intervals provide for early detection of recurrent tumor. Shortening the delay between a definitive elevation of CEA and reoperation resulted in an increase in the per cent of resectable recurrent tumor encountered from 26% in the retrospective group to 81% in the prospective group.

Serial CEA assays should be performed every 4 to 6 weeks after the primary operation. The physician must recognize not only the significance of the CEA level, but also the limitations of the assay. He must rely heavily on his clinical judgment, and all benign inflammatory conditions that cause CEA elevation must be searched for and ruled out before reoperation is decided upon. However, if our results continue to be substantiated and longer survival time accrues, the CEA assay will have made a significant contribution to control of gastrointestinal cancer.

REFERENCES

(1) Gold,P. and Freedman, S.O. (1965): J. Exp. Med. 121:439.
(2) Hansen, H.J., Lance,X.P., and Krupey, J. (1971):
      Clin.Res. 19:143.
(3) Martin, E.W., Jr., Kibbey, W.E., Minton, J.P. et al. (1976)
      Cancer 37:62.
(4) Martin, E.W., Jr., James, K.K., Hurtubise, P.E., Catalano P.,
      and Minton, J.P. (1977) Cancer 39:440.
(5) Minton, J.P. et al.: In Press. Cancer
(6) Roche Procedure Manual. Hoffman-LaRoche, 1974.
(7) Wangensteen, O.H., Lewis, F.J., and Tongen, L.A. (1951):
      Lancet 71:303.
(8) Wangensteen, O.H., Lewis, F.J., Arhelger, S.W., Muller, J.J.,
      and MacLean, L.D. (1954): Surg. Gynecol. Obstet. 99:257.
(9) Zamcheck, N. (1975): Cancer 36:2460.

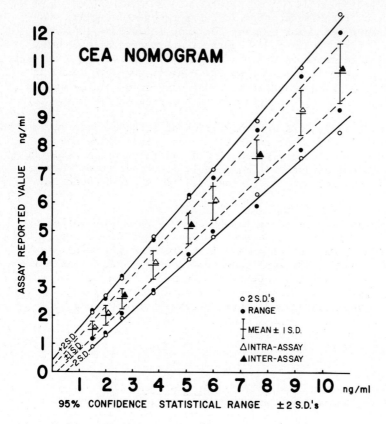

Fig. 1 CEA NOMOGRAM to be used for comparing serial CEA levels to determine if the change is significant (2 SD) to indicate recurrent gastrointestinal cancer (4).

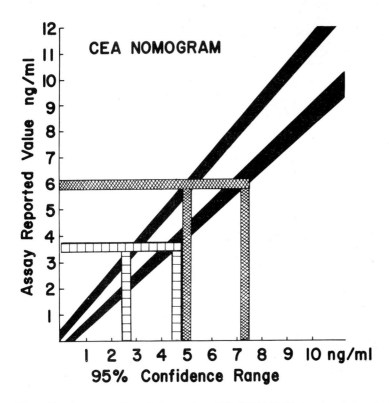

Fig. 2 An example of how the CEA NOMOGRAM is used to indicate a significant CEA change. See Text.

SECOND-LOOK SURGERY OF GASTROINTESTINAL CARCINOMA AND THE POTENTIAL
VALUE OF CEA MONITORING

H.J.Staab, F.A.Anderer, E.Stumpf*, R.Fischer*

Friedrich-Miescher Laboratorium der Max-Planck-Gesellschaft,
Spemannstraße 37-39, 7400 Tübingen, F.R.G.

*Chirurgische Klinik Bad Cannstatt,
Theodor Veiel Straße 90, 7000 Stuttgart 50, F.R.G.

INTRODUCTION
       Postoperative serial CEA determinations have been found of great
value in detecting disease progression in gastrointestinal cancer
before objective evidence of tumor recurrence can be demonstrated by
other clinical diagnostic methods (1-12). The early selection of
patients for second-look operation or other therapeutic treatment,
based on a careful CEA followup in connection with other diagnostic
methods, has become one of the most important tasks in the management
of patients with gastrointestinal carcinomas. We now present our preliminary results on the validity of CEA monitoring for selecting
patients for second-look surgery, which is part of a long term CEA
follow up study presently carried out by us with patients having
undergone resections of primary adenocarcinomas of the gastrointestinal tract. CEA monitoring is based on the analysis of computerized CEA surveillance diagrams.

METHODS AND PATIENTS
       CEA was determined in patients'sera using the Hansen assay with
the CEA Roche RIA test kit. Optimal test conditions were accomplished
by automatically controled dialysis of the perchloric acid extracts.
       Blood samples were drawn a few days before and 8-14 days after
operation and then routinely every 2 months connected with physical
examinations of the patients. In case of a suspected recurrence of
disease the patients underwent routinely other diagnostic methods
such as endoscopy, radiographic methods, radioisotopic scanning or
computer tomography.
       A computerprogram was developed (13) which covered all the work
of calling up the patients under surveillance by letter either
routinely every 2 months or in case of increasing CEA values without
delay. After a 2 years'followup patients were checked in intervals of
4 months. Electronic data processing was also used for the plotting
of the CEA surveillance diagrams every month, for printing all medical
records and all kind of files of specifications as well as for the
medical statistics. The slopes of the CEA surveillance diagrams were
calculated from the regression lines of the postoperatively ascending
CEA curves.

RESULTS
       Up to now 421 patients with histologically proven adenocarcino-
mas of the gastrointestinal tract have been registered in our study.

Surveillance diagrams were only plotted when at least 2 postoperative CEA values have been recorded. So far, surveillance diagrams have been established for 201 patients. However, our main interest was directed to only 144 patients with curatively resected primary carcinomas in order to derive parameters which could be used for early detection of disease progression and would allow a qualified selection of patients for second-look surgery or other therapeutical treatments. Essentially three main types of CEA surveillance diagrams have been observed (10,11).

The first type showed persistently falling CEA values and could be correlated with patients having undergone complete tumor resection without recurrence so far. The second type was characterized by a transient fall of the CEA level followed by slowly increasing CEA values thereafter. The third type of CEA surveillance diagrams showed frequently a transient decrease of the CEA level, too, but passed into a period of rapidly increasing CEA values. The second and the third type of the CEA surveillance diagrams with continuously increasing values were found to be only connected with patients developing recurrent disease. Besides these main tendencies one could observe transient elevations of the CEA level in some patients without any disease progression as well as in healthy control persons, lasting at most 3 months.

As has been shown previously (14) computerized CEA surveillance diagrams can be used not only to detect recurrent disease but also provide information on the type of relapse a patient starts to develop. The differentation of a local tumor recurrence or of metastatic disease progression can be achieved by slope analysis of the postoperative CEA time course. (Fig.1 flat slopes; Fig.2 steep slopes).

From the group of patients with "curatively" resected carcinomas up to now 36 patients developed recurrent disease and were potential second-look cases but only 28 patients which gave their consent were reoperated. More than 90% of our relapse cases could be correlated with increasing CEA values. The CEA rises always preceded a positive clinical diagnosis up to 10 months. Second-look surgery was performed as soon as clinical diagnosis was established or after an adequate interval had passed necessary to confirm the CEA rise (15). Nine of 36 patients have had steadily rising CEA values as the only indication of disease progression and were reoperated without any other diagnostic confirmation. Up to now we did not have a false positive case.

In the relapse cases mentioned above the analysis of the CEA surveillance diagrams of type 2 and 3 with respect to the ascending slopes led to numerical parameters which could, in most cases, differentiate distinct types of disease progression, i.e. metastatic progression and local tumor recurrence. The clinical significance of the numerical slope values can be seen from table 1 and 2, where flat CEA slopes with a mean of 0.16 ng CEA increase/10 days correspond mainly with local tumor recurrence and in only 3 cases with peritoneal carcinosis and cutaneous metastasis. Steep CEA slopes, with a mean increase of 1.8 ng CEA/10 days were only found with metastatic disease progression, mainly with liver metastases. All relapse cases were proven by second-look operation and histological examination, and in cases, where the patients'consent for second-look surgery could not be obtained, by other diagnostic methods or autopsy.

Table 1:Diagnosis of patients with disease progression, exhibiting flat ascending CEA slopes ranging from 0.05 - 0.3 ng CEA increase/10 days with a mean of 0.16 ± 0.09 ng CEA increase/10 days.

Diagnosis	mean slope	cases	location of the prim.carcinoma
local rec.	0.13 ± 0.05	4	stomach,sigma,rectum(2)
local rec.+ ly.n.met.	0.19 ± 0.09	5	stomach,pancreas(2),rectum(2)
perit.carc.	0.18	2	stomach,sigma
cut.met.	0.08	1	stomach

Table 2:Diagnosis of patients with disease progression, exhibiting steep ascending CEA slopes ranging from 0.6-3.8 ng CEA increase/10 days with a mean of 1.8 ± 0.9 ng CEA increase/10 days.

Diagnosis	mean slope	cases	location of the prim.carcinoma
liver met.	2.4 ± 0.7	13	stomach,sigma(7),rectum(5)
perit.carc.	1.2 ± 0.6	7	stomach,sigma(4),rectum(2)
lung met.	0.6	1	lung met.

The numerical slope values do represent therefore, a basis for the prognosis whether another resection is possible. Thus the clinican can select an appropriate therapy without delay and therefore may improve the survival rates of patients. As can be seen from table 3, flat slopes are indicating a high chance for a second resection as

Table 3:Resectability and mortality* of second-look cases according to CEA slopes (*death occurring 2-20 months after sec.-look surgery)

	steep slopes	flat slopes
resectable cases	6/21(28%)	9/12(75%)
mortality (total)	13/21(62%)	5/12(41%)
mortality (resect.cases)	3/ 6(50%)	2/ 9(22%)

judged from the number of resectable cases as well as from the pre-liminary mortality data. Patients exhibiting steep slopes, however, have only a minor chance for another resection. In this group the resectable cases were predominantly cases with solitary liver metas-

96

tases. The overall mortality of the patients who had a minor chance for another resection was 62% as compared to the group of patients who had a good chance for a second resection with a mortality of 41% only. The differences in the mortality rate of patients having undergone a second resection was 50%, in cases of steep CEA slopes and in cases of flat CEA slopes 22%.

COMMENTS AND DISCUSSION
(1) CEA followups with bimonthly determinations are a reliable basis for detection of early tumor recurrence.
(2) Slope analysis of CEA surveillance diagrams helps to discriminate metastatic disease from local tumor recurrence. Slopes differ by roughly one order of magnitude.
(3) A high chance for a second resection is indicated in all cases exhibiting flat CEA slopes whereas in cases with steep CEA slopes there is only a minor chance.
(4) The mortality is lower in the group of patients with flat CEA slopes than in the group with steep CEA slopes.
The number of our cases does not justify generalization. However, a significant trend indicates that resectability is improved by early second-look surgery. A CEA rise should therefore always be a signal for intensive search for tumor recurrence. The CEA slope tendency can be established within 2-4 months and may give, in most cases, valuable aid to a detailed diagnosis and an adequate therapy.

REFERENCES
(1) Sorokim, J.J., Sugarbaker, P.H., Zamcheck, N., Pisick, M., Kupchick, H.Z., and Moore, F.D.(1974): JAMA, 288, 49-53.
(2) Mach, J.P., Jaeger, P.H., Bertholt, M.M., Ruegsegger, C.H., Loosli, R.M., and PeHavel, J.(1974): Lancet, 2, 535-540.
(3) Booth, S.N., Jamisson, G.C., King, J.P., Leonard, J., Oates, G.D., and Dykes, P.W. (1974):Br.Med.J.,4,183-187.
(4) MacKay, A.M., Patel, S., Carter, S., Stevens, U., Laurence,D.J.R., Cooper, E.H., and Neville, A.M. (1974): Br.Med.J.,4,382-385.
(5) Herrera, M.A., Chu, T.M., and Holyoke, E.D. (1976): Ann.Surg., 183, 5-9.
(6) Sugarbaker, P.H., Skaring, A.T., and Zamcheck, N. (1976):J.Surg. Oncol., 8, 523-537.
(7) Ravry, M., Moertel, C.G., Schutt, A.J., and Go, V.L.W. (1974): Cancer, 34, 1230-1234.
(8) Holyoke, E.D., Chu, T.M., and Murphy, G.P. (1975): Cancer, 35, 830-836.
(9) LoGerfo,P., and Herter, F.P.(1975):Ann.Surg., 181, 81-84.
(10) Staab, H.J., Anderer, F.A., Stumpf, E., and Fischer, R. (1976): Z.Gastroenterol., Supplem. 11, 85-89.
(11) Staab, H.J., Anderer, F.A., Stumpf, E., and Fischer, R.(1977): Dtsch.med.Wschr., 102, 1082-1086.
(12) Martin, E.W., James, K.K., Hurtubise, P.E., Catalano, P., Minton, J.P.(1977): Cancer, 39, 440-446.
(13) Wehrle, E. (1977): Meth.Inform.Med., 16, 182-186.
(14) Staab, H.J., Anderer, F.A., Stumpf, E., Fischer, R. (1977): Proceedings of the 5th IRGCP meeting, Copenhagen
(15) Staab, H.J., Anderer, F.A., Stumpf, E., Fischer, R. J.Surg.Oncol. accepted July 1977

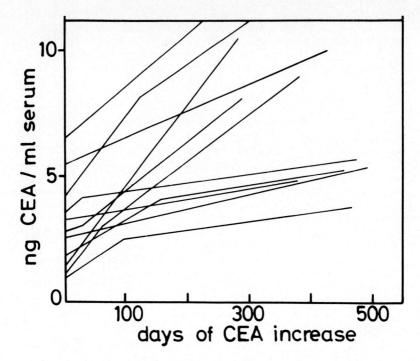

Fig. 1.Flat CEA slopes of cases given in table 1. Slopes, partly bi-
phasic, start with that CEA value preceding the CEA increase.

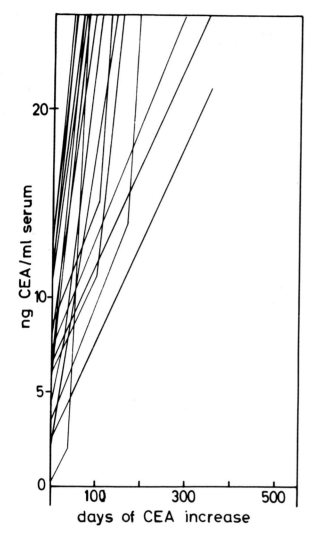

Fig. 2. Steep CEA slopes of cases given in table 2. Slopes, partly bi-phasic, start with that CEA value preceding the CEA increase.

DISCUSSION

COOPER E.H. (Leeds): We found that flat slope occurs 4 or 5 years after resection of primary colorectal cancer. Do you think this is a good indication for second-look surgery.

STAAB H.J. (Tubingen): I have to admit we do not have patients with 5 years follow-up in our programme. I always want to stress that we do not rely only on CEA values as an indication for second-look surgery.

MARTIN E.W. (Columbus) : I am not disagreeing with Staab. I think that delay of second-look surgery is not very interesting.

MACH J.P. (Lausanne): In summary, I think that in presence of a moderate rise of CEA level without any clinical evidence of tumour relapse one should repeat the CEA assay at least three times during a period of three months. If the CEA increases to a level at least two times higher than the base line of the particular patient and also two times higher than the normal value observed for a given CEA assay method, then a second-look surgery can be seriously considered.

CLINICAL APPLICATIONS OF SERUM CEA MONITORING
IN THE FOLLOW UP OF COLORECTAL CANCER.

J. Mouiel, Birtwisle Y., Chabannes B., Bus J.J., Krebs B.
Service de Chirurgie Générale. Professeur Ag. J. Mouiel.
Hôpital St-Roch, 5, rue Paul Devoluy 06000 NICE. FRANCE.

Carcinoembryogenic antigen (CEA) was measured in blood
taken from 30 cases of colorectal cancers, before and after
surgical resection of the tumour and during systematic chemotherapy (except DUKES A cases). The follow up consists of
monthly blood sampling, in accordance with the chemotherapy
schedule.

MATERIAL AND METHODS.
Table 1 shows the patients submitted to analysis.

TABLE 1

DUKES	A	B	C	D	TOTAL
Colonic cancer	1	12	3	2	18
Rectal cancer	2	2	7	1	12
TOTAL	3	14	10	3	30

CEA was measured in blood taken on EDTA with reagents commercialised by the french "Commissariat à l'énergie atomique"(1)
In this technic, the normal value is 5 ng/ml (2). But, in this
study, 10 ng was taken as the cut off level.

RESULTS

Preoperative levels and Dukes staging.
Out of 17 stage A and B, only one had more than 10 ng/ml CEA;
12 colonic carcinomas and all 4 rectal carcinomas were below
this level. In contrast 10 patients out of the 13 C and D Dukes
colorectal carcinoma presented high levels of CEA (fig. 1).
So, here exists a close relationship between the tumour extension and CEA preoperative level (Ref.3, 4) when one grouped
together on the one hand Dukes A and B, and Dukes C and D on
the other hand.

Postsurgical CEA levels.
CEA levels were measured during the period between surgery and
beginning of chemotherapy. For Dukes A and B, due to the low
level before surgery, no significative decrease was observed.
On the other hand, in Dukes C and D cases, decreasing of CEA
level was more clear without necessarily returning to normal
levels. This observation is simply explained in stage D cases,
where all metastatic disease was not removed at operation,

but is less easy to explain i stage C patients where complet
surgical extirpation should be followed by return to normal of
the serum CEA.
Thus it would seem that the Dukes classification is not apparently altogether satisfactory, since it fails to take into
account undetectable visceral metastases which retain their
secretary fonction. (fig.2)

EVOLUTION OF CEA DURING CHEMOTHERAPY.

We do not undertake chemotherapy in stage A cases. Among
14 cases stage B colorectal cancer, 3 cases were not given
chemotherapy due to age and have benn lost to view. 11 cases
were followed up regularly with investigations for metastatic
dissemination (liver enzymes, liver scan). 9 out of these 11
cases presented serum CEA levels always below 10 ng/ml for an
average period of 12 months. 2 patients had raised levels at
the 10 th month, correlated with certain local recurrence or
metastase.

Only one case out of the 10 stage C and D tumours retained
a serum CEA level below 10 ng/ml, without appreciable metastatic
dissemination. (fig.3) The other patients had variable but raised level, a progressive rise in serum CEA was well correlated
with the apparition of metastases or an approaching fatal outcome.

CONCLUSION.

In the follow up of patients during chemotherapy monitoring of CEA is of great value in stage B cases. All confirmed
elevated levels should be taken as danger signs, and should
lead to a comprehensive scaner for recurrence or metastases,
in order to facilitate intervention at an early stage. (5)

In stage C and D cases, CEA levels serve at the moment
only to confirm the clinical evolution, but it is to be hoped
that in the future they will enable the clinican to modify his
chemotherapy approach.

REFERENCES.

(1) Meriadec B., Martin F., Guerin J., Henry R., Klippling C.
    Description d'une méthode de dosage de l'antigène carcino-
    embryonnaire. Bull. Cancer 1973, 60, 403.

(2) Krebs B.P., Knecht J.T. et Coll,
    Communication personnelle.

(3) Mach J.P., Bertholet M.M., Jeager P., Pettavel J.,
    Wuilleret B.
    Bull. Cancer 1976, t.63, n°4, pp.551 à 562.

(4) Zamcheck M. D.
    Bull. Cancer 1976, t.63, n°4, pp.463 à 472.
(5) Martin Edward W. The use of CEA as an early indicator for
    gastrointestinal tumor recurrence and second-look procedures
    Cancer 39 : 440-446, 1977.

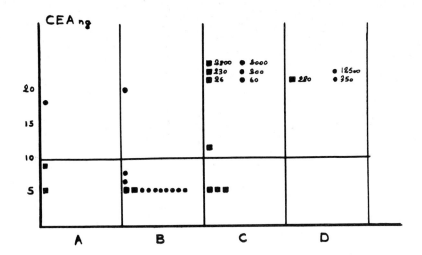

FIG. 1

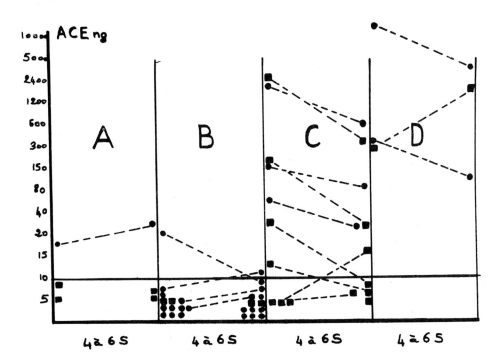

FIG. 2

103

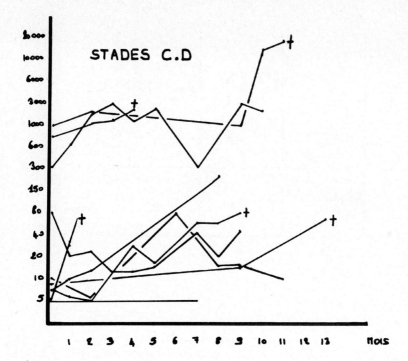

FIG. 3

VALUE OF CEA DETERMINATION IN POST OPERATIVE FOLLOW UP OF
COLORECTAL CARCINOMAS. DETECTION OF RECURRENCE AND SECOND
LOOK PROCEDURES.

Ph. SEGOL*, G. TRAVERT**, F. DUPUIS*, J.M. OLLIVIER*,
M. GIGNOUX*.

  * Service de Chirurgie Digestive, Pr. Ag. M. GIGNOUX
 ** Laboratoire de Radio-Immunologie, Pr. FERNANDEZ
    Centre Hospitalier Universitaire de CAEN, FRANCE.

We started serial determinations of CEA plasma levels
in all the cases of colorectal carcinomas we operated on
since the beginning of 1976 when this test was available
in our hospital.
    At the present time 71 patients with histologically
proven adenocarcinoma of the colon and rectum are followed
up by CEA determinations, routine clinical, radiological
and endoscopic examinations. Among these patients 27 had a
clinically complete resection of their lesion and 4 a second look procedure. The purpose of this paper is to illus
trate the practical application of the CEA test in a clinical setting.

MATERIAL AND METHODS.
    Plasma samples were analyzed for CEA content by the
Radioimmunoassay method (Kit Cis) described by B. MERIADEC
(1). The normal value has been established under 10 ng/ml,
20 ng/ml is considered as a certainly abnormal level. Between these limits interpretation is difficult mainly if
the patient is a smoker and the determination is repeated
after a period of abstinence.

Preoperative CEA values.
    On the 71 patients followed up 44 patients had a pre-
operative determination of CEA plasma level. All the patients underwent a laparotomy and diagnosis was confirmed
by histological examination. On the basis of operative findings patients were classified in three groups according
to BOOTH (2). Group 1 consisted in 27 patients with apparent localized disease (Dukes A, B or C) when curative
surgery was performed. Group 2 consisted in 10 patients
in whom the growth was apparently localized but advanced.
In these cases the tumour was unresectable or only palliative procedure was performed. Group 3 consisted in 7 patients with metastatic disease in the liver. The CEA levels
range are shown in Table 1.
    In 70 % of the cases classified in group 1 CEA plasma
level was over 10 ng/ml. In group 2 the incidence of positivity was slightly increased. No significant difference
could be noted between these two groups since the average
CEA value was similar in both. On the contrary in group 3

the average CEA value was very high and confirmed the value of CEA mesurement as index of metastatic disease (2).

TABLE 1 CEA levels in three groups with colorectal carcinoma before operation :

	Nº of patients	Nº with CEA 10ng/ml	Nº with CEA 10ng/ml	Average CEA value
Group 1	27	8	19 (70%)	42ng/ml
Group 2	10	2	8 (80%)	30ng/ml
Group 3	7	2	5	290ng/ml

We observed a marked difference between right and left colon tumour CEA plasma levels. Carcinoma of the caecum showed the lowest average CEA level and incidence of CEA positivity (3). Rectal carcinoma 's CEA levels were inter-
vening between the CEA values observed in Right colon carcinoma and Left colon tumour as shown in Table 2.

TABLE 2 CEA positivity peroperatively in Left colon Right
colon and rectal cancer (DUKES A, B, C).

CEA level ng/ml	Right colon carcinoma	Left colon carcinoma	Rectal carcinoma
0-10ng/ml	2	2	4
10ng/ml	3	8(80%)	8(66%)

Among the 27 patients submitted to curative resection the
preoperative CEA level related to DUKES'staging showed a
difference between the three groups as shown on Table 3.

TABLE 3 CEA level in localized COLO RECTAL cancer.

CEA level ng/ml	Dukes'A	Dukes'B	Dukes'C	All stages
0-10ng/ml	2	5	1	8
10ng/ml	2	10(66%)	7(87%)	19(70%)

In the preoperative follow up this last group is the only
one to have a practical interest, but only 70% of the patients can be followed up by serial determinations of CEA
to detect early tumour recurrence.

Postoperative CEA values.
In 27 patients who had a clinically complete resection
CEA plasma level was abnormal in 19 preoperatively. Among
these 19 patients 18 returned to normal value in the post
operative follow up. However, we have observed that CEA
levels may be elevated for as long as 3 months in patients
clinically free of disease before returning to normal.
In 10 patients postoperative CEA estimation was made
one month after the surgical resection : 5 patients returned to normal value, 2 had increased CEA plasma level which returned to normal value 3 to 5 months later, 3 had decreased CEA plasma levels but reached normal values only
at 4 to 8 months. The frequency of CEA estimations in our
follow up has been certainly inadequate to appreciate with
accuracy the exact time of return to normality, however
our data suggest that absence of early decline in CEA level to normal may not imply incomplete surgical resection
(4). The third postoperative month is considered in postoperative follow up as the best time to define the CEA
base line value, using it as a reference to further CEA
estimations.
At the present time 5 patients have had a tumour recurrence. In 4 cases CEA plasma level was over 10ng/ml at
least 3 months before clinical evidence of recurrence or
before recurrence could be proven. In the fifth case the
recurrence was discovered by systematic endoscopy and CEA
determination done simultaneously.
A patient demonstrated a second primary colon cancer
producing elevated CEA level. This patient had a right colectomy for a DUKES C carcinoma, her preoperative CEA estimation showed normal value. In the postoperative follow
up CEA level raised to 10ng/ml one year after resection.
A colonoscopy was done showing a polyp at 20cm from the
anal line, the patient refused endoscopic resection. Four
months after she had a resection showing a degenerated a-
denomatous polyp invading the muscularis mucosae. She underwent a laparotomy for segmental colectomy and lymphatic
clearance. This exploration was negative, no lymph node
involvement could be found on the surgical specimen and
the liver was normal.
On these 5 patients 2 are dead from the disease, death occured 10 months after recurrence in one case and 2
months in the other.
In 3 patients followed at least 9 months to 16 months
CEA estimations are abnormal but so far no evidence of recurrence has been proven. One of these patients is an heavy smoker. CEA values in these 3 patients are around 20ng/
ml. In one case preoperative level was normal. A second
look procedure is indicated and will certainly be performed as soon as patient's consent is obtained.

Second look procedure.
Abdominal reexploration indicated on maintened elevation of CEA was performed on 4 patients and showed recur-

rent tumour in 2. In 1 patient who had a left colectomy
for a DUKES'C carcinoma the second look procedure was negative, but certainly not satisfactorily performed. 3
months later the patient had acute small bowell obstruction and emergency operation showed an unrescectable lymphatic recurrence invading the first jejunal loop. A jejunal by-pass was performed. The other negative second
look is a case of postoperative second primary colonic can
cer, where liver palpation and specimen examination failed
to prove any metastatic disease.
    In two cases the reexploration was positive. The first
patient is a 63 years old man who had a localized resection of a degenerated rectal villous polyp associated with
radiotherapy. CEA plasma level returned to normal after
the excision. A local recurrence was found 6 months after
and abdominal-perineal resection was performed. The tumour
was classified DUKES'C. 2 months after resection, CEA estimation showed 130ng/ml and 320ng/ml fifteen days later.
A bone scan demonstrated abnormal aspect in the upper part
of the right femur. A second look laparotomy and bone biopsy were performed. 2 hepatic metastasis were found and
resected in the right lobe of the liver. Bone biopsy was
positive. This patient is at the present time under treatment with chemotherapy .
    The last patient is a 55 yearsold woman who had in
june 1974 a left colectomy for a DUKES'C carcinoma and resection of 2 little hepatic metastases. She received for
18 months a chemotherapy (5 FU). In 1976 serial CEA estimation showed maintened elevated values, the patient was
doing very well. A second look procedure was performed in
may 1976 and a left hepatectomy performed. CEA plasma level returned to normal (Figure 1) after the operation.
She had a chemotherapy since the second look procedure
and is still asymptomatic. At the present time CEA is again
abnormal and we tried to get her consent for a third look
procedure. She refused reoperation.

COMMENT.
    This series confirms the usefulness of the CEA assay
done preoperatively to appreciate the metastatic spread
of the disease. On the contrary, frequency of positivity
and average values are similar in localized and advanced
disease. It is impossible de predict the lesion's resectability by this test. We found as others (3) a significant difference between frequency of positivity in right,
left and rectal cancer. One of our patient had a right
colon cancer not producing CEA and a second primary cancer on the left colon producing elevated CEA plasma level.
This data suggest that CEA determinations are usefull pre-
operatively even if the resected lesion was not producing
CEA preoperatively.
    Persistent raised CEA more than 3 months after surgi-
cal resection should be assumed to indicate residual mal-
gignancy (2). However a fall of CEA to normal value does

not rule out the possibility for reccurrence. We found
that the postoperative base line value is best defined
3 months after the surgical procedure. In our date maintened CEA elevation has always been followed by a recurrence
histologically or clinically proven.

Second look procedure may permit a surgical treatment
with benefit for the patient in some cases. The time inter
val between the primary operation and second look procedure ranged from 8 to 18 months.

Serial CEA determination in patients submitted to curative resection of a CEA producing lesion is usefull to
detect early recurrence. This test is performed one month
after the resection and every 3 months during long term
follow up. The finding of a maintened increased CEA above
the base line value combined with clinical, radiological
and endoscopic examination leads to second look procedure in asymptomatic patients. Much problems can be encountered to obtain the consent for a reintervention on asymptomatic patients.

REFERENCES.
(1) MERIADEC B., MARTIN F., GUERIN J., HENRY R. et KLEP-
PING C. Description d'une méthode de dosage de l'Antigène
Carcino-Embryonnaire. Bull. Cancer, 60, 403-410, 1973.
(2) BOOTH S.N., JAMIESON G.C., KING J.P.G., LEONARD J.,
OATES G.D. and DYKES P.W. Carcinoembryonic antigen in management of colorectal carcinoma. Br. Med. J.,4,183-187,
1974.
(3) EDWARD W., MARTIN Jr., MD, WILLIAM E., KIBBEY, MD,
LORETTA DI VECCHIA, MS, GREGG ANDERSON, MD, PHILIP CATA-
LANO, MD, and John P. MINTON, MD, Ph. D. Cancinoembryonic
antigen. Clinical and historical aspects. Cancer, 37, 62-
81, 1976.
(4) B.A. BIVINS, MD, Carl R. BOYD; B.A. WILLIAM R. MEEKER,
Jr., MD, and Ward O. GRIFFEN, Jr., MD, Ph. D. CEA level
and prognosis in colon carcinoma. J. Surg. Oncol. 6, 413-
421, 1974.

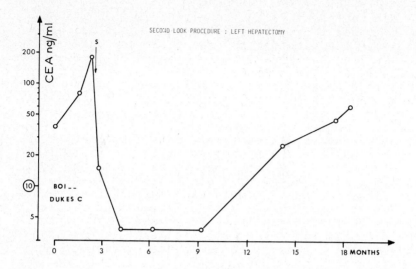

Fig. 1 Serial CEA levels before and after a left hepatectomy performed 18 months after a radical resection for
left colon carcinoma. Third look refused by the patient.

C.E.A. and 99m-Tc-sulphur colloid liver scan in the diagnosis and follow up study of malignomas.

E. Turba +, A. Fini +, D. Conighi °, and A. Abbati +

Servizio di Medicina Nucleare + e di Fisica Sanitaria°
Ospedali di Bologna - 40133

Follow up study of hepatic metastases of malignomas is
indispensable to therapy planning: as proposed by W.B.
Van Der Pompe   since October '76   104 cancer patients
referred to us for the investigation of the presence and
spread of hepatic metastases, have undergone C.E.A. pla
sma measurement and 99m-Tc sulphur colloid liver distribu
tion study by rectilinear scan and Phogamma III HP Anger camera, in an attempt to achieve a reduction of the
frequency of false positive and negative cases.

METHODS:

C.E.A. radioimmunoassay was performed using Gold's techni
que with reagents obtained from S.OR.IN (Saluggia, Ita-
ly): preliminar extraction by perchloric acid is not necessary with this kit and final separation B/F is obtained by the technique of a second antibody supported on
cellulose.
    Radioisotopic liver study was performed injecting
intravenously 2 mCi of 99m-Tc sulphur colloid Hoechst;
its liver distribution was investigated 30 min. later by
a Phogamma III HP Anger Camera with a diverging collima
tor and by an El Scint rectilinear scanner connected to
a VDP-2 processing unit, in anterior, right lateral and
posterior positions.

RESULTS

    The cases investigated had previously undergone a
complete clinical study with surgical and biopsical evidence of colonic (53) gastric (30) mammal (15) pancreas
(2) uterus (2) ileus (1) and ovarian (1) carcinomas.

99m-Tc sulphur colloid scans were classified as:

a) Positive (+), when presenting single or multiple cold or hypoactive central areas on the liver map.

b) Doubtful (?), when hypoactive and non-homogeneous areas were observed along the lower edge of the liver and/or in the free edge of the left liver lobe.

c) Negative (-), when no cold of hypoactive area was remarkable in the whole liver image.

C.E.A. levels were considered positive (+) when above 12 ng/ml and negative (-) when equal to or below this limit: this cutoff equals 3 standard deviations of mean values obtained in our laboratory from 30 normal human subjects.

Tables 1-5 show the distribution of results obtained.

It appears that a part of all of the doubtful or negative scans showed positive C.E.A. values, with a higher frequency in the group of colonic cancers.

This observation on a selected group of cancer patients provides the opportunity to use together these diagnostic techniques in order to reduce the number of liver metastasis cases which cannot be identified by liver scan, being below the resolution limits of the technique and/or situated in marginal areas of the organ, where only the association of colloid and positive radioactive compounds allows the recognition of their presence.

Moreover, as is well known, cold areas are not specific to metastases, but occur also in many other space occupying lesions, and C.E.A. can be positive also in pathological conditions different from metastatic tumours: a final diagnosis can be obtained in many of these cases by liver biopsy localised on the cold areas indicated by the scan.

REFERENCES:

(1) Pompe W.B., Cox P.H., Treurniet-Donker A.D., a. Boulis-Wassif S. (1976): Eur. J. Nucl. Med. 1, 141

(2) Gold P. Freedmann S.O. - (1965) J. Clin. Invest. 44, 1057

(3) Douglas Hoyoke E. a. Cooper E.H. (1976): Semi. Oncology 3/4, 377

(4) Martin E.W., James K.K., Hurtubise P.E., Catalano P., Minton J.P., (1977): Cancer, 39/2, 440

(5) Lamerz R. u. Riuder H. (1976): Münch. Med. Wschr. 118/12, 371

(6) Mor C., Orefice S., Rocco F., Accini R., Bartorelli A. (1977) Atti Convegno "Aggiornamenti in Endocrinologia", Trento 1976 pp 199-218.

TABLE 1

FINDING IN 104 SCREENED PERSONS

	CEA −	CEA +	TOTAL
99 m Tc S.C. +	11	35	46
99 m Tc S.C. ?	12	14	26
99 m Tc S.C. −	26	6	32
TOTAL	49	55	104

TABLE 2   COLON RECTUM

	CEA −	CEA +	Total
99 m Tc S.C. +	3	23	26
99 m Tc S.C. ?	5	9	14
99 m Tc S.C. −	11	2	13
TOTAL	19	34	53

TABLE 3 STOMACH

	CEA −	CEA +	TOTAL
99 m Tc S.C. +	3	6	9
99 m Tc S.C. ?	5	3	8
99 m Tc S.C. −	10	3	13
TOTAL	18	12	30

TABLE 4 BREAST

	CEA −	CEA +	TOTAL
99 m Tc S.C. +	3	4	7
99 m Tc S.C. ?	1	2	3
99 m Tc S.C. −	4	1	5
TOTAL	8	7	15

TABLE 5

	99mTc S.C.+ CEA +	99mTc S.C.+ CEA −	99mTc S.C. ? CEA −	99mTc S.C. − CEA −	TOTAL
PANCREAS	1	1			2
UTERUS	1			1	2
ILEUS			1		1
OVARY		1			1

C.E.A. activity in pure pancreatic juice

J.F. REY[+], B.P. KREBS, J. DELMONT

Centre d'Hépato-Gastro-Entérologie de Cimiez, Centre Antoine
Lacassagne (Nice)

A great abnormality of plasma C.E.A. has been demonstrated
in patients with carcinoma of the pancreas. Unfortunately this elevation was not always specific. There was an important overlap between the values in patients with benign pancreatic disease and those
with malignant disease. Some people showed a very conserable elevation without any real known cause, however in some cases with
malignant disease the plasma C.E.A. was normal.

Since this cancer is usually of duct cell origin and pancreatic
juice is in direct contact with malignant cells, high concentrations
of C.E.A. in pancreatic juice might be expected. With endoscopic
retrograd cholangio-pancreatography (ERCP) it is possible to study
with comparative ease the pancreatic duct system and collect the
juice. The object of our study is to estimate the diagnostic importance of C.E.A. values in particular where the interpretation of ERCP
pictures are not clear.

MATERIALS AND METHODS

We have collected with simple pre-medication (intravenous dia-
zepan 5-10 mg) pure pancreatic juice using a specially designed catheter. After checking the position of the catheter by aspiration of a
clear fluid, we stimulate the pancreas using Boots Secretin (1 clinical unit per kg body weight). Firsty we separate the samples into
different aliquots placed in storage at freeling point either alone of
employing different inhibitors. The results were not conclusive and
we shall assess the sample on pure ice. The radioimmunological
assay of C.E.A. was described by MERIADEC and MARTIN.

We thus have measured the C.E.A. values in 40 patients who
were hospitalised in the Centre d'Hepato-Gastro-Enterologie de
Nice.

We had 8 patients with cancer of the pancreas, 15 chronic pancreatitis, 3 different types of proven benign pancreatic pathology, 3
secondary cancers of the liver and 11 control cases.

RESULTS

In the pure pancreatic juice our results are markedly different
in various groups (table I).

The patients with pancreatic carcinoma had medium elevation
up to 461.75 ng/ml. The least elevated was 160 ng/ml, and the

[+]Present address : INSERM Unité 145 Dr P. FREYCHET (Nice)

greastest elevation was 1700 ng/ml.

In the chronic pancreatitis group the mean value was only 42.84 ng/ml. In the control group the mean value was 23.16 ng/ml. The highest level was 60 ng/ml. Finally we have found a measurement slightly above 150 ng/ml in three patients with metastatic liver cancer, without any evidence of carcinoma of the pancreas ; and in one patient with an embryological disorder called ventral pancreas.

On the other hand the measurement of plasma C.E.A. did not show a significative difference between the three groups.

TABLE I   Measurement of C.E.A. in pure pancreatic juice and plasma

Diagnosis	Pure pancreatic juice ng/ml			Plasma ng/ml
	mean	minimal level	maximal level	mean
Pancreatic carcinoma	461.75	160	1700	9
Chronic pancreatitis	42.84	10	350	20
Control	23.16	8	60	4.75

DISCUSSION

We would like to make some observations :

1° The difference between the various groups namely cancer and chronic pancreatitis is highly significant ($P < 0.01$). If we fix a limit at 150 ng/ml (this is arbitrarily fixed) we observe only one patient in the group of carinic pancreatitis overlapping with the malignant group.

2° On the contrary it is not possible to distinguish the level in a patient with chronic pancreatitis from the controls, because of the complete overlapping.

3° In the last column of figure 1 we have put 3 patients with congenital abnormalities of the pancreas. One of these patients had an inexplicable level at 183 ng/ml. But recently COTTON (2) has shown chronic pancreatitis of the body and the tail of the pancreas, in patients with separate drainage from the main and accessory pancreatitis ducts. Perhaps this patient had undiagnosed chronic pancreatitis ?

4° Finally these 3 patients showed secondary carcinoma of the liver and as far as we could tell abnormal pancreas. We have seen a level higher than 150 ng/ml. Whatever the cause of this elevation of C.E.A. be it primary or secondary tumour a raised level in the pancreatic juice could be explained by an excretion of plasma C.E.A. by the pancreas. This finding must be confirmed and we suggest studies on pancreatic juice in patients showing elevated C.E.A. and in patients with proven liver metastasis. We ourselves will use a more specific method by employing the perchloric extraction technique.

TABLE II   Comparative studies of C.E.A. levels in pure pancreatic juice

	Pancreatic carcinomas ng/ml	Chronic pancreatitis ng/ml	Controls ng/ml
Kawanishi et al	109	6,4	2
McCabe et al	100	27,5	14,5
Sharma et al	309	18,6	8,1
Rey et al	461,75	42,8	23,1

Our results are confirmed by other workers : H. KAWANISHI et al (3) McCABE et al (4) and SHARMA et al (5). They showed a significant difference between the chronic pancreatitis group and carcinoma patients (table 2). The difference between the absolute level in these studies is really on account of the different methods used.

Only ESCOURROU (6) did not find any real difference but his work was only carried out on a very small number of patients, and he stimulated the exocrine pancreatic secretion with caeruleine which has a cholecystokinin-like action, of wich the action on the volume is less important.

CONCLUSION

This method is in itself limited by the technical difficulties of recoverey of the juice ; it is not possible because of the time consuming factor to perform at the same time E.R.C.P. and pancreatic juice collection. If the X-ray studies are not certain we think that the measurement of C.E.A. pancreatic juice should be extremely useful.

In effect pancreatic diseases are amongst the most difficult to diagnose for the clinician. In these doubtful cases the collection of pancreatic juice which allows assessment of C.E.A. and also lactoferine in pancreatitis, affords the clinician further possibilities for diagnosis without resorting to such methods as laparotomy.

REFERENCES

(1) Rey J.F., Salmon P., Ljunggren B. and Delmont J. (1977) : Journal Med Lyon, 1311, 15-19

(2) Cotton P.B., Kizu M. (1977) : Gut, 18, A 400

(3) Kawanishi H., Sell J.E., Pollard H.M. (1976) : Gastroentero-logy, 70, 1033

(4) McCabe R.P., Kupchick H.Z. and Zamcheck N. (1974) : Federation Proceedings, 33, 637

(5) Sharma M.P., Gregg J.A., Loewenstein M.S., McCabe R.P. and Zamcheck N. (1976) : Cancer, 38, 2457-2461

(6) Escourrou J., Ribet A. (1977) : IIIe international symposium on digestive endoscopy, Brussels, 24-26 feb. 1977

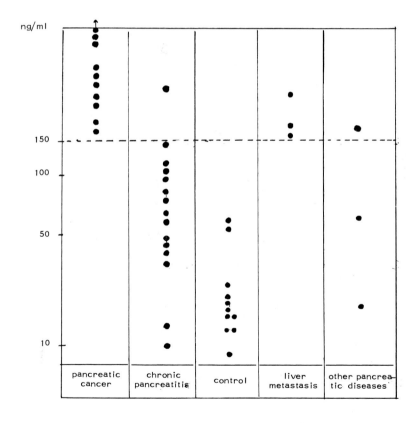

Fig. 1 : datas of the measurement of C.E.A. in pure pancreatic juice.

119

DISCUSSION

ZAMCHECK N. (Boston): The authors should be congratulated on this
work. We found pancreatic cannulation to be a difficult procedure.
There are pitfalls in CEA assay. You need to know the time of collection of pancreatic juice, otherwise you have no real basis for
measuring the actual amount of CEA that comes out of the pancreatic
duct. I think it may be more useful to look for a pancreatic cancer
marker, more specific than CEA.

REY J.F. (Nice): I think the procedure is easy to perform if you
have good practice. To-day, we can stay half an hour in the
pancreatic duct, even after injection of secretin or cholecystokinin,
if the catheter is deeply placed; the motricity of the duct is out
of importance.

PROGNOSTIC INTEREST OF CARCINOEMBRYONIC ANTIGEN (CEA) ASSAYS IN OESOPHAGEAL CANCERS - A STUDY OF 102 PATIENTS IN THE CENTRE FRANCOIS BACLESSE OF CAEN

J.E. Couette, J. Goussard, A. Roussel, J. Robillard and J.S. Abbatucci

Centre François Baclesse - Route de Lion-sur-Mer
14018 CAEN CEDEX - France

The CEA assays were determined in patients with oesophageal cancers. The majority of these patients is tobacco and ethylic consumer, and had precarious hygienic and alimentary conditions. Thereby, we are entitled to expect results of assays entirely abnormal. Nevertheless, we cannot show significant difference about the frequency of chronic bronchitis and cirrhosis between patients with rates above 30 ng and other patients with rates below 5 ng.

CHATAL could not find relationship between CEA levels and age, site of tumor, macroscopic form of tumor, presence of metastases, sites of metastases. On the other hand, he showed the possibility of a supervision by CEA level.

To us, it seemed that the patients with high CEA levels had more often secondary sites, but it was impossible to argue from it some prognosis. Therefore, we thought it could be interesting to make a retrospective study in order to show :

1) Correlations being able to guide to the origin of CEA in oesophageal cancers

2) A prognostic factor of the assay

3) An eventual indication of the progress of the disease.

METHOD

CEA assay is performed directly on the serum according to the method of the double antibody developed by the "Commissariat à l'Energie Atomique".

We selected the records of patients having had CEA assay :

1) In our Laboratory

2) At the time of the first medical consultation

3) In oesophageal tumors with histological verification

4) In patients having had a checkup including : clinical examination, oesophageal radiography, esophagoscopy, lung radiography.

Every time the level notion was found in the record, we noted : age, time of follow-up, tumor site in the oesophagus, aspect, apparent size of the lesion (cm), histology, state of satellite nodules, presence of metastases with site, other neoplastic site, CEA level and survival after the first medical advice.

121

For patients who had two assays (the first one done at the beginning and the second one 1-12 months after) we noted : the interval, the new level, the treatment received and the clinical state in the second treatment (improved, constant, worsened).

MATERIAL

Two hundred and eleven patients with oesophageal cancers were submitted to CEA assays. But, we are obliged to exclude from this study :
- patients who did not fall into this category (other digestive cancers and patients without histology)
- patients who had assay only after or during the progression of the treatment, or who had, before oesophageal cancer, another cancer being able to increase CEA.

At the end of this classifying, it remains 102 patient's records (18 with 2 assays).

Among the 102 patients, we find :
- N 1 : 13 patients
- M 1 : 6 patients (lung : 4, bone : 1, liver : 1)
- Seven patients have a second neoplastic site during the first month after the medical advice (hypopharynx : 4, larynx : 1, tonsil : 1, rectum : 1).

Levels are rarely elevated, but more often mean (Table 1).

TABLE 1 : Oesophageal cancer - CEA level

CEA ng	$\leqslant$ 10	11 - 20	21 - 30	> 30	Total
	45 *	32	17	8	102

*($\leqslant$ 5 ng = 28)

RESULTS

1) Origin of CEA in oesophageal cancer :

We can confirm that : the age and the lesion aspect do not explain CEA level (Table 2 and Table 3).

Table 2 : Oesophageal cancer - CEA - Age

CEA ng \ Age	30 - 50	51 - 60	61 - 70	$\geqslant$ 71	Total
$\leqslant$ 10	5	11	9	20	45
> 10	10	14	24	9	57

TABLE 3 : Oesophageal cancer - CEA - Macroscopic aspect

Aspect	Number	Mean level	$\leqslant$ 10	> 10
Vegetating	42	13,9	18	24
Ulcerating	9	7,5	6	3 *
Infiltrating	16	11,2	9	7
Unspecified	35	18,7	12	23

*1 patient > 500 not included for the calculation of the mean level

We thought that the histology could explain some elevated CEA, particularly for lesions near glandular aspect (Table 4). We could also think that, at the level of the lower third, the proximity of glandular mucous membrane whould involve more elevated CEA levels (Table 5), but it is not obvious. On the other hand, for lesions poorly differentiated, we find mean level a little lower.

TABLE 4 : Oesophageal cancer - CEA - Histology

Histology	Poorly differentiated	Malpighian	Glandular
Number	19	81	2
CEA ng mean level	9,7	16,2	15

TABLE 5 : Oesophageal cancer - CEA - Tumor level

	Number	CEA ng mean level	≤ 10	> 10
Upper third	17	11,6	7	10
Middle third	47	14,4 *	23	24
Lower third	38	16	15	23

* 1 patient > 500 not included for the calculation of the mean level.

It remains the extent of the disease :
- The size of the primary tumor gives no explanation (Table 6)
- Node involvement, no more (Table 7)
- Presence of secondary distant tumor or other neoplastic site (Table 8) seems to be well correlated, although not statistically significant.

TABLE 6 : Oesophageal cancer - CEA - size of lesion

Size (cm)	Number	CEA ng mean level	≤ 10 ng	> 10 ng
< 5	22	18	10	12
6 - 10	36	14	13	23
≥ 11	13	10,6	8	5
Unspecified	31	13,5	14	17

TABLE 7 : Oesophageal cancer - CEA - Node involvement

	Number	CEA ng mean level	≤ 10	> 10
No Mo	80	13,5	35	45
N1 Mo	13	12,5	6	7

TABLE 8 : Oesophageal cancer - CEA - Metastases or other neoplastic sites

CEA	> 30	> 20	≤ 5
M1 or 2 nd neoplastic site	3/8 37,5 %	8/25 29 %	4/28 14,2 %

$0,10 < p < 0,15$

Lung metastases involve high CEA levels but especially other neoplastic sites involve notable increases (Table 9).

TABLE 9 : Oesophageal cancer - Metastases - Other neoplastic sites

	Number	CEA ng mean level	≤ 10	> 10
M1 lung	4	19,2	2	2
M1 other	2	6,5	2	
2nd neoplastic site	7	28,5 *	1	5 *

*patient with rectal cancer   (CEA level : 500)   not included

2) CEA, prognostic factor :

If CEA level is higher in case of secondary sites, prognosis should be worst (Table10).

TABLE 10: Oesophageal cancer - CEA - Survival after 6 months

CEA ng	Survival after 6 months	
> 20	11/18	(61 %)
11 - 20	12/21	(57 %)
0 - 10	13/23	(59 %)

But it is nothing of the king if the prognosis is evaluated on the survival after 6 months.

Is an increasing level a worse prognosis ? (Table 11). It does not seem because the survival after 6 months is the same when CEA increases or decreases.

TABLE 11 : Oesophageal cancer - Evolution of CEA level - Survival after 6 months.

CEA	Increased	Constant	Decreased
Number	8	2	8
Survival after 6 months	7/8	2/2	6/7 *

*It is too soon to evaluate the 6 months survival for one patient

3) <u>Can CEA be an eventual indication of the progress of oesophageal</u>
<u>cancer</u> ?

If the second assay is higher than the first one, we except a worsened clinical state. An evaluation is made in 18 patients : 7 patients are
improved, 7 are unchanged and 4 worsened (Table 12).

TABLE 12 : Oesophageal cancer - Evolution of CEA level - Clinical
state in the second treatment

Clinical state	2 nd CEA	
IMPROVED	Decreased	5
	Increased	2
	Constant	0
UNCHANGED	Decreased	2
	Increased	3
	Constant	2
WORSENED	Decreased	1
	Increased	3
	Constant	0

Although the number of patients is small, it seems that the evolution of the clinical state is correlated with the increased of CEA level.
The correlation between level and clinical state is not better if
patients with initial pathological levels are only concerned (Table 13).

TABLE 13 : Oesophageal cancer - Evolution of CEA level according to
the initial level

Initial level	Final level	Clinical state
47	21	constant
26	16	worsened
54	17	improved
40	15	improved
36	56	constant
25	32	improved
19	17	improved
15	0	improved
16	10	unchanged
13	19	unchanged
17	76	worsened
12	22	improved
10	0	improved
0	0	unchanged
4	5	unchanged
9	20	unchanged
0	8	worsened
5	23	worsened

In conclusion : we found CEA level above 10 ng/nl in 56 % of our patients. The origin of this CEA seems to be particularly related to the presence of metastases. The evolution of the assays seems to be correlated with the clinical progress. But, actually therapeutic decision in the progress of oesophageal cancer, based on this assay, is not possible.

REFERENCE

(1) Chatal, J.F., Dedieu, P.R., Le Mevel,B.P., Helary, J., Guihard, D. and Salard, J.L. (1976) : Bull. Cancer, 63, 531.

THE LEUKOCYTE ADHERENCE INHIBITION ASSAY FOR THE DETECTION OF
COLORECTAL CANCER*

A.T. Ichiki, Y.P. Quirin, I.R. Collmann, T. Sonoda and S. Krauss

University of Tennessee Memorial Research Center and Hospital,
Knoxville, Tennessee 37920, USA

The objective of this paper is to demonstrate that the leukocyte adherence inhibition assay (LAI) does have value in assessing
cell-mediated anti-tumor immunity in colorectal cancer patients.

METHODS AND MATERIALS

The leukocyte adherence inhibition assay was performed by the
test tube method which was described by Grosser and Thomson (1).
Colorectal tumors were extracted by 3 M KCl according to the methods
of McCoy et al. (2). The resulting extract was considered to contain the colorectal tumor associated antigen. Nonspecific antigens
included preparations of normal colon tissues and melanoma which
were similarly extracted.

RESULTS

The results of the LAI assay was expressed by the nonadherence
index (NAI) which was calculated by the following formula:

$$NAI = \frac{\% \text{ nonadherent cells in presence of specific antigen} - \% \text{ nonadherent cells in presence of nonspecific antigen}}{\% \text{ nonadherent cells in presence of nonspecific antigen}} \times 100$$

The NAI was calculated with both the normal colon extract and melanoma extract. The specificity of the assay for colorectal cancer
was determined by testing peripheral blood leukocytes from normal
subjects, patients with chronic nonmalignant diseases, unrelated malignant diseases and colorectal cancer. The results found in Figure
1 were calculated with normal colon extract (circles) and melanoma
extract (triangles). The average NAI for the control subjects,
patients with chronic nonmalignant diseases, and patients with non-
related cancers was less than 30, which was considered a positive
value. Repeated positive NAI was observed with a normal subject and
a patient with malignant melanoma. A patient with chronic ulcerative
colitis was also positive. The colorectal cancer patients were
grouped according to the Dukes' classification. The average NAI for

*Supported by General Research Support Funds (USPHS) and The Physic-
ians Medical Educational and Research Foundation.

127

the Dukes' A and B patients was 28.3 with normal colon and 16.2 with melanoma, was 35.1 with normal colon and 22.1 with melanoma for the Dukes' C patients, and was 68.2 with normal colon and 35.8 with melanoma for the patients with metastatic disease. A considerable spread of the NAI was noted with the PBL from the patients with metastatic disease which could be due to the effects of the chemotherapeutic regimen. A difference in the NAI values could be discerned when the calculations were made with the two different nonspecific antigens. A higher NAI was observed with the normal colon antigen. Unfortunately, we did not have sufficient newly diagnosed patients to test prior to surgical resection at the time this study was initiated.

A summary of the 30 colorectal cancer patients included in this study are found in Table 1. All patients had histologically proven adenocarcinoma of the large bowel. Patients who were staged Dukes' C received 5-fluorouracil adjuvant chemotherapy, while patients with metastatic disease received 5-fluorouracil and mitomycin C chemotherapy as described by Sonoda and Krauss (3). The LAI assay was performed at least 28 days after the completion of the last course of chemotherapy. The patients were also separated according to their prognosis.

TABLE 1 Summary of the colorectal patient population

Group	Dukes' Classification	Prognosis Favorable	Unfavorable	Total
(Patients studied prior to surgical resection)				
I	C	2(1)[+]	1(1)	3(2)
				3
(Patients studied post-surgical resection)				
II	A	1	0	1
III	B	1(1)	0	1(1)
IV	C	8(5)	0	8(5)
V	Metastatic Disease	1	16(10)	17(10)
				30

+ = number of female patients appear in parenthesis.

When the results of the LAI assays were summarized according to the staging and by prognosis (Table 2), we noted that the mean NAI with normal colon extract was the highest for the patients who had metastatic disease who had an unfavorable prognosis. Therefore, it was concluded that an increasing NAI reflected a decrease in the efficacy of the cell-mediated anti-tumor immunity in the colorectal cancer patient.

TABLE 2 Summary of mean NAI values for colorectal cancer patients
according to prognosis

Group	Favorable		Unfavorable	
	Mel	NCE	Mel	NCE
I	42.8± 34.8 N=2, NT=2	45.21± 21.7	34.6 N=1, NT=1	ND
II,III,IV	46.7± 16.6 N=10, NT=20	35.1± 10.2		
V	7.2± 38.9 N=1, NT=3	-1.72± 4.1	39.3± 11.3 N=16, NT=29	105.1± 37.5

N = Number of patients; NT = Total number of tests performed; ND =
Not done; NCE = Normal colon tissue extract; Mel = Melanoma tumor
extract; NAI = Nonadherence index.

Sequential LAI studies have been performed usually at 3 to 4
month intervals. The results of one of our patients, a 72 year old
male staged as Dukes' C, are found in Figure 2. The LAI study was
initiated 3 months after surgical resection and after the patient had
been given two courses of 5-FU chemotherapy. A positive NAI was observed; however, a negative NAI was determined when the patient was
retested 9 months later. It was further observed that the carcinoembryonic antigen (CEA) level was negative at the time of the initial
study, but increased dramatically (greater than 25 ng/ml) when the
NAI dropped. The results with this patient and others we have studied have strongly indicated that a decrease in the NAI was reflected
by an unfavorable clinical course of the patient. Our results led
to the reevaluation of the patient to determine the possibility of
recurring disease.

In order to substantiate the existence of a colorectal tumor-
associated antigen (CTAA), we prepared antisera with a colon tumor
extract which had been subjected to gel filtration to remove the high
and low molecular weight macromolecules. The remaining material was
then subjected to affinity chromatography with antibodies against
normal human serum proteins covalently linked to Sepharose 4B beads.
The unbound proteins were used to immunize the rabbits to produce
antibodies against the CTAA. The anti-CTAA activity was determined
by the capacity to abrogate the CTAA activity in the LAI assay. The
results found in Table 3 indicated that the antiserum affected the
percent nonadherence with the tumor extract but not the normal colon
extract when tested with peripheral blood from colorectal cancer patients. Normal rabbit serum, on the other hand, did not affect the
activity of either extracts. The antisera did not affect the activity of melanoma associated antigen when tested with peripheral
blood leukocytes from melanoma patients. Therefore, the antisera
prepared against CTAA was useful in substantiating the specificity
of our assay.

TABLE 3 Immune and non-immune sera pre-incubated with CTAA and NCE

% Nonadherence	Patients with Colorectal Cancer		Patients with Melanoma	
	N.C.	S.P.	D.D.	A.G.
CTAA	20.4 ± 1.8	60.3 ± 6.4	34.8 ± 4.3	14.5 ± 2.8
NCE	9.0 ± 1.2	34.8 ± 3.5	47.3 ± 1.2	19.1 ± 3.4
NRS + CTAA	24.3 ± 3.8	61.7 ± 0.0	45.7 ± 0.4	22.7 ± 2.4
Anti-CTAA + CTAA	14.3 ± 2.8	43.0 ± 3.9	42.8 ± 1.7	20.5 ± 1.5
Anti-CTAA + NCE	13.3 ± 1.0	53.9 ± 2.4	50.8 ± 0.8	25.8 ± 2.6

SUMMARY

    In summary, the extraction of colorectal tumor materials by 3 M
KCl yielded a colorectal tumor associated antigen which could be demonstrated by the leukocyte adherence inhibition assay. This assay
appears to be most valuable in assessing the cell-mediated anti-tumor
immunity of individual cases, since the LAI results reflected the
clinical course of the patient.

REFERENCES

(1) Grosser, N. and Thomson, D.M.P. (1975): Cancer Res., 35, 2571.
(2) McCoy, J.L., Jerome, L.F., Dean, J.H., Cannon, G.B., Alford,
     T.C., Doering, T. and Herberman, R.B. (1974): J. Nat. Cancer
     Inst., 53, 11.
(3) Sonoda, T. and Krauss, S. (1977): Clin. Res., 25, 411A.

ABBREVIATIONS USED

NAI - Non-adherence index
LAI - Leukocyte adherence inhibition
PBL - Peripheral blood leukocytes
CTAA - Colorectal tumor associated antigen

130

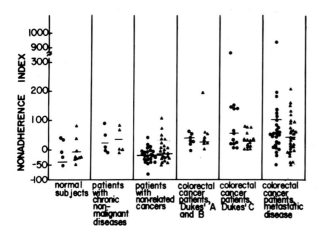

Fig. 1 The nonadherence index of all of the patients tested were calculated with the normal colon extract (●) and melanoma extract (▲). The mean NAI values were indicated by the horizontal lines.

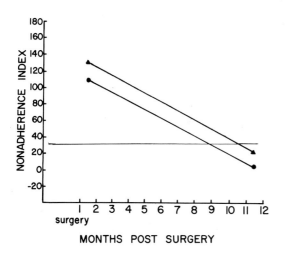

Fig. 2 The sequential NAI values of patient JM who was studied following surgical resection and 2 courses of 5-FU chemotherapy. The NAI was calculated with normal colon extract (●) and melanoma extract (▲).

131

DISCUSSION

HERBERMAN R.B. (Bethesda): I wonder why you are refering to this test as reflecting cell-mediated immunity in the patient. I thought that it was supposed to be a serum antibody mediated test.

ICHIKI A.T. (Knoxville): Well, we have looked at other immunological parameters in our studies including CEA. We have also looked at the antigen by the leukocyte migration inhibition assay. It appears that our results with this assay reflect the cell-mediated immunity of the patients as has been indicated by the other assay method.

IDENTIFICATION AND PURIFICATION OF A GASTRIC GOBLET CELL ANTIGEN IN INTESTINAL METAPLASIA AND GASTRIC CANCER

W.Rapp und K.H.Wurster

Medizinische Universitätsklinik Heidelberg, Pathologisches Institut der Universität Heidelberg und Institut für Nuklearmedizin am Deutschen Krebsforschungszentrum Heidelberg

In intestinal metaplasia normal gastric epithelium is substituted by striated columnar cells and by goblet cells, normally present in the small and large gut. Goblet cells stain with PAS and more specifically with alcian blue (AB) at pH 2.5. Antigenic substances of human goblet cells have already been identified (1,2,3) and purified (3). More recently gastric goblet cells have been reported to contain carcinoembryonic antigen (CEA) and normal intestinal glycoprotein NCA2 crossreacting with CEA (4,5).

This paper describes the purification and immunohistochemical demonstration of an antigenic AB-staining component of gastric goblet cells (GO-Ag) which is devoid of any immunochemical relationship with CEA and other normal gastric antigens hitherto identified.

METHODS

Purification

A resected gastric tumor composed of signet ring cells and of intestinalized adjacent tissue was homogenized in PBS and extracted by 0.2M perchloric acid (PCA). After neutralization and dialysis the extract was applied on a DEAE cellulose column. Discontinuous eluation was performed at rising molarities at 0.01, 0.04, 0.1, 0.2 and 0.3M at pH 7.0. The pooled eluates were then applied to a Sephadex G 200 column. Pooled fractions containing AB-staining substances were then applied to preparative polyacrylamide gel electrophoresis (PAGE) at pH 9.0 using 7% separation gel. Strips of 3mm were eluted, dialysed and concentrated as described (6).

Analytical PAGE according to ALLEN (6), gel system no.2, was used for monitoring of proteins, glycoproteins and AB substances.

Two rabbits were immunized with complete Freund's Adjuvant and boostered at two weeks interval using 4 x 100 µg/ml protein of purified material.

Immunohistochemistry

The indirect immunoperoxidase method was used. Per-
oxidase conjugated anti rabbit IgG (goat; Miles Laboratories) were applied at 1/20 working dilution. Immunoglobulin fractions directed against GO-Ag were used at 1/10 to
1/100 working dilutions.

Resected gastric tissue specimens (12 blocks per
specimen) were fixed in 96% alcohol – 1% acetic acid,
cleared in benzol and embedded in paraplast (7). Serial
sections of 4μ were made and stained routinely with HE,
PAS and AB at pH 1.0 and pH 2.5 and with the immunoperoxydase method.

Antibodies directed against CEA (10 to 100 ug/ml protein) were obtained by solid immunoadsorbents (PCA extract
of liver metastasis) after complete absorption of common
site antibody by solid immunoadsorbents of lung PCA extracts (8). CEA antibodies did not react with granulocytes,
erythrocytes and normal gastric and intestinal tissue.

RESULTS

In vivo neutralized gastric juice of patients with
intestinal metaplasia and gastric extracts of intestinal
metaplasia demonstrate several AB staining components in
analytical PAGE, the main component being found in the 6%
anodic gel zone. This AB staining main component (AB-MC)
was soluble in 0.2 to 1.0M PCA. Upon DEAE chromatography
AB-MC was eluted from 0.04 to 0.2M, the highest concentration was found in 0.2M. By Sephadex G200 gel filtration
AB-MC of DEAE fractions were eluted with a void volume. By
subsequent preparative PAGE of 20mg protein starting material AB-MC could be further purified and eluted in a
cathodic zone of approx. 2cm length in the 7% gel. The
total gain of MC-AB by one preparative PAGE was 1mg. The
end product demonstrated electrophoretic microhetereo-
genity upon analytical PAGE.

After immunization with purified AB-MC we obtained
antisera which were contaminated by antibodies directed
against one plasma protein and against one antigenic constituent of normal gastric epithelium. After absorption
with lyophilized plasma (10mg/ml) and normal gastric mucosa (20mg/ml) followed by DEAE chromatography (0.04 – 0.08M,
pH 7.0) the antiserum was specific for AB-MC. In gel diffusion extremely weak precipitin bands were observed when
reacted with starting material.

In immunhistology goblet cells of the duodenum, small
and large gut stained extremely well with the antiserum,
giving rise to an excellent immunological contrast. Normal
gastric mucosa of corpus and antrum showed no reaction.
However, gastric specimens with intestinal metaplasia
showed specific staining of goblet cells but not of the
striated border. The distribution of the goblet cells was

134

either diffuse, focal or minimal (staining of one single
goblet cell within the whole field could be observed)
(fig.1a). Typical staining of the goblet cells was observed in the cytoplasma, in the secreted mucus and in the
lumen of the foveolae (fig.1b).

When 30 gastric cancer out of 100 resected specimens
were studied in immunhistology the following results were
obtained (table 1).

TABLE 1   Immunhistological demonstration of goblet cell
antigen in CEA-positive and negative tumors

	Tumors n	Tumor cells +	Mucus only +
	30	3	4
CEA+	21	3	4

The three cancer specimens staining with the antiserum were of the mucus producing signet ring cell type.
They also stained for CEA. In other CEA positive or negative tumors interdispersed rests of goblet cells or
trapped masses of mucus did stain, but not the tumor cells
proper.

In 19 of these 30 gastric cancers we observed diffuse
or focal accumulation of staining goblet cells in the tumor adjacent tissue. In 11 of these specimens we found
a small percentage of 1 to 5% of the total goblet cell
mass staining for CEA.

DISCUSSION

Gastric mucosal goblet cells contain a PCA soluble
immunogenic substance of high molecular weight which stains
with AB at pH 2.5, sharing thus the properties of a non-
sulfated acidic glycoprotein. This substance does not stain
with protein stains and PAS. In electrophoresis it migrates
in the cathodic zone of high molecular proteins analogous
to CEA and results in weak precipitin lines in immuno-gel-
diffusion. From our findings we can conclude that there
exists an antigenic identity between goblet cells of
normal intestine and intestinalized gastric mucosa, but we
have no evidence for any immunological relationship with
CEA or CEA-like substances. GO-Ag is present in the cytoplasma of AB positive signet ring cell carcinoma, but not
in other gastric carcinoma studied in this present series.
From this we assume that there must be a histogenetic
relationship between gastric goblet cells and signet ring
cell carcinoma. The fact that some goblet cells in tumor
adjacent tissue contain CEA can be considered as malignant

associated changes demanding further elucidation. The substance described here as GO-Ag might be identical with the intestinal mucosa specific glycoprotein (2,3).

REFERENCES

(1) Nairn,R.C., Fothergill,J.E., McEntegart,M.G., and Porteous,I.E. (1962): Brit.Med.J.1, 1788.
(2) DeBoer,W.G.R.N., Forsyth,A., and Nairn,R.C. (1969): Brit.Med.J.3, 93.
(3) Kawasaki,H., Imasato,K., Kimoto,E., Akijama,K., and Takeuchi,N. (1972): Gann 63, 231.
(4) Denk, H., Tappeiner,G, Davidovits,A., and Holzner,J.H. (1973): Virschoff Arch.Path.Anat.360, 339.
(5) Burtin,P., Sabine,M.C., and Chavanel,G. (1977): Int.J.Cancer 19, 634.
(6) Rapp,W., and Lehmann,H.E. (1976): J.Clin.Chem.Clin. Biochem.14, 569-576.
(7) Kuhlmann,W.D. (1975): Histochemistry 44, 1, 155.
(8) Primus,F.J., Newman,E.S., and Hanson,H.J. (1977): J.Immunology 118, 55.

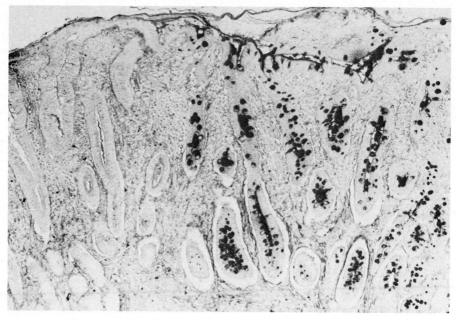

Fig.1a Immunhistological demonstration of goblet cell antigen in goblet cells of focal distribution in gastric antral mucosa x 54.

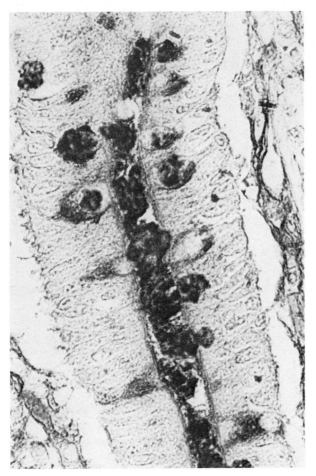

Fig.1b Typical cytoplasmatic localization and secretion
pattern of goblet cell antigen, normal mucosa of colon
x 440.

DISCUSSION

RAMPAL P.(Nice): Did you check the enzyme equipment of your gastric
metaplasia.

RAPP W. (Heidelberg): No, we did no enzymatic studies but the diagnosis was very easy.

RAMPAL P.(Nice): Have you any further data on the biochemical composition of your glycoprotein.

RAPP W. (Heidelberg): Yes, first it is a very unusual substance; it does not stain as a protein. According to gel filtration and polyacrylamide gel electrophoresis its molecular weight is over 200 000 daltons. In agar gel electrophoresis it migrates as a beta protein but in DEAE chromatography it is eluted at high ionic strength of the eluent.

ZAMCHECK N. (Boston): Have you tested colorectal or lung cancers? Have they a lot of goblet cells?

RAPP W. (Heidelberg): We started recently with the colonic cancer and we speculated that we would find the same protein on several occasions, in intestinal goblet cells of normal colon as well as in some mucus producing cancers.

TISSUE POLYPEPTIDE ANTIGEN IN COLORECTAL CARCINOMA

Å. Andrén-Sandberg and S. Isacson

Department of Surgery, Central Hospital, Halmstad, Sweden

A tumor-associated antigen, tissue polypeptide antigen (TPA), was originally described by Björklund and co-workers in 1957 (1). Some of the present knowledge of the chemical structure and immunochemical properties of TPA is presented by dr Björklund in this volume (2). TPA is not a tumor-specific antigen. It has been found transiently in patients with inflammatory diseases and to some extent (2-5%) in apparently healthy persons. TPA has also been found in fetus and placenta (3). The antigenic specific determinant of TPA has also been found in species other than the human one (4).

At our department of surgery we have for the last 4 1/2 years investigated the clinical value of the TPA-test (5, 6). We have found it useful in the diagnosis of urinary bladder carcinoma in patients with haematuria (7, 8).

This paper will present a longitudinal study of patients operated for colorectal carcinoma with special regard to the correlation between TPA in serum and histopathological staging and other laboratory parameters. We also want to discuss the value of serum-TPA determinations in the follow-up of those of the patients who were radically operated.

METHODS

TPA-determinations were performed with an assay technique (9) based on the classical haemagglutination inhibition reaction. Determinations of TPA were made in serum. According to Björklund TPA-values equal to or above 0.09 U/ml were considered pathological.

MATERIAL

The material consists of 137 patients; 51 with rectal and 86 with colon carcinoma. The diagnoses have been verified by histopathological examinations.

RESULTS AND DISCUSSION

TPA correlated to tumor stage

Figure 1 shows the preoperative values of TPA in serum correlated to the classification of Duke. Unfortunately, it was not possible to get preoperative test results from all the patients. Patients

with distant metastases are classified as "Duke D". Pathological
TPA-values ($\geq$ 0.09 U/ml) were seen in 50% of the patients belonging to Duke´s group A, in 38% of Duke´s group B, in 40% of Duke´s
group C, and in 90% of Duke´s group D. The group of patients with
distant metastases has significantly higher values of serum-TPA
compared to the other groups. This means that even a single high
preoperative value of serum-TPA may be of a prognostic value.

TPA correlated to tumor differentiation

The grade of malignancy according to the histological picture
has been established by the same pathologist in all cases. The
correlation of the preoperative values of serum-TPA showed no
difference between the tumors of high and intermediate grade of
differentiation. Compared to these groups the TPA-values are higher in the group of patients with poorly differentiated tumors.
This does not necessarily mean that poorly differentiated tumors
produce more TPA than highly differentiated ones, but shows that
tumors with a low grade of differentiation release more TPA into
the blood stream.

Single determinations of serum-TPA are not suitable for screening purposes, since the preoperative TPA-values in patients with
potentially curable stages of colorectal carcinoma are pathological only in about 50% of the cases. Preoperatively high serum-TPA
levels can indicate that the tumor is poorly differentiated or widely spread and therefore also indicate an unfavourable prognosis.

TPA correlated to other laboratory parameters

We have also been interested in studying how TPA is correlated
to routinely used laboratory parameters. Fig. 3 shows the preoperative values of serum-TPA correlated to the erythrocyte sedimentation rate (ESR). ESR is known to be tumor-associated, with a low
specificity and a rather high sensitivity. TPA and ESR measured
jointly give a higher yield of pathological values than we would obtain by measuring each of these parameters alone. Nearly 1/4 of the
patients has normal ESR and TPA-values. There are no patients classified as belonging to Duke´s group D with normal TPA and ESR, but
there is an overrepresentation of patients belonging to Duke´s
group D among the patients with both positive TPA and ESR. Correlation of TPA to fibrin and fibrinogen degradation products (FDP),
to lactate dehydrogenase (LD), and to alkalic phosphatases (ALP)
shows the same tendency. This might imply that TPA measures other
biological events than what could be measured by routinely used laboratory parameters. Since more preoperative information is obtained by combining tests as ESR, LD, ALP, FDP, and TPA, this can be a
reason for including TPA-determinations in a panel of routinely u-
sed laboratory tests in order to evaluate the staging of patients
with colorectal carcinoma.

TPA correlated to survival

Our study shows that where the preoperative value is 0.36 U/ml or more, only 3 patients of 13 are alive after 12 months. In the group with very low preoperative values, 0.03 U/ml or less, 32 patients out of 36 are alive after the same period of time. In radically operated patients, who are free from disease after a 24 month follow-up, we notice that, although there are 17 patients out of 46 with pathological TPA-values before the operation, there is only 1 out of 46, who has pathological values after 1 year (Fig. 4). This shall be compared to the TPA-values of those patients, where a radical operation was not possible (Fig. 5). It is evident that a rising TPA-value after an operation for colorectal carcinoma is correlated to a bad prognosis.

TPA correlated to time for clinical evidence of recurrence

13 patients got a recurrence in spite of a clinically radical operation according to the surgeon and to the pathologist (Fig. 6). The patients have been followed regularly with laboratory examinations including TPA-tests. Recurrence is confirmed either by hepatic metastases shown by angiography or isotope scanning, by pulmonary metastases shown by X-ray, by a palpable local growth or by other obvious clinical evidences. In 10 out of 13 patients the TPA-levels reached supra-normal values several months before the clinical evidence of recurrence was seen. In one case TPA became positive at the same time as the recurrence became clinically evident and in 2 cases TPA failed to rise to a pathological level until the recurrence was already clinically established. ALP and FDP have in these cases shown a high specificity, but the levels reach a pathological stage somewhat later in the development of the recurrence than TPA. LD is in this respect somewhat more promising. ESR seems to have a higher sensitivity than the other parameters, but 4 of the recurrences are completely missed, and ESR also has a high rate of false positives.

CONCLUSION

Our results indicate that a single determination of tissue polypeptide antigen (TPA) in serum is not suitable for screening colorectal carcinoma in its potentially curable stages, since the test is pathological only in about 50% of these cases.

However, if the TPA-test is combined with the determination of other laboratory parameters more preoperative information is obtained than if we measure each of the parameters alone.

The TPA-test can also be useful when assessing the prognosis of patients radically operated for colorectal carcinoma and is a valuable tool in the follow-up of these patients.

REFERENCES

(1) Björklund, B. and Björklund, V. (1957): Int. Arch. Allergy
     Appl. Immunol. 10:153-184
(2) Björklund, B. (1978): Proceedings of the Symposium on Clinical
     Application of Carcinoembryonic Antigen and Other Antigenic
     Markers Assays. Nice, 1977.
(3) Lundström, R., Björklund, B. and Eklund, G. (1973): Immunolo-
     gical Techniques for Detection of Cancer. Stockholm, Bonniers,
     1973, pp. 243-247.
(4) Björklund, B., Björklund, V., Lundström, R. and Eklund, G.
     (1976): Advances in Experimental Medicine and Biology: The Re-
     ticuloendothelial System in Health and Disease. Plenum Press,
     1976, pp. 357-370, Vol. 73 B.
(5) Isacson, S., Lindblad, C., Nistor, L. and Risholm, L. (1974):
     XI International Cancer Congress. Florence, 1974. Abstract.
(6) Andrén-Sandberg, Å. and Isacson, S. (1976): Third Internatio-
     nal Symposium on Detection and Prevention of Cancer. New York,
     1976. In press.
(7) Isacson, S. and Andrén-Sandberg, Å. (1976): Third Internatio-
     nal Symposium on Detection and Prevention of Cancer. New York,
     1976. In press.
(8) Isacson, S. and Andrén-Sandberg, Å. (1978): Proceedings of the
     Symposium on Clinical Application of Carcinoembryonic Antigen
     and Other Antigenic Markers Assays. Nice, 1977.
(9) Björklund, B. and Paulsson, J.E. (1962): J. Immunol. 89:759-
     766.

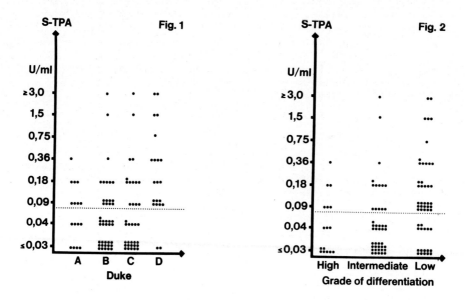

Fig. 1 Preoperative serum-TPA values in patients with colorectal
carcinoma classified according to Duke.

Fig. 2 Preoperative serum-TPA values in patients with colorectal
carcinoma classified according to the grade of tumor differentiation.

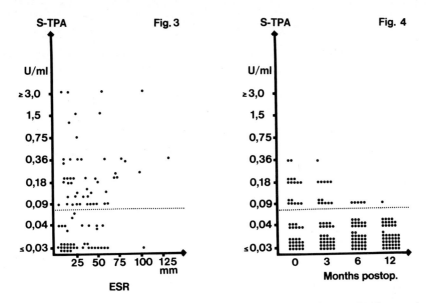

Fig. 3 Preoperative serum-TPA values correlated to ESR in patients with colorectal carcinoma.

Fig. 4 Pre- and postoperative serum-TPA values in patients radically operated for colorectal carcinoma (Duke´s groups A, B, and C).

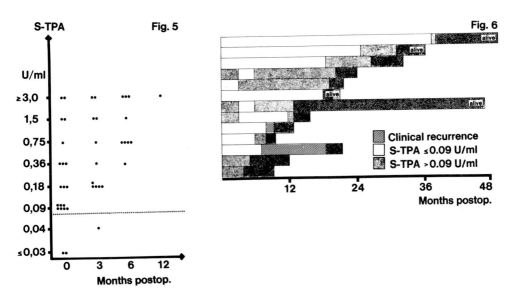

Fig. 5 Pre- and postoperative serum-TPA values in patients not radically operated for colorectal carcinoma (Duke´s group D).

Fig. 6 Pathological serum-TPA values correlated to time for clinical recurrence in 13 patients radically operated for colorectal carcinoma.

DISCUSSION

DELMONT J. (Nice): Have you done any study concerning control group with benign polyps or inflammatory bowel diseases, like ulcerative colitis?

ANDREN-SANDBERG A.G. (Halmstad): We have had very few patients with polyps . They do not show high values of TPA. Some of the patients with inflammatory bowel disease have high values of TPA, but not so elevated as in patients with advanced cancer.

DIAGNOSTIC AND PROGNOSTIC SIGNIFICANCE OF THE MAKARI INTRADERMAL TEST
IN PATIENTS WITH COLON CANCER.

K. Blake,[*] J. Concannon,[†] M. Dalbow,[†] and A. Panahandeh[*]

Department of Surgery[*] and Clinical Radiation Therapy Research
Center,[†] Allegheny General Hospital, Pittsburgh, PA 15212, USA

The Makari Intradermal Test (MIT) was first described in 1960(1)
as a tumor detection test. Several additional studies (2-7) using
the materials isolated and purified by Makari indicate that the test
may be a valuable adjunctive test for the diagnosis of cancer. A
recent study by Tee (8) indicates that the MIT may be of prognostic
value as well. Our studies indicate that the test is positive in
nearly 90% of patients with untreated primary tumors of the colon and
in 60% of patients with recurrent or metastatic disease. The test
has also been shown to become negative in the post surgical period
suggesting that it may have prognostic as well as diagnostic significance in following patients with colonic tumors. Although the incidence of false positive tests is approximately 15% in healthy volunteers, it has a very high incidence of positive reactors among
patients with benign disease of the colon; especially in those associated with a higher than expected incidence of cancer.

METHODS

The methods for the preparation of the Makari tumor polysac-
charide substances (TPS) have been described (2) as have the methods
for the preparation, administration, and interpretation (6) of the
test. The carcinoembryonic antigen (CEA) studies reported here were
performed by the technique of Hansen (9) using the CEA-Roche reagents.

RESULTS

We have previously reported that the MIT was positive in ∿70%
(6,7) of all patients who had an untreated malignant disease. The
test was positive in all patients with a primary colonic tumor, but
also was positive in 42% of the patients with benign diseases of the
gastrointestinal system. Since the time of these early reports we
have confined our testing to patients with various GI disorders and
healthy volunteers.
Table 1 shows the results of the MIT studies in a group of patients with a primary malignancy of the lower bowel. The results of
the radioimmunoassay for plasma levels of CEA are also shown.
The Makari test was positive in all patients (12/12) with carcinomas in situ and in 63 of 71 patients (89%) for all stages combined. The plasma CEA value was positive at the >2.5 ng/ml significance level in 37 of 71 patients (52%). Twenty-four of the patients
(35%) had CEA levels >5 ng/ml and 12 had levels >10.0 ng/ml.

TABLE 1 Comparison of the MIT with the CEA assay for the detection of patients with primary cancer of the large bowel.

Disease Stage	No. Patients	MIT Positive	$\leq$2.5	CEA ng/ml		
				>2.5	>5.0	>10.0
CA In Situ	12	12	9	3(25%)	2(18%)	0
Duke's A	4	3	4	0	0	0
Duke's B	18	16(89%)	11	7(39%)	1(6%)	0
Duke's C	28	25(89%)	8	20(74%)	15(56%)	7(26%)
Duke's D	9	7(78%)	2	7(78%)	6(67%)	5(56%)
Totals	71	63(89%)	34(48%)	37(52%)	24(35%)	12(17%)

The CEA plasma level was elevated above 5 ng/ml in 3 of the patients and above 10 ng/ml in 2 of the patients who were MIT negative. The two tests combined, using the CEA at a significance level of >5 ng/ml, indicated a positive diagnosis of cancer in 93%(66/71) of the patients in this series.

The CEA assay was also shown to be a valuable adjunct in pre-operative staging of these patients. Twenty-one of 24 patients (88%) who had CEA levels >5.0 ng/ml were found to have either remote disease or regional lymph node envolvement. These results are shown in Table 2.

TABLE 2 Pre-surgical plasma CEA levels in relation to extent of disease for patients with colonic tumors.

Disease Stage	No. Patients	MIT Positive	CEA (ng/ml)		
			$\leq$5 ng	>5.0 ng	>10 ng
In Situ-Duke's A&B	34	31(91%)	31	3(7%)	0
Duke's C (Neg.nodes)	10	9(90%)	10	0	0
Duke's C (Pos.nodes)	18	16(89%)	3(17%)	15(83%)	7(39%)
Duke's D (Remote)	9	7(78%)	3(33%)	6(67%)	5(56%)
Totals	71	63(89%)	47	24	12

The results of the MIT for patients with various benign diseases tested before and after treatment are shown in Table 3. The data are divided into three disease categories: 1) benign neoplasms; 2) inflammatory GI disease, and 3) ulcers. There is a high incidence of false positive reactors (65%) in patients with benign neoplasms and in patients with benign inflammatory disease (48%). The incidence of positive reactors was also high in patients with benign gastric ulcers.

After polypectomy the proportion of positive responders to the Makari test materials is greatly reduced in patients with adenomatous polyps. The 5 positive responders were all tested within 6 months after polypectomy, and we have observed that the MIT frequently remains positive up to 6 months after surgery in patients who have had a definitive colon tumor resection and are apparently free of disease. Although the number of patients with other benign diseases, tested after therapy, is small there were a few positive responders.

TABLE 3 Results of the MIT in patients with benign diseases of the gastrointestinal system.

BENIGN DISEASE	PRETREATMENT No. Patients	No. MIT+	POST TREATMENT No. Patients	No. MIT+
Adenomatous Polyps	28	18(64%)	23	5(22%)
Carcinoid Tumor	1	0	. . .	. . .
Gardener's Syndrom	1	1	. . .	. . .
Pseudo Polyps	2	2	. . .	. . .
Villous Adenoma	2	1	2	0
Biliary	12	2(17%)	. . .	. . .
Crohn's	4	3	5	1
Diverticulitis	1	1	1	0
Gastritis	2	0	. . .	. . .
Irritable Bowel	2	0	1	0
Pancreatitis	2	2	. . .	. . .
Ulcerative Colitis	4	4	7	2
Anal Ulcers	2	0	. . .	. . .
Duodenal Ulcers	2	0	. . .	. . .
Gastric Ulcers	5	3(60%)	. . .	. . .
Totals	70	38		

Serial followup MIT studies were performed in a number of patients with primary tumors of the colon after surgical resection. The results are shown in Table 4.

TABLE 4 The MIT results for serial studies in patients who had a colonic tumor resection with no evidence of recurrent disease.

MONTHS AFTER Surgery	No. Tested	No. MIT +	No. MIT Positive by Stage In Situ	A	B	C
<1	1	1	---	---	1/1*	---
1 – 6	10	6(60%)	3/3	0/2	2/4	1/1
6 – 12	20	5(20%)	0/4	0/2	3/8	2/6
12 – 18	11	3(27%)	0/1	1/2	1/4	1/4
18 – 24	3	2	---	2/3	---	---
>24	5	3	---	---	1/2	2/4

*No. MIT Positive/No. Tested

The MIT test remains positive in the majority of patients tested up to 6 months after treatment even in patients with localized cancer. The test becomes negative in the majority of patients with no evidence of disease after 6 months. The 3 patients (1 Duke's B, 2 Duke's C) who tested MIT positive at >24 months had at least 1 negative test between 6 and 24 months. There is no clinical evidence of recurrent or metastatic disease in these patients at this time. The 2 patients who were MIT positive in the Duke's A group at 18 to 24 months also previously tested negative. The 2 patients are clinically free of disease at this time.

A similar time related analysis of serial MIT studies was made for data from patients who have developed recurrent or metastatic disease. The MIT test was positive in 12 of 19 patients (63%) who had clinical evidence of recurrent or metastatic disease at the time of the Makari test or within one month after the MIT. A similar incidence of positive tests was observed in patients tested between 1 and 6 months before clinical evidence of progressive disease was found. Three of 3 patients tested 6 to 12 months before recurrent disease was detected were MIT positive while 4 of 4 patients tested more than 15 months before detection of progressive disease were MIT negative.

A scatter diagram of the MIT ratios determined preoperatively for the patients with colon cancer and the healthy volunteers is shown in Figure 1. As with all diagnostic tests the MIT has a gray zone of positive and negative (hatched area) where individuals with cancer are close to negative and healthy volunteers are close to positive.

ACKNOWLEDGEMENTS

The authors wish to gratefully acknowledge the technical and clerical contributions of Judith Conway, Elaine Callery, Michael Debes, James Headings, Dru Ann Heath, Cindy Kline, Ann Lanious, Electra Markopoulos, and Joann Perri. Supported by Grant Q-67 from the Health Research and Services Foundation, Pittsburgh, PA.

REFERENCES

(1) Makari, J. (1960): J. Am. Geriat. Soc.,8, 675.
(2) Makari, J. (1969): J. Am. Geriat. Soc., 17, 755.
(3) Honda, K., Hoshishima, K., Kato, K., et al. (1973): Trans. N.Y. Acad. Sci., 35, 368.
(4) Boisivon, A. (1973): Trans. N. Y. Acad. Sci.,35, 380.
(5) Tee, D. (1973): Trans. N. Y. Acad. Sci., 35, 387.
(6) Concannon, J., Blake, K., Brodmerkel, G., et al. (1976): Ann. N. Y. Acad. Sci., 276, 97.
(7) Concannon, J., Dalbow, M., and Emg, C. (1976): Third Int. Symp. Detection Prevention Cancer, New York, 1976. pp 574.
(8) Tee, D. and Munson, K. (1977) Lancet ii, 480.
(9) Hansen, H., Snyder, J., Miller, E., et al. (1974): Human Pathol.,5, 139.

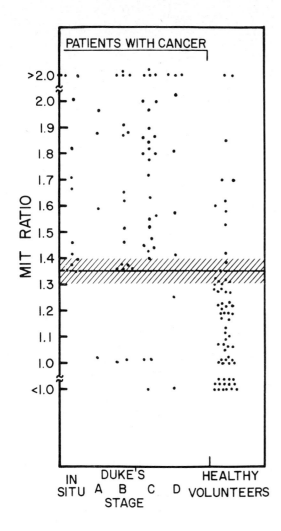

Fig. 1 Scattergram showing the distribution of MIT ratios for patients with colon cancer and healthy volunteers.

DISCUSSION

RAPP W. (Heidelberg): Do you have any idea about the immune pathological process in your intradermal Makari reaction. The problem with the Makari test is that you have difficulties in standardisation. We have shown that the purification of mitochondries and microsomes from gastric tissues is impossible. Have you any idea about reactive substances?

BLAKE K.E. (Pittsburgh): We are not certain of the immune mechanism of the Makari reaction, but it is not unlike the evanescent passive cutaneous reaction. We have suggestive evidence that the test is immunological in nature. Anergic patients react negatively to the MIT and so do patients on steroid therapy. We have absorbed our substance with normal tissue antigens and the false positives reactions decrease.

BJORKLUND B. (Halsmtad): Does repeated use of the Makari test change the patient's reactivity? Have you some experience on that?

BLAKE K.E. (Pittsburgh): This is a distinct possibility. We had one patient who had an anaphylactic reaction after being tested for the fourth time and several of our patients who appear to be free of disease have reacted positively upon retesting the third or fourth time after previously testing negative.

MACH J.P. (Lausanne): Do you know if the material you inject is soluble and do you have any idea about the molecular weight of this material?

BLAKE K.E. (Pittsburgh): The Makari materials are soluble. We have no data on the physical characteristics of these substances, but they are mucopolysaccharides.

HERBERMAN R.B. (Bethesda): How do you feel the test can help the clinician in differential diagnosis of gastro-intestinal cancer since you have about 50% positive in normal population and 2/3 of people with benign polyps.

BLAKE K.E. (Pittsburgh): The incidence of false positive tests is only 15% in the healthy volunteer group. This we feel is acceptable for a diagnostic test. The high incidence of positive reactors referred to by Dr. Herberman in patients with benign disease may be due to the premalignant nature of those diseases. Many of these conditions are thought to be premalignant and although the subject is controversial, there is substantial evidence to suggest that adenomatous polyps may also be premalignant.

CARCINOID SYNDROME MONITORED BY 5HIAA IN RESPONSE TO STREPTOZOTOCIN THERAPY*

M.J. O'Halloran, G.M. Mullins, F.X. O'Connell and H.R. Browne.

Radiotherapy and Clinical Oncology Centre,
Saint Luke's Hospital, Dublin, Ireland.

The optimal approach to the chemotherapy of metastatic progressive carcinoid syndrome remains uncertain. Some authorities believe that the most promising therapy is regional arterial perfusion with agents such as 5 Fluorouracil (1). Others consider that the combination of cyclophosphamide and methotrexate is the most effective treatment (2).

Streptozotocin has been shown to be an effective agent in carcinoid syndrome (3,4.) However, the role of Streptozotocin in this condition has not been adequately accessed.

Using 5HIAA measurements as a marker may indicate a clinical response to Streptozotocin Therapy.
Primary carcinoids are not all benign tumours (5) and when they metastasize show a high selectivity for the liver. Other sites for metastases occur chiefly in bone, lung and pancreas.

The syndrome is mediated by the release of one or more biologically active agents by the tumour. Tryptophan, a normal end product of protein synthesis is acted upon by one of these agents producing in turn 5-Hydroxytryptophan (5HTP), 5 - Hydroxytryptamine(Serotonin) and 5-Hydroxyindolacetic Acid (5HIAA). This latter substance is rapidly excreted in the urine and most of the circulating Serotonin can be accounted for as urinary 5HIAA (6).

Substances identified as producing the syndrome include Serotonin, Bradykinin, Histamine, ACTH, Substance P. (7).
The syndrome may produce one or all of the following symptoms - Cutaneous flushes, Telangiectasia, Diarrhoea, Cardio Valvular lesions, Bronchial Constriction, Arthropathy.

* Streptozotocin supplied by courtesy of Drs. S. Carter, and S. Legha of the Cancer Therapy Evaluation Branch, National Cancer Institute, Md., U.S.A.

TABLE 1. Findings in 5 patients who had primary
carcinoids.

Patient and Site		5 HIAA	Metastases	Symptoms
1	Lung	↑	Liver, Bone	+ + +
2	Rectum	Normal	Liver, Pancreas	+ +
3	Ascending Colon	↑	Liver, glands	+ +
4	Appendix	Normal	None	-----
5	Unknown	↑	Lymph Glands	+ +

Two patients were treated with Streptozotocin.

PATIENT NO. 3

Female, married, age 65.   In 1969 she had an
inoperable growth of the ascending colon, with multiple
secondary deposits in the liver.   Histopathology -
Anaplastic Adeno-Carcinoma.   An Ileocolostomy bypass
was undertaken.   Patient returned in 1976 complaining
of diarrhoea, weight loss, flushes and abdominal cramps.
5HIAA was markedly raised.   A (R) Hemiscolectomy was
undertaken and the Histopathology was Carcinoid.   Patient
received Streptozotocin and Urinary 5HIAA levels fell to
normal limits, only to rise again after an interval
(Fig.1) and patient again refused to return for review.

PATIENT NO. 1

Female, married, age 60.   In January 1975
Thoracotomy and right Lobectomy was undertaken for
histopathologically confirmed Carcinoid.   February 1976
patient complained of diarrhoea, flushes, telangiectasia.
Her liver was enlarged and biopsy in April 1976 confirmed
secondary carcinoid.   5HIAA levels were 404mg./24 hr.
Streptozotocin was commenced and 5HIAA levels have
fallen to normal (Fig.2) with minimal symptoms from July
1976 to August 1977.   Liver scan shows significant
decrease

in size from July 1976 to September 1977, and the amount
of functioning liver has increased.
Routine skeletal survey in December 1976 showed sclerosis
in L2, S1, S2, and the patient was asymptomatic. Routine
biochemical assays and blood count remain normal.

SUMMARY

5HIAA monitoring might be considered as an index
of response to treatment in patients with carcinoid
syndrome treated with Streptozotocin, should studies
presently under investigation show this Drug to be
effective in this Syndrome.

REFERENCES

(1) Principles of Internal Medicine. Eds: Wintrobe,
     M.M. et al. McGraw Hill, New York, 1974 (seventh
     edition) p.607.
(2) Cancer Medicine. Eds: Holland, J.F. and Frei, E.
     Lea and Febiger, Philadelphia. 1973 p.1593.
(3) Iweze, F.I. et al. Carcinoid syndrome treated with
     Streptozotocin. Proceedings of Royal Society of
     Medicine, 65: 164-5, 1972.
(4) Personal communication by G.M. Mullins.
(5) Pearson, C.M., Fitzgerald, P.J., Cancer 1949,2,
     1005.
(6) J.A. Oates, in Harrison Textbook of Medicine.
     Chap. 105, page 593.
(7) P. Skrabanek., D. Cannon, J. Kirrane, D. Legee and
     D. Powell.   Irish Journal of Medical Science, Vol.
     145, No. 12, December 1976, pp 399-408.

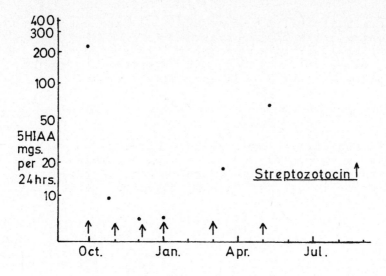

Fig. 1. Response to Streptozotocin in Patient No. 3.

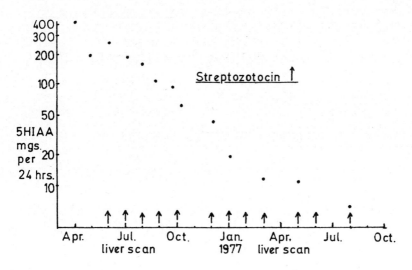

Fig. 2. Response to Streptozotocin in Patient No. 1.

DISCUSSION

TALERMAN A. (Rotterdam): You have found a good correlation between the values of 5 H1AA and the progress of the disease. We have studied this in carcinoids of the small intestine, the lung and ovary treated in the same way and our results are similar to yours.

EVALUATION OF DIFFERENT ANTIGEN SOURCES FOR LEUKOCYTE MIGRATION TESTING OF GASTROINTESTINAL CANCER PATIENTS

M.Zöller[1], S.Matzku[1], W.Lernhardt[1] and U.Schulz[2]

[1]Institute of Nuclear Medicine, German Cancer Research Center, and
[2]Department of Surgery, University, Heidelberg

In animal tumour models it was found, that spontaneously arising tumours carry tumour-associated antigens of fetal origin, which in the fetus arise at a well defined gestational age (1). These antigens, being immunogenic to the host, are located mainly in the cytoplasm and only to a lower degree in the plasma membrane (1,2). Spontaneously arising animal tumours are considered to show the highest degree of analogy to the human cancer situation. One should therefore expect to meet similar characteristics of antigen expression in man. We especially wanted to find out, whether tumour-associated antigens in human tumours are of fetal origin and whether those antigens are located in the cytoplasm or the plasma membrane. As a test system we have used the LM reactivity of gastrointestinal cancer patients.

MATERIAL AND METHODS

40ml blood samples were taken from patients with malignant and benign gastrointestinal disease (Department of Surgery) and from out door patients and members of the Institute of Nuclear Medicine. The LMT is described in detail elsewhere (3). As antigen sources 3M KCl extracts (3), papain digests from isolated membranes and cytoplasmic fractions (4) of tumours and normal tissue were used. Fetuses of 2 1/2, 3, 3 1/2 and 6 1/2 months of gestational age were extracted by the 3M KCl method. All patients were tested with a normal tissue extract and with five 3M KCl tumour extracts. Simultaneously, patients' lymphocytes were tested either against isolated membrane fractions and cytoplasmic fractions, originating from the same tumours as the 3M KCl extracts or against 3M KCl extracts of fetuses.
The evaluation of LM reactivity by the panel test mode is described elsewhere (3).

RESULTS

Patients' lymphocytes were tested against 3 types of
extracts, containing exclusively membrane proteins (limited papain digestion of isolated membranes), exclusively
cytoplasmic proteins (soluble cytoplasmic fraction) or
both constituents (3M KCl extracts). As a control the
different extract types of a normal gastric mucosa were
tested in several groups of patients in order to exclude
unspecific reactivities due to artefacts, being caused by
the extraction procedures themselves. The results are
shown in Table 1.
Gastric cancer patients were to some degree reactive with
the normal gastric mucosal extracts, but in all other
groups an abnormal MI only occasionally was observed. No
significant difference (chi square test) was found between
the reactivities of the 3 extract types tested. So, after
all, unspecific reactivities due to the extraction procedures seem to be excluded.

TABLE 1   Leukocyte migration reactivity with different
extract types of normal gastric mucosa

Leukocyte donor	Patients with abnormal MI Total number of patients		
	3M KCl[1]	Cytoplasm[1]	Papain digest[1]
Malignant disease:			
Gastric cancer	9/44 (20%)	8/44 (18%)	6/18 (33%)[2]
Non-gastric ca.	9/91 (10%)	6/91 (7%)	2/29 (7%)
Benign disease:			
Gastric	2/23 (9%)	2/23 (9%)	0/7 (0%)
Non-gastric	3/96 (3%)	2/96 (2%)	1/44 (2%)
Healthy donors	1/30 (3%)	0/30 (0%)	0/30 (0%)

[1] Protein concentration during incubation: 1mg/ml
[2] Chi square test: $p \leqslant 0.05$

However differences were observed, when tumour extracts
obtained by the three extraction procedures were tested.
The frequencies of "positive" reactivities (abnormal MI
with 3 out of 5 tumour extracts) are shown in Table 2.

TABLE 2   Leukocyte migration reactivity with different
types of gastric tumour extracts.

Leukocyte donor	Patients with "positive" reactivity		
	Total number of patients		
	3M KCl	Cytoplasm	Papain digest
Malignant disease:			
Gastric cancer	62/72 (86%)	59/72 (82%)	25/39 (64%)[1]
Non-gastric ca.	28/91 (31%)	23/91 (25%)	7/29 (24%)
Benign disease:			
Gastric	2/23 (9%)	2/23 (9%)	1/7 (14%)
Non-gastric	5/96 (5%)	4/96 (4%)	1/44 (2%)
Healthy donors	1/30 (3%)	0/30 (0%)	0/30 (0%)

[1]Chi square test: $p < 0.05$

While again in healthy donors and patients with benign
disease with either tumour extract type "positive" reactivity rarely was observed, patients with non-gastric cancer
were found to be reactive to some degree and gastric
cancer patients were highly reactive.There was no difference in reactivity between 3M KCl extracts and cytoplasmic
fractions, but "positive" reactivity was less frequently
observed with isolated membrane fractions (p 0.05).
The question whether fetal specificities are contained in
tumour extracts, inducing LM reactivity, was tested by exposing patients' lymphocytes to a panel of tumour extracts
and a panel of fetal extracts simultaneously (Table 3).
Lymphocytes of healthy donors and patients with benign
disease were rarely reactive with tumour extracts and with
fetal extracts, while in gastrointestinal cancer patients
an abnormal MI with tumour extracts was observed in 77%
of tests (not shown in Table 3) and with fetal extracts
in 64% of tests, corresponding to a "positive" reactivity
with tumour extracts in 92% of patients and with fetal
extracts in 80% of patients.

TABLE 3 Migration reactivity with fetal extracts and with tumour extracts.

Leukocyte donor	Number of patients	Abnorm.MI with fetal extr.+				"Pos." reactivity with tumor extr.	"Pos." reactivity with fetal extr.
		1+	2+	3+	4+		
Gastroint.ca.	45	26	32	27	30	42	36
			64%			92%	80%
Benign disease	18	1	1	2	2	2	2
Healthy donor	10	3	1	0	0	0	1
			9%			7%	11%

+ Age of extracted fetuses: 1=2 1/2m, 2=3m, 3=3 1/2m, 4=6 1/2m.

No conclusive evidence can be presented pointing to a specific gestational age of fetal extracts being reactive in the test, since reactivities of individual extracts, differing in developmental stage, did not show significant differences in reactivity.

When comparing "positive" reactivities of fetal extracts and tumour extracts (Table 4), a good correlation of unreactivity was found in healthy donors, only one individual being reactive with 2 out of 4 fetal extracts and none being reactive with 3 out of 5 tumour extracts. In the group of gastrointestinal cancer patients discrepancy was mainly caused by a rather large portion of patients being "negatively" reactive with the fetal panel but "positively" reactive with the tumor panel. Further insight in individual reactivities revealed, that within this portion 3 patients did not react with any fetal extract, but still responded to 3-5 out of 5 tumour extracts. Conversely, all three tumour patients with "negative" reactivity in the tumour panel, but "positive" reactivity in the fetal panel did in fact respond to 2 tumour extracts and thus had to be considered as "negatives".

TABLE 4 Correlation of "positive" reactivities with fetal extracts and tumour extracts.

	Fetal / Tumour		Leukocyte donor Gastrointest.ca.	Healthy
Concordant	+	+	33/45	–
	–	–	–	9/10
Discordant	+	–	3/45	1/10
	–	+	9/45	–

DISCUSSION

Our experiments aiming at the elucidation of cellular localization of LM reactive tumour antigens could not define a single compartment of the tumour cell. Reactivities were equally often observed with 3M KCl extracts and with cytoplasmic preparations, but consistent reactivity was observed with membrane digests too. It is common knowledge, that 3M KCl extracts, when performed on homogenized tumour material, will contain cytoplasmic constituents and solubilized membrane constituents as well. A predominance of reactivities with 3M KCl extracts and cytoplasmic fractions can thus be interpreted in the sense, that the major part of antigens stay inside the plasma membrane and outside the nuclear membrane. The presence of antigenic material on, or attached to the cell membrane could be explained by assumption of antigen secretion. Such an interpretation would agree with results in animal tumour models. There the major source of cross reacting antigens is the cytoplasm, although tumour cells can be stained by corresponding antibodies (1). Our findings confirm, that 3M KCl extracts are most appropriate for LMT studies. They contain the most comprehensive spectrum of antigens and they can be sterilized by filtration - unlike crude - tumour homogenates. This point seems trivial, however it is of enormous importance for tests like the LMT.

The type of antigen localization we observed fits very well with the fetal specificities of (at least a part of) the antigens expressed in gastrointestinal tumours. TSTA-like antigens clearly would have occured in papain digests and in KCl extracts, since they are expressed only at the membrane. However, tumour extracts must contain additional, non-fetal specificities. This is judged from the fact, that we found patients, which were completely unreactive with fetal extracts, but responded well to tumour extracts. Furthermore, the panel method, which intends to present a spectrum of antigens as comprehensive as possible to the lymphocytes, definitely was more effective with tumour extracts than with fetal extracts. It will be interesting to see, whether the relation of tumour panel "positivity" to fetal panel "positivity" will change, when tumours of other organ localization or tumours of different histological types will be tested.

REFERENCES

(1) Baldwin,R.W., Glaves,D. and Vose,B.M. (1974): Br.J. Cancer 29, 1.
(2) Parker,G.A. and Rosenberg,S.A. (1977): J.Immunology 118, 1590.
(3) Zöller,M., Matzku,S. and Schulz,U. (1977): J.Nat. Cancer Inst.58, 897.
(4) Zöller,M., Price,M.R. and Baldwin,R.W. (1976): Int.J. Cancer,17, 129.

DISCUSSION

VON KLEIST S.(Villejuif): You only counted positive a patient reacting with 3 out of 5 different tumour extracts. Would your results
change if you dropped the rather high level until 2 out of 5 extracts
or if you counted each positivity. Did you apply the same limit for
normal controls. In other words,would you say there is no reaction
when less than 3 out of 5 extracts are positive.

MATSKU S. (Heidelberg): For the first question : if we analyse our
data with respect to one single antigen extract, we get the same
results that Dr. HERBERMAN showed us and similar to those which have
been published by others.
For the second question : if we would cut off at one out of 5, of
course, we would have more positive results in normals. We do not
know whether the criterion of 3 out of 5 reduces the technical faults
in the system or if there is occasionally a true reactivity in normal
patients.

GROPP C. (Marburg): We made the same test as yours with extracts of
lung cancer and we were worried about the high amounts of false
positive reactions in normal patients or volunteers. We have seen
about 30% false positive results in normal people with the microcapil-
lary tube method and with the CLAUSEN test. And if you look at the
several antigens in these extracts you can understand this. There are
many antigens and lot of proteins in these extracts and I think this
may be an explanation.

CALMETTES C.(Paris): Just a comment : in bronchogenic carcinoids,
CEA levels are similar to those observed in intestinal carcinoids,
never above 30 ng/ml. But a significant diminution of CEA is observed
after surgery.

HERBERMAN R.B. (Bethesda): In your results, the difference between
the KCl and papain digest is possibly related to some papain degradation of the antigenic site rather than a difference between cytoplasmic and membranes antigen. And also a point of clarification :
is your material human or rat foetus.

MATSKU S. (Heidelberg) : We have not checked this point of degradation . Foetuses used were of human origin.

THE LEUKOCYTE MIGRATION TEST AND THE CEA-RIA IN POST SURGICAL CONTROL OF COLORECTAL CANCER PATIENTS

S. Matzku[1], M. Zöller[1], and U. Schulz[2]

[1]Institut für Nuklearmedizin, Deutsches Krebsforschungszentrum, and [2]Chirurgische Universitätsklinik, Heidelberg

The benefit of assessing plasma CEA levels in post surgical control of colorectal cancer patients is commonly accepted. Much less data is available for the leukocyte migration test, which is thought to monitor the sensitization of peripheral lymphocytes to tumour associated antigens. In our hands, this test proved to be a sensitive indicator of colorectal cancer in a preoperative situation and to reflect to a certain degree the development of disease after surgical removal of the primary tumour (1). Here we report first results of a study, wherein both assay systems were compared in patients undergoing radical as well as palliative surgery.

PATIENTS

Patients hospitalized for colorectal surgery were tested preoperatively and in at least semiannual intervals thereafter.

METHODS

Twenty ml of heparinized blood were processed in LMT 1-3 hrs after venous puncture. EDTA-Plasma was collected simultaneously and stored frozen at -20°C until use. Plasma CEA levels were determined by the CEA Roche assay (cut-off level 2.5ng/ml). Direct LMT was performed according to (2), a panel of 5 different 3M KCl extracts of colorectal tumours being used as antigen source. Patients showing an abnormal migration index (0,8 MI 1,2) with 3 out of 5 extracts were considered as positives.

RESULTS

According to the data shown in Table 1, the panel test mode of LMT results in a high degree of positivity in colorectal cancer patients irrespective of the stage. The reactivity in patients with nonmalignant colorectal disease can be ascribed to patients with M.Crohn. Some cross-reactivity is observed in other gastrointestinal

TABLE 1   LMT reactivity in patients with colorectal cancer and other diseases against colorectal tumour extracts

Leukocyte donors	n	Positive reactivity (definition see text)	
Colorectal cancer	179	158	88%
nonmalign. colorectal disease	51	8	16%
other GI cancer	23	3	13%
non GI cancer	78	2	3%
healthy volunteers	40	0	0%

(GI) cancer patients, but virtually no reactivity is found with nonmalignant, non-GI disease and in healthy volunteers.

The diagnostic potential of LMT prompted us to look at patients undergoing surgical treatment and to compare the test to the CEA-RIA (Table 2).

TABLE 2   Comparison of LMT and CEA-RIA (cumulative results)

Patients	Positive reactivity	
	LMT ($\geqslant$ 3/5 ext)	CEA ($>$ 2.5ng/ml)
Colorectal cancer Preop. radical	51/59 (86%)	24/59 (41%)
palliative	12/13 (92%)	12/13 (92%)
Postop. sympt. free 6 months	8/22 (36%)	4/22 (18%)
6 months[+]	6/57 (11%)	11/57 (19%)
local recurrence[+]	8/ 9 (89%)	5/ 9 (56%)
metastasis[+]	4/ 5 (80%)	5/ 5 (100%)
Nonmalign. colorectal disease	2/14 (14%)	3/14 (21%)
Healthy volunteers	0/17 (0%)	2/17 (12%)

[+] some of these patients were not tested before operation

Besides the well known features of the CEA assay
(low degree of positivity with primary tumours, post surgical decline, high degree of positivity in patients with
metastases), we face a somewhat complementary performance
of the LMT. The test is more frequently positive before
operation, reactivity declines p.o. in a quite similar
manner and it reappears with local recurrence and metastases.

When analizing individual patient's data with respect
to concordance versus discordance of LMT and CEA-RIA
(Table 3), we observe a high incidence of discordance
(mainly LMT+, CEA-) with primary tumours as opposed to a
high frequency of concordance in patients with advanced
disease (LMT+, CEA+) and in healthy volunteers (LMT-,
CEA-).

TABLE 3 Comparison of LMT and CEA-RIA in individual
patients

Patients	n	Concordance		Discordance	
		LMT+CEA+	LMT-CEA-	LMT+CEA-	LMT-CEA+
Colorect.cancer					
Preop.radical	59	22	6	29	2
palliative	13	11	0	1	1
Postop.sympt.free					
6 months	22	1	11	7	3
6 months[+]	57	3	43	3	8
rec./metast.[+]	14	8	0	4	2
Healthy volunteers	17	0	15	0	2

[+] see above

In conclusion we may state that monitoring of colo-
rectal cancer patients looks promising with the LMT, but
especially with a combination of LMT and CEA-RIA. The further pursuit of our follow-up study will give insight into the prognostic potential of both assays, i.e. their
respective diagnostic lead time, as well as into the clinical significance of discrepant readings.

REFERENCES

(1) Zöller,M., Matzku,S. and Schulz,U. (1977): Cancer
     Immunol. Immunother., in press.

(2) Zöller,M., Matzku,S. and Schulz,U. (1977): J. nat.
     Cancer Inst., 58, 897.

DISCUSSION

MACH J.P. (Lausanne): I am not too surprised by the discrepancy,
because one test concerns a tumour marker with no immunological reaction of the patient and the other is supposed to test his immunological reaction.
May I ask you a short question? In your non malignant diseases,
what is the percentage of positive leukocyte inhibition tests?

MATSKU S. (Heidelberg): We must discriminate between colorectal
disease (20% false positive) and non colorectal disease (4% false
positive).

Antigenic Markers Associated with Lung Cancer

Ronald B. Herberman, K. Robert McIntire, James Braatz, S. Gaffar,
James L. McCoy, Jack H. Dean, and Grace D. Cannon, Laboratory of
Immunodiagnosis, National Cancer Institute, and Litton-Bionetics,
Inc., Bethesda, Maryland   20014 U.S.A.

Many important problems related to the biology, diagnosis and
management of lung cancer require the accurate assessment of the
presence of tumors and of their size and extent of growth. In recent
years, a variety of antigenic substances have been found to be specific for lung cancer, or quantitatively altered in tumor-bearing
patients, and these therefore may aid in the identification of tumors
and in the assessment of tumor burden. However, it is important to
note that only a few of these markers have been shown to have a place
in clinical oncology. Most tests for antigenic markers still need to
be evaluated for their possible utility for several distinct clinical
applications: 1) Detection of cancer cases by screening of general
populations or of groups of high risk of developing cancer; 2) Aid in
differential diagnosis of patients with lung diseases; 3) Aid in
determining stage of disease and prognosis; and 4) Serial monitoring
for early detection of recurrences.

A variety of types of antigenic substances have been associated
with human lung cancer (Table 1). Some are normally present in the
tissues of the fetus or placenta and then disappear or are much reduced in amount after birth. Some antigens have been associated
particularly with lung cancer and have been undetectable, or present
in lower amounts, in normal lung tissues. Most tumor markers are
characterized only by their immunologic properties, but some have
functional activities or are variants of normal functional products.
These include hormones, enzymes, and metal-binding proteins. Lung
cancers have been particularly associated with ectopic production of
a variety of hormones. In addition to detection of circulating
tumor markers, measurement of the immune response of patients to lung
cancer associated antigens may be quite sensitive and useful.

In this paper, we will briefly summarize the available information on the various types of antigens, particularly those which
appear most promising as markers for diagnosis or monitoring of lung
cancer.

The marker which has been studied most extensively for its
clinical usefulness in lung cancer is CEA. This antigen has been
shown to be produced by lung tumors as well as by colorectal cancers
and elevated levels have been detected in the circulation of many
patients with all histologic types of carcinoma of the lung (1-3,
5-7) and this has necessitated the use of higher cut-off values to

TABLE 1 Types of antigenic markers associated with lung cancer

I.   Oncofetal
        Carcinoembryonic antigen (CEA)
II.   Placental
        Human chorionic gonadotrophin (HCG)
        Human placental lactogen
        Placental alkaline phosphatase
III. Other Ectopic Hormones
        Pro-ACTH
        Calcitonin
        Antidiuretic hormone (ADH)
        Parathormone
        β-Lipotropin
IV.   Organ associated Antigens
        Lung tumor associated antigens (HuLTAA)
V.   Normal Antigens and Their Variants
        Ferritin
        Lactoferrin
        K-Casein
        β_2-Microglobulin
        Ceruloplasmin
VI.   Antigens Detected by Immune Responses of Patients
        Cell-mediated immunity
            Delayed cutaneous hypersensitivity
            Leukocyte migration inhbition
            Lymphoproliferative responses
        Antibodies
        Antigen - antibody complexes

discriminate patients with lung cancer from these controls. With
such higher cut-offs, the sensitivity of the assay has been rather
low, with the majority of values in patients with localized disease
being below the cut-off and even in with metastatic disease 20% or
more had negative results (5,8,9). In contrast, measurement of CEA
has appeared more promising for assessing prognosis and detecting recurrences in lung cancer patients. Preoperative CEA values have
shown some correlation with stage of disease (2,8,9) and elevated
values have been associated with poor prognosis. However, few
studies have analyzed the prognostic significance of elevated CEA
levels within a particular stage, and the available evidence on this
is somewhat conflicting (8,9). Therefore, it is not clear whether
measurement of CEA levels will provide the clinician with additional
information beyond that gained by careful clinical and pathologic
staging. Measurement of CEA within a few months after resection of
tumor may provide somewhat better information. Patients with persistent CEA elevations have usually developed recurrent disease
(8,10). Similarly, serial determinations of CEA levels have appeared
useful. Rising CEA levels may precede clinical recurrence by up to
12 months and long term survivors usually had persistently normal
levels (10). However, even in this area, the degree of predictive
value has not been completely documented. In addition, serial
measurements of CEA levels have not appeared to be a good guide to

responses to chemotherapy or radio therapy (8,10).

In recent years, increasing attention has been directed toward the association of lung cancer with elevated levels of various hormones. A prohormone form of adrenocorticotropic hormone (ACTH), termed "big ACTH" and which normally does not enter the circulation, was found to be produced by a large proportion of lung cancers (11). Recently, Wolfsen and Odell (12) reported that, in a prospective study of patients with abnormal chest X-rays, all patients with benign diseases had normal levels of ACTH and 75% of cancer patients had elevated levels. These results are very encouraging, and if confirmed, such assays should play an important role in the initial diagnosis of lung cancer. The value of ACTH determinations for monitoring has not yet been reported. Elevated calcitonin levels have been particularly associated with oat cell cancers, being found in 35-75% of patients studied (13-15). Some patients with other types of lung cancer have also had detectable calcitonin production (16) but not enough patients have been studied to allow an estimate of frequency. All of these studies have been on basal levels of calcitonin and it seems likely that stimulation by pentagastrin or other agents could increase the sensitivity of detection. In addition, it has been suggested that the hormone produced from lung tumor cells is larger and has some immunological differences from thyrocalcitonin (17); this might also lead to a more sensitive detection assay. HCG and human placental lactogen have been found in some patients with lung cancer, but the frequency appears to be less than 10% (18-22). Several groups have reported elevated ADH levels in either urine or plasma of 17-40% of patients (15,22-24). Hypercalcemia due to ectopic production of parathormone has been reported to be the most common form of endocrinopathy in lung cancer, occurring in 7% of new cancer patients (25), but the frequency of elevated levels by radioimmunoassay and its specificity for cancer is not clear.

A number of attempts have been made to produce antisera in heterologous species against lung tumor associated antigens (TAAs) (26-32). These antigens have been separated and characterized to various extents but none have yet been applied clinically. A major problem with this approach is to clearly distinguish between lung TAAs and normal tissue components. For example, Veltri (32) developed antisera which was initially thought to be directed against 3 different lung TAAs, but each was later shown to be a normal serum antigen: ferritin, lactoferrin, and an unidentified component of Cohn fraction 4 of normal serum.

For the past few years, our laboratory has pursued this approach and a new human lung cancer antigen, termed HuLTAA, has been identified (28,33,34). Rabbits were immunized with a perchloric acid extract of homogenates of pooled primary lung cancers. After absorptions with normal human plasma, saline extracts of normal lung tissues and ABO erythrocytes, the antisera gave a single precipitin line in agar gel double diffusion with extracts of lung tumors but not with normal lungs (Table 2). Eighty-five percent of primary lung cancers tested gave positive results and a similar proportion of tumors of all histological types were found to contain the antigen.

TABLE 2 HuLTAA in various tissue extracts, as detected by agar gel double diffussion

Tissue	No. Tested	No. Positive	% Pos.
Lung Cancer	92	78	85
Normal Lung	12	0	0
Fetal Lung	5	0	0
Other Cancer	13	1	8
Sarcoma	5	1	20

In contrast, the antigen was not detectable in normal or fetal lung, and was found in only a small proportion of other types of tumors. HuLTAA has been shown to be different from a variety of other known TAAs and normal serum antigens, including CEA, alphafetoprotein, placental alkaline phosphatase, ferritin, lactoferrin, normal cross-reactive antigen (NCA), ceruloplasmin, and β-oncofetal antigen. As the initial purification step, antigen was eluted from an antibody-affinity chromatographic column. This resulted in a 25-50 fold increase in specific activity, but there were still five distinct protein bands on polyacrylamide gel electrophoresis. Isolation of the antigen was facilitated by radioiodination of partially purified antigen, with subsequent following of radiolabel. Two dimensional radioimmunoelectrophoresis indicated that the fourth band was the antigen. After elution of this band from the gels, this was shown by a variety of criteria to be a homogenous protein with a molecule weight in the range of 80,000. Using the trace labelled and isolated HuLTAA as a marker, we have been able to purify larger quantities of the antigen from a second tumor and we are in the process of developing a radioimmunoassay which can be used to test for circulating antigen. In a double antibody radioimmunoassay, a 1:10,000 dilution of absorbed antiserum still precipitates 25-30% of the labelled antigen. Addition of known amounts of HuLTAA gives a linear dose responsive inhibition of precipitation, over a range from 1.5 to 1,500 nanograms/ml. Attempts to utilize the assay to look for serum antigen have been impeded by some problems with nonspecific inhibition by normal serum. Some factors contributing to this have been identified and we hope to have a working assay for serum antigen in the near future. Only then will we be able to tell whether HuLTAA will be a useful marker for lung cancer.

Studies of the immune response of patients with lung cancer against autologous or allogeneic tumors would also be expected to be useful in identifying lung TAAs. There have been very few detailed studies of sera of patients for antibodies against lung cancer antigens. In contrast, several groups of investigators have demonstrated cell-mediated immunity against lung TAAs. As summarized in Table 3, we have found that the lymphocytes of a majority of lung cancer patients had proliferative responses to autologous tumor cells or crude membrane extracts of their tumors (35). In contrast, only one extract of autologous normal lung elicited a significant response.

168

Virtually all of the reactions were from patients with localized disease. Some of the negative reactions have been attributable to the presence of adherent suppressor cells, and after their removal reactivity could be detected.

TABLE 3 Lymphoproliferative responses to autologous lung cancer cells and to crude membrane extracts of tumor cells

Stimulant	No. Positive/ No. Tested(%)	Mean SI of Responder Cultures[1]	Mean nCPM (±SD) in Responder Cultures[2]
Intact tumor cells	8/13 (62%)	11.3	5,178 (1,300)
Membrane extracts			
Cancer lung	30/63 (48%)	15.8	9,745 (1,870)
Normal lung	1/17 –	– –	– –

[1] SI (stimulation indices) were considered positive if ^{3}H-thymidine incorporation was increased 2-fold or more and different from control cultures at $p < 0.01$. The concentration of extract or tumor cells giving the highest level of proliferation selected for calulation of the mean.

[2] Net counts per minute (nCPM) of responding cultures = experimental CPM - control CPM.

Most of the other studies of cell-mediated immunity in lung cancer have utilized extracts of allogeneic tumor cells. Some patients were found to have specific reactivity in delayed cutaneous hypersensitivity tests (36,37) and in leukocyte migration inhibition (LMI) assays (38-42), indicating that at least some of the cell-mediated immunity is directed against lung TAAs which are shared by a variety of lung tumors. The studies in LMI have indicated that the various histologic types of lung cancer share common antigens, since similar proportions of patients with the various types of disease reacted to extracts derived from adenocarcinoma and squamous cell carcinoma of the lung (42). A summary of our LMI data is given in Table 4. In addition to reactions by about half of the lung cancer patients, an appreciable number of patients with cancers of other types reacted. However, the degree of reactivity was significantly less than that of lung cancer patients. In serial tests of patients after resection of tumor, there has been a trend toward higher reactivity among patients who developed recurrent disease than among those who remained free of detectable disease.

TABLE 4   Leukocyte migration inhibition reactions to soluble extracts
of lung cancer cells

Antigen	Sources	No. positive tests/ total individuals tested (%+)		
		Lung Cancer	Other Cancers	Normal Donors
7661	adenoca., pleural effusion	40/63(59%)	13/37(35%)	4/40(10%)
CaLu-1	epidermoid ca. cell line	21/38(55%)	2/10(35%)	1/11(9%)

In studies of delayed cutaneous hypersensitivity reactions,
several different antigens appeared to be involved. Hollinshead et
al (36) described reactivity to an antigen restricted to epidermoid
lung cancer, as well as more broadly distributed lung TAAs and a
normal lung antigen. At least one of the antigens may be present in
fetal lung, since extracts of fetal lung elicited delayed hypersensitivity reactions in some lung cancer patients (37).

Most of the tests described above have depended on the specific
detection of circulating antigens or immune reactants. If antibodies are being produced against circulating antigens, then antigen-
antibody complexes may be formed. Recently, sensitive tests have
been developed to detect such circulating immune complexes and preliminary tests with these procedures have indicated elevated levels
in the sera of an appreciable proportion of lung cancer patients
(43,44).

There have been a few studies which have tested sera from lung
cancer patients for more than one antigenic marker, to determine
their possible additive or synergistic value for diagnosis. Several
reports have indicated that lung tumors may produce more than one
ectopic hormone (15,19,20,22,23,45-47). Sussman et al (19) measured
two placental hormones, HCG and HPL, as well as placental alkaline
phosphatase in the sera of 5 lung cancer patients and detected elevated levels of one, two or all three markers. They also found that
the same tumor could produce α and β subunits of HCG as well as the
complete hormone (20). Franchimont et al (47) measured CEA along
with HCG, βHCG and casein and found at least one elevated marker in
most patients with advanced lung cancer. Similarly, Gailani et al
(21) have found a low proportion of patients with elevated HCG
levels at the time when they had normal CEA values. Odell et al
(22) measured a variety of hormones in the sera of a larger number
of lung cancer patients. The majority of specimens had elevated
big ACTH and β-lipotropin levels and about 40% had elevations in
ADH. Hansen and Hummer (15) found elevated ACTH and ADH levels in a
lower proportion of patients with small cell carcinoma and noted
elevated calcitonin levels in about one-third of the patients. The
overlap or correlation among these markers was not indicated in

170

these preliminary reports, but it seems likely that the measurement
of all these markers will have some additive value for diagnosis and
monitoring in lung cancer.

Among the many antigenic markers which have been examined, there
are several promising leads for the application to the diagnosis and
management of lung cancer. From the data collected thus far, it
is possible to select a number of antigens for more detailed and extensive clinical studies. The very promising circulating markers
might include CEA, pro-ACTH and calcitonin. To these might be added
the measurement of HuLTAA, antigen-antibody complexes, and of
cell-mediated immune reactivity to lung tumor antigens. It seems
quite likely that some combination of these markers could provide
high levels of specificity and sensitivity. It would also be very
helpful if simpler tests could be developed for detection and
monitoring of lung cancer. The radioimmunoassays are probably the
most practical tests of large scale application and many of the
other procedures, like skin tests or leukocyte migration inhibition,
present considerable logistical and technical problems. One approach
would be to use tumor-associated antigens, which have been identified
by the current techniques, for the production of heterologous antisera and the eventual development of a radioimmunoassay. The data
accumulated thus far are sufficiently encouraging to lead to a
search for new lung cancer-associated antigens and to more extensive
evaluation of currently available markers.

REFERENCES

(1) Logerfo, P., Herter, F.P., Braun, J and Hansen, H.J. (1972):
    Ann. Surgery, 175, 495.
(2) Laurence, D., Jr., Stevens, U., Bettelheim, R., Darcy, D.,
    Leese, C., Turberville, C., Alexander, P., Johnsen and
    Neville, A.M. (1972): Brit. Med. J., 3, 605.
(3) Vincent, R.B. and Chu, T.M. (1973): J. Thor. Cardiovasc. Surg.,
    66, 320.
(4) Vincent, R.B., Chu, T.M., Fergen, T.B. and Ostrander, M. (1975):
    Cancer, 36, 2069.
(5) Concannon, J.P., Dalbow, M.H., Liebler, G.A.,Blake, K.E.,
    Weil, C.S. and Cooper, J.W. (1974): Cancer, 34, 184.
(6) Stevens, D.P. and Mackay, I.R. (1973): Lancet, 2, 1238.
(7) Pauwels, R. and Van Der Straeten, M. (1975): Thorax, 30, 560.
(8) Dent, P.B., McCullogh, P.B., Wesley-James, O., McLaren, R.,
    Muirhead, W. and Dunnett, C.W. (1977): Cancer, in press.
(9) Concannon, J.P., Dalbow, M.H., Hodgson, S.E., Headings, J.J.,
    Markopoulos, E., Mitchell, J., Cushing, W.J. and Liebler, G.A.
    (1977): Cancer, in press.
(10) Vincent, R.B., Chu, T.M., Lane, W.W., Gutierrez, A.C.,
    Stegemann, P.J. and Madajewicz, S. (1977): Proceedings, Second
    Conference on Lung Cancer Treatment, in press.
(11) Gewirtz, G. and Yalow, R.S. (1974): J. Clin. Invest., 53, 1022.
(12) Wolfsen, A. and Odell, W. (1977): Clin. Res., 25, 502A.
(13) Silva, O.L., Becker, K.L., Primack, A., Doppman, J and
    Snider, R.H. (1974): New Eng. J. Med., 290, 1122.

(14) Coombes, R.C., Hillyard, C., Greenberg, P.B. and MacIntyre, I. (1974): <u>Lancet, 1,</u> 1080.

(15) Hansen, M. and Hummer, L. (1977): <u>Proceedings, Second Conference on Lung Cancer Treatment,</u> in press.

(16) Hillyard, C.J., Coombes, R.C., Greenberg, P.B., Galante, L.S. and MacIntyre, I. (1976): <u>Clin. Endocrinol., 5,</u> 1.

(17) Neville, A.M., Coombes, R.C., Hillyard, C.J. and MacIntyre, I. (1976): <u>Cancer Related Antigens, 1976. pp. 151-162.</u>

(18) Braunstein, G.D., Vaitukaitis, J.L., Carbone, P.P. and Ross, G.T. (1973): <u>Ann. Intern. Med., 78,</u> 39.

(19) Sussman, H.H., Weintraub, B.D. and Rosen, S.W. (1974): <u>Cancer, 33,</u> 820.

(20) Rosen, S.W., Weintraub, B.D. Vaitukaitis, J.L., Sussman, H.H., Hershman, J.M. and Muggia, F.M. (1975): <u>Ann. Int. Med., 82,</u> 71.

(21) Gailani, S., Chu, T.M., Nussbaum, A., Ostrander, M. and Christoff, N. (1976): <u>Cancer, 38,</u> 1684.

(22) Odell, W., Wolfson, A., Yoshimoto, Y., Weitzman, R. and Fisher, D. (1977): <u>Clin. Res., 25,</u> 525A.

(23) Hamilton, B.P.M., Upton, G.V. and Amatruda, T.T., Jr. (1972): <u>J. Clin. Enocrinol. Metab., 35,</u> 764.

(24) Haefliger, J.M., Dubied, M.C. and Vallotton, M.B. (1977): <u>Clin. Res., 25,</u> 295A.

(25) Rassam, J.W. and Anderson, G. (1975): <u>Thorax, 30,</u> 86.

(26) Yachi, A., Matsuura, Y., Carpenter, C.M. and Hyde, L. (1968): <u>J. Natl. Cancer Inst., 40,</u> 663.

(27) Schlipkoter, H.W., Idei, H., Barsoum, A.L. and Vollmer, U.J. (1973): <u>Zbi. Bakt. Hyg., 158,</u> 109.

(28) McIntire, K.R. and Sizaret, P.P. (1974): <u>Proceedings, XI International Cancer Congress, Cell Biology and Tumor Immunology, 1974. pp. 295-29 , Vol. 1.</u>

(29) Sega, E., Natali, P.G., Ricci, C., Minnco, C.T. and Citro, G. (1974): <u>I.R.C.S., 2,</u> 1278.

(30) Frost, M.J., Rogers, G.T. and Bagshawe, K.D. (1975): <u>Br. J. Cancer, 31,</u> 379.

(31) Bell, C.E., Jr., Seetharam, S. and McDaniel, R.C. (1976): <u>J. Immunol., 116,</u> 1236.

(32) Veltri, R.W., Mengoli, H.F., Maxim, P.E., Westfall, S., Gopo, J.M., Huang, C.W. and Sprinkle, P.M. (1977): <u>Cancer Res., 37,</u> 1313.

(33) McIntire, K.R., Adams, W.P., Braatz, J.A., Gaffar, S.A., Kortright, K.H. and Princler, G.L. (1977): <u>Proceedings, Second Conference on Lung Cancer Treatment,</u> in press.

(34) Braatz, J.A., McIntire, K.R., Princler, G.L., Kortright, K.H. and Herberman, R.B. (1977): Submitted for publication.

(35) Dean, J.H., McCoy, J.L., Cannon, G.B., Weese, J.L., Oldham, R.K. and Herberman, R.B. (1977): <u>Proceedings, Third International Symposium on Detection and Prevention of Cancer,</u> in press.

(36) Hollinshead, A.C., Stewart, T.H.M. and Herberman, R.B. (1974): <u>J. Natl. Cancer Inst., 52,</u> 327.

(37) Wells, S.A., Jr., Burdick, J.F., Christiansen, C., Ketcham, A.S. and Adkins, P.C. (1973): <u>Natl. Cancer Monogr., 37,</u> 197.

(38) Alth, G., Denck, H., Fischer, M., Karrer, K., Kokron, O., Korizek, E., Micksche, M., Ogris, E., Reider, C., Titscher, R. and Wrba, H. (1973): Cancer Chemother. Rep., 4, 275.
(39) Boddie, A.W., Holmes, E.C., Roth, A. and Morton, D.L. (1975): Int. J. Cancer, 15, 832.
(40) Oldham, R.K., Weese, J.L., Herberman, R.B., Perlin, E., Mills, M., Heim, W., Blom, J., Green, D., Reid, J., Bellinger, S., Law, I., McCoy, J.L., Dean, J.H., Cannon, G.B. and Djeu, J. (1976): Int. J. Cancer, 18, 739.
(41) Vose, B.M., Kimber, I. and Moore, M. (1977): J. Natl. Cancer Inst., 58, 483.
(42) McCoy, J.L., Jerome, L.F., Cannon, G.B., Weese, J.L. and Herberman, R.B. (1977): J. Natl. Cancer Inst., in press.
(43) Theofilopoulos, A., Wilson, C.B. and Dixon, F.J. (1976): J. Clin. Invest., 57, 169.
(44) Rossen, R.D., Reisberg, M.A., Hersh, E.M. and Gutterman, J.U. (1977): J. Natl. Cancer Inst., in press.
(45) Bailey, R.E. (1971): J. Clin. Endocrinol. Metab., 32, 317.
(46) Rees, L.H., Bloomfield, G.A. and Rees, G.M. (1974): J. Clin. Endocrinol. Metab., 38, 1090.
(47) Franchimont, P., Zangerle, P.F., Nogarede, J., Bury, J., Molter, F., Reuter, A., Hendrick, J.C. and Collette, J. (1976): Cancer, 38, 2287.

DISCUSSION

MATZKU S. (Heidelberg) : Can you exclude that your bronchogenic antigen derived from host cell?

HERBERMAN R. (Bethesda) : Well, there is no evidence for that. We have looked at extracts of other tissues including spleen and leukocytes after absorption. We noticed no reactivity with these.

ZAMCHECK N.(Boston) : Did you show a relationship between CEA and early detection of lung cancer ? How early will elevated CEA pick up lung cancer metastasing to the liver.

HERBERMAN R. (Bethesda) : I do not have too much details about that. My own impression as regard to early detection of lung cancer is that it would probably not play much of a role and that among the patients who have been described with resectable disease, only a small proportion of these patients showed elevated levels of CEA. I put much more optimism in some of these other markers that are coming along, for instance big ACTH, and ceruleoplasmin and other markers which have been elevated in a majority of patients with Stage I carcinoma of the lung.

VINCENT R.G. (Buffalo) : In conclusion, do you know of any other tumours that provide as many metabolic markers as does lung cancer.

HERBERMAN R. (Bethesda) : I think this a fascinating question in regard to why the lung tumour is making so many different markers. Dr. SHUSTER raised a question of possible similarity to the pituitary. I am not sure that this is an explanation, because the type of ectopic hormones is often placental as well as pituitary. Other cancers may have a fair proportion of cases with elevated ACTH, HCG and other markers.

CARCINOEMBRYONIC ANTIGEN AS A MONITOR OF SUCCESSFUL SUR-
GICAL RESECTION IN 130 PATIENTS WITH CARCINOMA OF THE
LUNG

R. Vincent, T. Chu, W. Lane, A. Gutierrez, P. Stegemann,
S. Madajewicz

Roswell Park Memorial Institute, 666 Elm Street, Buffalo,
New York U.S.A. 14263
In lung cancer CEA has been shown to be elevated in
all cell types but not with sufficient consistency or
magnitude to be used for screening purposes (4). CEA,
however, may well have value as a monitor of successful
surgical extirpation of lung cancer or presage the failure of surgery to totally ablate the tumor. If progression of the disease can be anticipated before it becomes
clinically evident, other therapeutic methods can be
instituted in a more timely and natural fashion.
     The technique of radioimmunoassay capable of detect-
ing plasma levels of CEA in an nanogram range was described by Thomson in 1969 (3). We use Hansen's modification of radioimmunoassay for CEA which employs the use of
zirconylphosphate gel (2).

RESULTS

     Following workup, each patient was staged according
to the methods of the American Joint Committee for Cancer
Staging and End Results Reporting (1).
     A blood sample is drawn from all surgical patients
prior to surgery. Upon confirmation of a histologic
diagnosis of carcinoma of the lung, additional blood
samples are drawn postoperatively and at 30 day intervals
for 3 months and then 3 month intervals until the patient
is lost to followup.
     The serial CEA levels were recorded in 130 patients
in which surgical resection of a histologically proven
carcinoma of the lung had been accomplished.
     For purposes of analysis and comparison these
patients are divided into four groups consisting of the
following.

Group 1

     Thirty-two (32) patients who have lived longer than
15 months and are currently alive without clinical evidence of progressive disease or who died at any time but

*Radioactive CEA and goat CEA antibody were kindly supp-
lied by Dr. Hansen of Hoffman-LaRoche Inc., Nutley, N.J.

were shown by a complete autopsy to be free of disease.

Most patients who are not cured by surgery will give clinical evidence of this fact within six to 15 months after surgery. For this reason the 32 patients in this group are regarded as having been cured by surgery.

The median preoperative CEA value for this group was 0.4 ng/ml. In the initial CEA evaluation, 4 patients exceeded 5 ng/ml with one of these values reaching 14.9 ng/ml. Of importance is the fact that the interval median CEA value for this group during a 36 month followup period never exceeded 1.5 ng/ml. Of all the interval samples collected in this group after the first 3 months of followup, 5 ng/ml was exceeded 3 times and 6.5 ng/ml only once (Fig. 1).

Group II

Of the 23 patients in this group, survival was greater than 15 months but in every instance surgery failed to control the disease. The median CEA value at the time of diagnosis was 3.7 ng/ml (Fig. 1), while the post-resection median value dropped to 2 ng/ml within six months of surgery, subsequently the median values continue to rise progressively to exceed 6 ng/ml by the 12th month of followup.

Four of these patients lived longer than three years. Two of these four were surgically explored because of an unexplained increase of CEA levels. One had recurrence in the lung and the second had a second primary of the kidney. In both patients, resection of the second lesion was accomplished.

Group III

All of these 39 patients died within 15 months of surgery and where it could not be shown that other causes were responsible for death it was presumed that death was secondary to persisting lung cancer and that surgery had failed to control the disease (Fig. 1). The median preoperative diagnostic value for this group was 5.6 and while CEA values generally decreased after surgical resection, within six months the values usually exceeded 6.0 ng/ml.

Group IV

Thirty-six (36) patients who are alive without evidence of disease but less than 15 months since surgery. Since these patients are not yet designated as either surgical "cures" or "failures" they are not included in subsequent statistical evaluations.

CEA As a Monitor

176

While it is apparent that there is a parallel between rising CEA values and progression of malignant disease, it is important to determine if there is sufficient correlation between these two factors to be able to use CEA values to detect or anticipate progressive disease before it becomes clinically evident.

A comparison is made in the median CEA values of patients cured by surgery and those who failed following surgery (Fig. 2). The date of last contact is used as the endpoint in the surgically cured patients and the median CEA value characteristically remained at 1.5 ng/ml or lower at all followup intervals.

Where clinical recurrence of disease became evident, a CEA value of 6 ng/ml preceeded this endpoint in 50% of the patients by 3 months with one case being followed with an elevated CEA for more than 24 months (Fig. 2).

Where death is used as an endpoint a CEA value of 8.0 ng/ml preceeded death by 9 months in 50% of the patients (Fig. 2).

DISCUSSION

It is evident from the data that CEA is not sufficiently sensitive to be used to screen high risk populations for the presence of lung cancer particularly for lesions that are deemed to be resectable (5). Sixty percent of those patients who were resected in this series did not have an initial CEA value elevated above 2.5 ng/ml.

The initial CEA value, however, can be of some help in suggesting the eventual clinical prognosis. In the clinical evaluation of the lung cancer patient, 2.5 ng/ml and 6.5 ng/ml represent important levels of discrimination. A patient with evidence of pulmonary disease that has a CEA concentration of less than 2.5 ng/ml may or may not have malignant disease but should be followed. A patient with CEA between 2.5 ng/ml and 6.5 ng/ml has very suggestive evidence of the presence of malignancy.

If the CEA concentration in this patient increases or does not decrease with effective treatment of concomitant benign conditions the diagnosis of possible malignancy must be taken seriously. In a patient with pulmonary disease and a CEA in excess of 6.5 ng/ml the clinician should be very reluctant to abandon a diagnosis of lung cancer. A CEA concentration of 15 ng/ml in a potential surgical candidate casts great doubt on the possibility of successful surgical resection.

Forty-nine percent of the patients with preoperative concentrations of 2.5 ng/ml or less remain disease free following the resection. On the other hand, 74% of patients that had CEA above 2.5 ng/ml preoperatively eventually developed disseminated disease and are regarded as treatment failures.

If CEA has any value as a monitor to reflect progression or remission of disease it will be in the event of the surgical patient where there is a sudden reduction of tumor volume with some possibility that there has been a total extirpation of the tumor. The data as herein presented suggest that CEA can serve as a clinical prognosticator in the surgically resected patient within certain limitations.

If during a postoperative followup period that has been greater than 3 months the CEA values exceed 2.5 ng/ml the surgeon should follow the patient carefully and hope for a lesser value upon the next examination. However, if the CEA rises during this period to 5 ng/ml a diagnostic evaluation of the patient is indicated with the intent of finding residual disease or a second primary. Where the CEA exceed 6.5 ng/ml in two measurements during the postoperative period, consideration should be given to the institution of additional antineoplastic therapy.

SUMMARY

In the lung cancer patient, CEA has limited value in screening for the early lesion, modest value in presaging a successful resection and considerable value monitoring the course of disease following resection.

CEA is a clinical tool that merits further investigation and has the potential of leading to the identification of a lung tumor specific marker.

ACKNOWLEDGEMENT

The authors acknowledge the efforts of Tona Flak and Gail Philbin in the tabulation of data and the preparation of the manuscript.

REFERENCES

(1) Anderson, W.A.D. et al (American Joint Committee for Cancer Staging and End Results Reporting) Clinical Staging System for Carcinoma of the Lung (1973).
(2) Hansen, H.J., Lance, K., Krupey, J.: Demonstration of an Ion Sensitive Antigen Site on Carcinoembryonic Antigen Using Zirconylphosphate Gel (1971) Clinical Research 19, 143.
(3) Thomson, D.M.P., Krupey, J., Freedman, O. et al: The Radioimmunoassay of Circulating Carcinoembryonic Antigen of the Human Digestive System (1969) Proc. Natl. Acad. Sci. 64, 161.
(4) Vincent, R.G. and Chu, T.M.: CEA in Patients with Carcinoma of the Lung (1973) J. Thor. Surg. 66, 320.
(5) Vincent, R.G., Chu. T.M., Fergen, T.B. et al: CEA in 228 Patients with Carcinoma of the Lung (1975) Cancer 36, 2069.

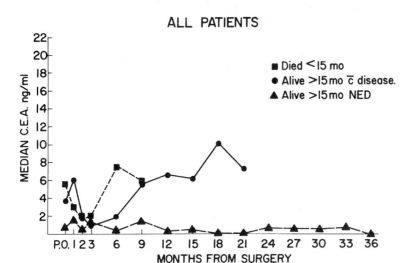

Fig. 1 The serial CEA value in patients following surgical resection of lung cancer contrasting the median CEA
values in the patients who were cured with values where
tumor recurrence became evident.

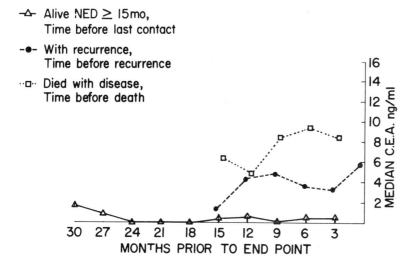

Fig. 2 A comparison of median CEA values at different
intervals prior to :
    (a)   the date of last contact in the patients with
           a totally disease free interval
    (b)   the date of first evidence of recurrent disease
    (c)   the date of death in all patients who failed
           surgical resection and died of disease

179

DISCUSSION

ZAMCHECK N. (Boston) : This is a fine demonstration of good clinical investigation. You actually have answered most of the questions. You have shown with lung cancer findings similar to those shown previously with colonic cancer; the difference being that lung cancer is a much more serious disease. Its course is much briefer. It is not even as uniform a CEA producer as is colonic cancer. Most colonic cancers are well differentiated adenocarcinomas which produce higher levels of CEA. It would be interesting to see whether your group "adenocarcinoma" is a better CEA producer and has a worse prognosis than your other categories.

VINCENT R.G. (Buffalo) : May I ask a question to Dr. ZAMCHECK : is it possible that the earlier forms of the reagents used by HOFMANN/LA ROCHE were more specific for lung cancer and became less specific as they made it more specific for colonic cancer.

ZAMCHECK N. (Boston): I do not know. You know that the CEA reagent used in test kits is derived from metastatic colonic cancer to the liver, so I can speculate that the marker could be more specific for liver metastases of colonic cancer than for primary colonic cancer. That is why I would like to see a lung cancer antigen used in the assay for lung cancer or at least an antigen to lung cancer metastases to the liver. The other problem relates to methodology and this is complicated. Methods have changed somewhat during the years .

HERBERMAN R. (Bethesda) : Do you feel that measuring the CEA in the preoperative period provides additional information beyond the TNM classification to the clinician?

VINCENT R.G. (Buffalo) : Yes, I do. If patients are in stage I, and if CEA is above 10, you are probably wrong in your staging and you need to go back and reassess the patient again.

ZAMCHECK N. (Boston) : I wonder if you had the opportunity to compare "adenocarcinoma" with "small cell" cancer or "squamous" cancer. Plasma CEA would be the best marker for the best CEA producer.

VINCENT R.G. (Buffalo) : Adenocarcinoma has consistently higher levels of CEA as compared to the other cell types of lung cancer.

THE CLINICAL SIGNIFICANCE OF THE CEA ASSAY IN PATIENTS WITH BRONCHO-GENIC CARCINOMA

J. Concannon, M. Dalbow, K. Blake, S. Hodgson,[†] J. Headings and
E. Markopoulos

Clinical Radiation Therapy Research Center, Allegheny General Hospital
320 East North Avenue, Pittsburgh, PA 15212, U.S.A.
[†]Radiation Therapy Department, Ohio State University, Columbus, OH
43210, U.S.A.

Preoperative plasma carcinoembryonic antigen (CEA) levels were
measured by radioimmunoassay for 172 patients with bronchogenic carcinoma. One hundred and forty-nine of these patients had serial CEA
studies. The data were used to determine the prognostic value of the
CEA assay in these patients.

METHODS

The CEA studies reported here were performed by the method of
Hansen (1) using the CEA-Roche reagents. The patients in this study
were staged with both pre and postoperative information by the method
outlined by the "American Joint Committee Clinical Staging System for
Carcinoma of the Bronchus"(2).

Survival curves were generated by the Life Table Technique (3)
and tested for statistical differences by the Generalized Wilcoxon
Test (4). Statistical differences in the mean survival of groups
of patients were tested by the student t test.

RESULTS

Concannon, et al. (5) have previously reported that patients
with bronchogenic carcinoma with preoperative plasma CEA levels
>6 ng/ml have a universally poor prognosis. All of the patients who
had such preoperative elevations in plasma CEA died in less than 3
years; the majority (93%) died within 1 year of surgery. Although approximately half of the patients with preoperative CEA levels $\leq$ 6
ng/ml die in a relatively short period all of the long-term survivors
were found to have preoperative CEA levels in this range. The results of Concannon, et al. indicated that the preoperative measurement of the plasma CEA level would have little prognostic significance for individual patients with values $\leq$ 6 ng/ml. However, all
long-term survivors had low CEA measurements and the > 6 ng level
would, therefore, indicate a poor prognosis. It was further suggested
that patients with such elevations in plasma CEA would benefit very
little from a surgical procedure and these patients should be thor-
oughly worked-up prior to surgery to rule out all possibilities of
metastatic disease. The results of the present study confirm these
earlier observations of Concannon, et al. (5), and also indicate that
serial measurements of the plasma CEA level may be of prognostic

value in the postoperative followup of patients with lung cancer. One hundred and forty-nine patients had serial CEA determinations within 9 months of death or within the past 3 months for surviving patients. Twenty-eight of 43 patients (65%) with preoperative CEA levels $\leq$ 6 ng/ml had an elevation in plasma CEA (>6 ng/ml) before death. Forty-eight patients with pre-operative CEA levels >6.0 ng/ml had persistently high CEA levels until death. Eight patients (pre-operative > 6 ng/ml) showed a post surgical decrease below 6 ng/ml but had an increase to >6 ng/ml before death. Forty patients who have died had persistently low CEA levels(< 6 ng/ml). Twenty-five patients who were alive for periods ranging from 20 to 68 months at the time of this analysis have had persistently low plasma CEA levels.

Survival curves generated for the survival of patients from the time of diagnosis are shown in Figure 1. The patients were divided into two groups based on their CEA determinations: 1) patients who had persistently low ($\leq$6 ng/ml) CEA levels; and 2) patients who had plasma CEA levels > 6 ng/ml at any period. There is an obvious stage of disease effect in the survival of these patients. The survival curve for the patients with Stages I and II disease who had persistently low CEA levels ($\leq$ 6 ng/ml) show a predicted survival of 73% at 5 years. All of the patients in Stages I and II who had a CEA determination > 6 ng/ml have died; the majority within 2 years post surgery.

The plasma CEA level does not have a similar prognostic significance for patients with Stages 3 or 4 disease. Although the survival curves for the two groups of patients categorized on the basis of CEA level are not statistically different for the patients with Stage 3 or 4 disease, the curve for Stage 3 patients ($\leq$ 6 ng/ml) predicted a survival of approximately 16% at 4 years.

All patients with Stage 1 and 2 disease had a definitive resection. Two patients had a wedge resection, 30 had a lobectomy, and 17 had a pneumonectomy. However the patients in Stages 1 and 2 constitute a rather heterogenous group relative to extent of disease; since patients who are treated by pneumonectomy generally have more extensive disease than patients treated with the less radical wedge resection or lobectomy. These patients were divided into two surgical groups. The mean survivals plotted for the two surgical groups, further subdivided into 3 groups based on CEA studies are shown in Figure 2. The mean survivals for the patients who had persistently low CEA levels ($\leq$ 6 ng/ml) were significantly greater for both surgical groups when compared with either of the groups who had elevated CEA levels before or after surgery (P < 0.01). The mean survival of the patients with persistently low CEA levels who had a wedge resection or lobectomy was not significantly different from the patients with persistently low CEA levels who had a pneumonectomy. However, a greater proportion of the patients treated by pneumonectomy have died indicating that survival is related to the extent of the disease at the time of thoracotomy.

Although these data indicate that serial measurements of the plasma CEA level in patients with lung cancer may have prognostic significance it is doubtful that such information will be of practical clinical value at this time since there is little that can be done therapeutically for these patients. However since there is always hope that new therapeutic modalities may prove effective, we

182

have examined these data to determine the lead time the CEA signal will provide the physician. Figure 3 shows the survival curves generated for the survival of patients from the time of their first elevation in plasma CEA titer > 6 ng/ml. Although many patients die within a short period following such elevations in CEA, the curve for the patients with Stage 2 disease shows that the time to median (50%) survival was 9 months and nearly 1/3 of the patients lived at least 1 year. The time to median survival for the patients with Stage 3 or 4 disease was approximately 6 months. Twenty percent (20%) of the patients in Stage 3 and 10% in Stage 4 lived for 1 year.

In summary we feel that these data indicate that the measurement of plasma CEA levels in patients with lung cancer who are being considered for thoracotomy will provide valuable information relative to the end results of this procedure. We have found that patients with preoperative CEA levels > 6 ng/ml invariably die.

Although the followup of patients with lung cancer with serial CEA measurements is of less practical value at this time, it may prove a useful adjunct for monitoring therapy in the future.

The authors wish to gratefully acknowledge the technical and clerical contributions of Michael Debes, Deanna Atzinger, and Dru Ann Heath. Supported in part by Public Health Service Research Grants 5 S015709 and CA 10438.

REFERENCES

(1) Hansen, H., Snyder, J., Miller, E., et al. (1974): Human Pathol., 5, 139.
(2) The American Joint Committee for Cancer Staging and End Results Reporting (1973): Clinical Staging System for Carcinoma of the Lung., Chicago, IL, U.S.A.
(3) Cutler, S. and Ederer, F. (1958): J. Chron. Dis., 8, 699.
(4) Gehan, E. (1965): Biometrika, 52, 203.
(5) Concannon, J., Dalbow, M., Hodgson, S., et al. Cancer - In press

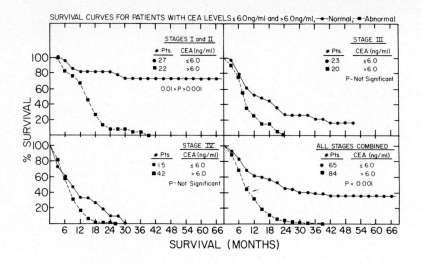

Fig. 1 Survival curves comparing patients with persistent CEA levels ≤ 6 ng/ml with patients having CEA levels > 6 ng/ml.

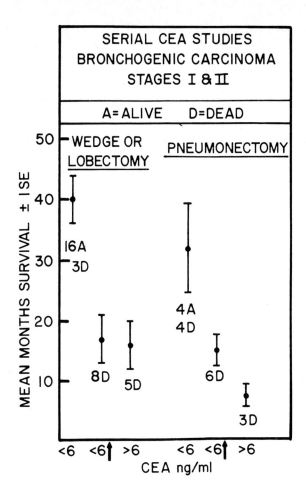

Fig. 2 Diagram of the mean ± 1 SE survival of patients (Stages I
and II categorized by surgical procedure) who had persistent CEA
levels < 6 ng/ml or CEA levels < 6 with a subsequent increase >6 ng/
ml (< 6 ng ↑) or had persistent CEA levels > 6 ng/ml.

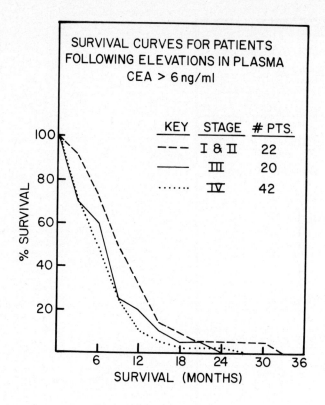

Fig. 3 Survival curves for patients who had a CEA determination
> 6 ng/ml. Survival taken from the time of the first CEA elevation
> 6 ng/ml.

DISCUSSION

HERBERMAN R. (Bethesda) : I would like to ask about the prognostic
value of CEA within a stage. You show that there was no significant
indication of the preoperative CEA value for stages III and IV and
you show prognostic value for combined stage I and II. Since there
is a prognosis difference between stages I and II, I wonder why the
two have been put together and in fact, if you analyse only the stage
I and only the stage II, would you have seen the same significant
prognosis indication for CEA?

BLAKE K.E. (Pittsburg) : We had only 3 patients with Stage I disease,
I do not feel this number would seriously affect the data and the
conclusions drawn from the data.

186

RADIOIMMUNOASSAY OF CARCINOEMBRYONIC ANTIGEN IN BRONCHIAL CARCINOMA

E.A.MacDonald[*], P.Chauvel[*], M.Namer[*], M.Schneider[*], H.Richelme[+], B.Blaive[+], J.M.Aubanel[*], G.Milano[*], B.P.Krebs[*] and A.Ramaioli[*]

[*] Centre Antoine Lacassagne, 36 Voie Romaine, 06054 NICE Cedex,France
[+] Hôpital Pasteur, 30 Voie Romaine, 06 NICE, France

This study aims to show the importance in prediction of prognosis and clinical follow up of the routine estimation of serum chorio-embryonic antigen in bronchial carcinoma.

At Centre Antoine Lacassagne since 1975, 112 cases of lung cancer have been included in the study.

POPULATION

The histological distribution of tumours is shown in Table 1. The proportions of each type are in keeping with national statistics, notably the largest group being squamous cell carcinoma. Almost half the patients 48/112 cases underwent surgery. Complementary treatment with irradiation chemotherapy or immunotherapy was given according to currently accepted practice.

TABLE 1 Histological classification of bronchial tumours:112 cases

Squamous cell carcinomas	64
Undifferentiated tumours	11
Small cell carcinomas	5
Adenocarcinomas	7
Bronchoalveolar carcinoma	2
Mesothelioma	5
Positive cytology only	8
Unknown	10

MONITORING BEFORE TREATMENT

In 36 cases CEA serum levels were estimated before the start of treatment. Correlation of these levels with survival revealed two apparently clearly distinct populations - those who presented abnormal serum antigen levels - and those who did not.

Table 2 shows the mean survivals in these two groups. Those patients who had a serum CEA level above 5 ng/ml before treatment had a mean survival af 3,87 months a compared with 9,24 months for those with CEA below this level at presentation.

TABLE 2 Correlation of survival with CEA plasma levels before treat-
-ment.

Level less than 5	12 cases	geometric mean 9,24 months	median 12 months
Level more than 5	20 cases	geometric mean 3,87 months	median 4 months
Total	32 cases	geometric mean 5,37 months	median 5 months

Figure 1 illustrates clearly the difference between the two
populations. We have drawn the cumulative percentage of death as a
fonction of actuarial survival expressed in probit log. For example
at 10 months 80 % of patients with CEA levels higher than 5 are already dead versus 50 % of those with normal CEA levels at presentation
In an attempt to establish the threshold of significance for
this test at this Centre, actuarial survival curves (Fig. 2) were
plotted for varying threshold values. It was found that the threshold
of 5 ng/ml most sensitively reflected the difference between the two
populations. Table 3 confirms that the maximum difference calculated
between each pair of slopes was most significant at the 5 ng/ml level.

TABLE 3 Table showing maximum relative difference[*] in survival between
CEA positive and negative populations according to thresholds of
positivity .(* = D)

CEA threshold of positivity	3 to 6 months	6 to 12 months	12 to 24 months	Summation D
5	33	27	35	95
10	28	16	29	73
20	17	7	21	45

Pretreatment levels were then assessed in the light of TNM
Classification. Extent of primary tumour did not appear to be reflected in CEA levels. On the other hand those patients presenting with
detectable mediastinal lymph node involvement,N1 or N2,more frequently also presented raised serum antigen.
Tables 4 and 5 demonstrate the correlation of raised serum CEA
levels with the presence of mediastinal involvement.

TABLE 4 Correlation of CEA serum level before treatment with mediastinal lymph node involvement (number of patients in each group)

	No (10)	N1-2 (13)
CEA < 5 (8)	5	3
CEA > 5 (15)	5	10

TABLE 5 Correlation of CEA serum levels before treatment with mediastinal lymph node involvement by survival (months)

	Survival No (10)	Survival N1.2 (13)	Mean survival with CEA level
CEA < 5 (8)	10.5 (5)	6.5 (3)	8.61
CEA > 5 (15)	4.6 (5)	3.5 (10)	3.57
Mean survival with N	6.84	3.72	

In this group of patients the majority of cases of clinical mediastinal involvement without apparent metastatic spread had raised serum CEA levels. The group of patients without evident mediastinal lympho node invasion was equally divided between those with normal and abnormal serum antigen levels. The mean survival of the group with clinical node involvement was as expected less than seen in patients with no node involvement. The demonstration of raised CEA levels in both groups reduced the mean survival. Naturally the best survival (10,5 months) was seen in No patients with CEA serum less than 5 ng/ml ant the worst (3,57 months) in N1, N2 patients with raised serum antigen.

CEA estimation at presentation thus shows some correlation with the clinical assessement of lymph node invasion. In our patients positive antigen levels did not accurately reflect the clinical assessement of dissemination at presentation possibly due to the presence of multiple non-detectable micro metastases. However during the course of the disease a strong correlation emerged between the presence of disseminated disease and abnormal antigen levels at presentation.Tab.6

TABLE 6 Correlation of serum CEA levels before treatment with metastatic dissemination at or after presentation.

Less than 5 ng/ml	58 %	M-
	42 %	M+
More than 5 ng/ml	33 %	M- *
	66 %	M+

* All dead within 4 months.

66 % of patients with rased CEA levels before treatment later developed overt metastases. The 33 % of cases apparently without métastases (7 cases) all died either of their primaty disease or from therapeutic accident within 4 months : perhaps before clinical appearance of dissemination.

It is interesting to note that antigen levels did not correlate with other factors affecting the clinical decision of operability. 7 cases in this group with raised CEA levels at presentation were considered operable as opposed to 6 cases without demonstrable serum levels.

No positive correlation was found between raised antigen level and either the histology of the tumour or age or sex of the patients.

CEA MONITORING AFTER INITIAL TREATMENT

The usefulness of CEA monitoring in bronchial carcinoma after definitive treatment is less easy to assess. Certain points are clear. Long survival is associated with consistently low levels of serum CEA. In our study 13 cases currently surviving more than 20 months have all had consistently low levels of CEA. Only 12 samples but of a total of 70 taken were above the threshold level of 5 ng/ml. The highest being 21 ng/ml.

On the other hand, figure 3 demonstrates that a steadily rising level of serum antigen predicts an approaching fatal outcome in the months before death. Study of the variation of CEA levels after treatment and their comparison with pretreatment levels reinforces our previous findings.
1. Patients with CEA below 5 before and after treatment have the longest survival (16 months, geometric mean).
2. Diminution of CEA levels raised before treatment does not result in increased survival (7 months).
3. On the other hand increasing CEA levels predict approaching death (mean geometric survival 4 months).

Finally we have studied the usefulness of CEA monitoring during the chemotherapy for known disease.

Three types of clinical event become apparent :
a- local recurrence or progression of primary disease
b- metastatic dissemination
c- clinical stability, either without tumour or with non-progressive disease.

Table 7 confirms the findings in the literature showing that with localised disease, half the patients have normal and half raised serum antigne levels (1,2).

TABLE 7 Correlation of CEA monitoring with clinical evolution during chemotherapy for known disease

	CEA always $<$ 5 ng/ml	CEA $>$ 5 ng/ml
Primary tumour increasing (19)	47.4%	52.6%

Table 8 illustrates that metastatic dissemination is correlated with a rise in serum CEA in 73% of confirmed metastases. This result reaffirms published data (1, 2).

TABLE 8 Correlation of CEA monitoring with clinical evolution during chemotherapy for known disease

	CEA always < 5 ng/ml	CEA > 5ng/ml
Metastatic Dissemination (26)	26.9%	73.1%

Table 9 illustrates the following main points.

TABLE 9 Correlation of CEA monitoring with clinical evolution during chemotherapy for known disease

	Clinically stable (20)		
35% always < 5	65% not always < 5		
No possible monitoring	CEA ↘	CEA stable	CEA ↗
	46%	38.5%	15.5% *
	84.5%		
	AGREEMENT		DISAGREEMENT

* 2 patients clinically stable, but latest level increasing perhaps predicting evolution?

35% of clinical remissions (7 cases) occured in patients whose tumours at no time produced detectable serum levels of CEA. Thus monitoring of these cases is impossible. Among the 13 cases with detectable variations in serum CEA 84.5% reflect clinical events. This high percentage confirms the potential value of CEA monitoring in bronchial carcinoma. The apparent discordance in 2 cases may be explained by the fact that it is the latest estimation which is elevated and may thus presage progression of disease.

Figure 4 represents one case in which CEA monitoring accurately reflects the clinical evolution, the effect of treatment and the prediction of clinical deterioration before death and exemplifies the role of CEA monitoring in clinical practice.

Finally our study brought to light two possible artefects in monitoring. Sudden isolated peaks in serum CEA levels were seen in samples taken immediately following bronchoscopy or in the days immediately following systemic chemotherapy.

191

CONCLUSION

  Throughout our study two distinct populations could be distin-
guished : those with detectable secretion of CEA into the serum and
those without.
  Elevated serum antigen levels are associated with decreased
survival and reflect with fidelity the clinical evolution.

REFERENCES

(1) Concannon,J., Dalbow,M.H., Liebler,G.A., Blake,K.E., Weil,C.S.,
  Cooper, J.W. (1974) : Cancer 34, 184.
(2) Vincent,R., Chu,T., Fergen,T., Ostrander, M. (1975) : Cancer 36,
  2069.

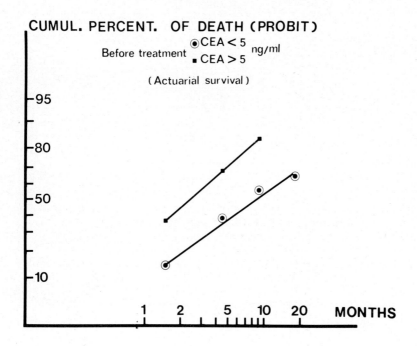

Fig. 1 Cumulative percentage of death (Probit)

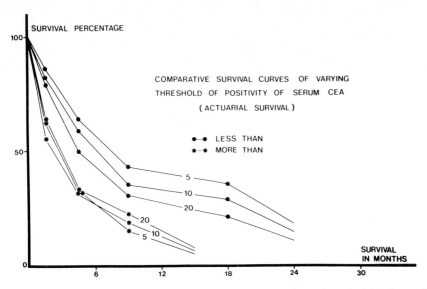

Fig. 2 Comparative survival curves of varying threshold of positivity
of serum CEA (actuarial survival)

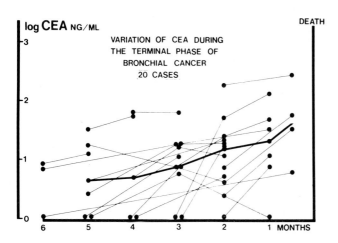

Fig. 3 Variation of CEA during the terminal phase of bronchial
cancer (20 cases)

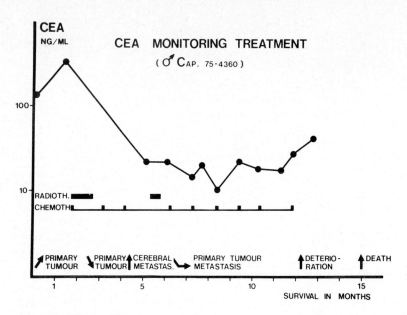

Fig. 4 CEA monitoring treatment.

DISCUSSION

RICHELME H. (Nice) : I am not a biologist, so I wonder why everybody uses different cut-off values.Is this a question of technique?

KREBS B.P. (Nice) : Methodology with perchloric acid extraction step will give results lower than assays performed directly on plasma. Thus, cut-off could be different. Nevertheless, for each cancer loca-lisation, the cut-off may be different. At least, for each proposi-tion - diagnosis, prognosis, recurrence, metastatic widespread - the statistician will, in retropective study, give you the threshold resulting in the best descrimination between two populations.

VINCENT R.G. (Buffalo) : A question related to mediastinal tumours : was this determination made on a clinical basis or was it made on an autposy basis.

MAC DONALD E.A. (Nice):It was made entirely on clinical basis.

ZAMCHECK N. (Boston) : No mention was made of metastases to the liver . Do you have any data about the relationship between the metastases to the liver and CEA.

MAC DONALD E.A. (Nice): Our figures were insufficient to be able to distinguish between the various kind of metastases.

VINCENT R.G. (Buffalo): In our experience, no relation was found between CEA and liver metastases.

INTEREST OF CARCINOEMBRYONIC ANTIGEN ASSAY IN BRONCHOGENIC CARCINOMA

J.P. Bisset⁺, F. Roux⁺, R. Sauvan⁺, J. Pasquier⁺, R. Poirier⁺⁺, J.P. Kleisbauer⁺⁺

+ Nuclear Medicine, Pr H. Roux, C.H.U. Timone, Marseilles France
++ Pneumology Department, Pr P. Laval, Michel Levy Hospital, Marseilles, France

Carcinoembryonic antigen (CEA), associated with colonic cancer was found by Gold and Freedman (1) ; later, this antigen was detected with elevated plasma values by numerous authors in patients with cancer of the lung, breast, and many other sites.

The purpose of our study was : to try to determine a level of discrimination between a positive and a negative test in patients with lung cancer, to correlate pretreatment CEA values with the histologic categories, the stage of the disease at time of diagnosis, the survival of patients, to compare initial CEA value with values in different periods of disease, to assess the effect of a therapy (surgical resection, radiation, chemotherapy).

PATIENTS AND METHODS

The reagents for CEA radioimmunoassays used in this study were prepared by the C.I.S. (CEA, IRE, SORIN).

Radioimmunoassay determinations were performed on the serum of three groups of subjects : 49 healthy subjects (H.S.), 225 patients with benign pulmonary disease (P.D.), 88 patients with carcinoma of the lung at time of diagnosis (L.C.).

In a serie of patients with bronchogenic carcinoma, several assays were performed and the value was correlated with the stage of disease and therapy.

RESULTS

Pretreatment values

Control population (n = number of subjects, $\bar{x}$ = mean value, S.D. = standard deviation, | | = limits) : 49 healthy subjects working in hospitals, from 20 to 60 years old, had a radioimmunoassay for CEA (Table 1) (n = 49, $\bar{x}$ = 2.9, S.D. = 4.1, | 0-17 |) ; 94 % had a serum level below 10 ng/ml as it was reported by several authors (2),(3),(4).

Benign pulmonary disease : Concannon (2), Cullen (5) demonstrated the CEA mean value was greater in benign pulmonary disease or in smokers ; we established it in

225 patients with benign pulmonary disease during their hospitalisation (Table 1) (n = 225, $\bar{x}$ = 15.3, S.D. = 11.4, | 0-80 |). These data showed that the minimum level of discrimination between positive and negative tests for diagnosis of lung carcinoma should be at least 40 ng/ml (CEA serum value is below 10 ng/ml in only 38 % and below 40 ng/ml in 97 % of benign disease).

TABLE 1   CEA serum values in three groups of subjects

CEA serum values (ng/ml)	$\leqslant$ 10	10-40	> 40
Healthy subjects	46 (94%)	3 (6%)	0
Benign pulmonary disease	85 (38%)	133 (59%)	7 (3%)
Lung carcinoma pretreatment value	32 (36%)	38 (43%)	18 (21%)

Bronchogenic carcinoma :
88 patients with histologically verified malignant lesion of the bronchus had a plasma CEA value performed before any treatment (Table 1) ; 64 % of subjects had a CEA level above 10 ng/ml and only 21 % above 40 ng/ml, our point of discrimination (Figure 1) ; CEA level could be used in diagnosis of lung cancer in 21 % of the cases.

The 88 patients were subdivided into various histologic categories (Table 2).

TABLE 2   Various histologic categories and initial CEA mean value (ng/ml)

	n	mean value	limits (ng/ml)	% of normal value ($\leqslant$ 40 ng/ml)
Squamous cell	53	24.5	0-310	89
Adenocarcinoma	9	65.9	1-212	56
Small cell	9	10.9	0-27	100
Anaplastic	4	—		—
Unknown	13	—		—

These data clearely indicate a significant difference between the histologic categories : adenocarcinoma had the greatest mean value with 44 % above 40 ng/ml, epidermoid only 11 % above 40 ng/ml ; on the other hand, small cell carcinoma had 0 % of pathological value although Vincent (3) recently established there was no relation to the cancer histology.

In the squamous cell carcinoma, two types of staging were used : the first method is the TNM system (Figure 2), the second method is based on limited or advanced carcinoma (Figure 3). These results indicate that at the time of diagnosis there was a slight correlation between CEA level and limited or advanced disease (6) and, several times, a low CEA value was observed as well in limited as in advanced carcinoma.

The figure 5 established that there was no evident relation between initial CEA value and survival since very low values were observed in patients who died after a few months and a high level could have a satisfactory surgical resection.

Values in various stages of disease

Table 3 shows that the % of patients having a CEA level above 40 ng/ml is about the same at the time of diagnosis (21 %) and at the time of recurrence (10 %) or metastasis (24 %) ; this percentage increases only in premortem (44 %).

TABLE 3   CEA levels in various stages of bronchogenic carcinoma

	n	% of CEA value $>$ 40 ng/ml
Initial value	88	21
Recurrence	20	10
Metastasis	42	24
Premortem value	51	44

The follow-up of patients before, during and after therapy showed (Figure 4) : the mean CEA level drops after surgical resection (25 ng/ml $\longrightarrow$ 5 ng/ml), it mounts during radiation (21 ng/ml $\longrightarrow$ 28 ng/ml) and drops after (28 ng/ml $\longrightarrow$ 12 ng/ml), it is inchanged before and during chemotherapy and mounts after (28 ng/ml $\longrightarrow$ 36 ng/ml) ; the mean value increases from 38 ng/ml to 112 ng/ml from the time of diagnosis to the month preceding death.

CONCLUSIONS

The CEA serum level was determined in three series of subjects : 49 healthy, 225 with benign pulmonary disease, 88 lung cancer. CEA values in patients with benign disease showed that the point of discrimination between positive and negative tests in bronchogenic carcinoma should be above 40 ng/ml. These data demonstrated that CEA assay, not selective or specific enough, is not a good in vitro screening test for bronchogenic carcinoma, but can be useful to diagnosis (21 % of the cases). The data also indicated that the CEA assay at time of diagnosis does not correlate with the stage of disease and has not a pronostic value. We found a significant difference of mean values between histological categories and we established a significant difference of mean values before and after surgery and radiation.

The main interest of CEA assay is to allow the follow up of the clinical course of a patient with lung cancer(7); furthermore it permits to observe the succes of surgery or another therapy ; besides, increasing values of CEA can anticipate a clinical or radiological evidence of evolution of the lung carcinoma.

REFERENCES

(1) Gold, P. and Freedman, S.O. (1965) : J. Exp. Med.,12, 439.
(2) Concannon, J.P., Dalbow, M.H., Liebler, G.A., Blake, K.E., Weil, C.S. and Cooper, J.W. (1974) : Cancer, 34, 184.
(3) Vincent, R.G. and Chu, T.M. (1973) : J. Thorac. Cardiovasc. Surg., 66, 320.
(4) Gautier, H., Huguenin, P., Lededente, A., Morin, P. and Parrot, R. (1976) : Bull. Cancer, 63, 699.
(5) Cullen, K.J., Stevens, D.P., Frost, M.R. and Mackay, I.R. (1976) : Aust NZ J. Med, 6, 279.
(6) Reynoso, G., Chu, T.M., Holyoke, D., Cohen, E., Nemoto, T., Wang, J.J., Chuang, J., Guinan, P. and Murphy, G.P. (1972) : J. Amer. Med. Ass., 220, 361.
(7) Poirier, R., Kleisbauer, J.P. and Laval, P. (1976) : Rev. Fr. Mal. Resp., 4, 589.

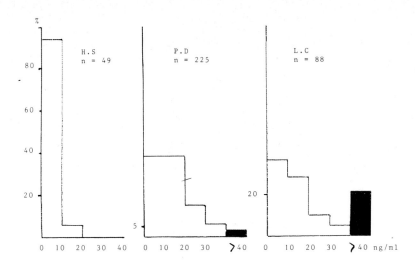

Fig. 1 The distribution of serum CEA values.

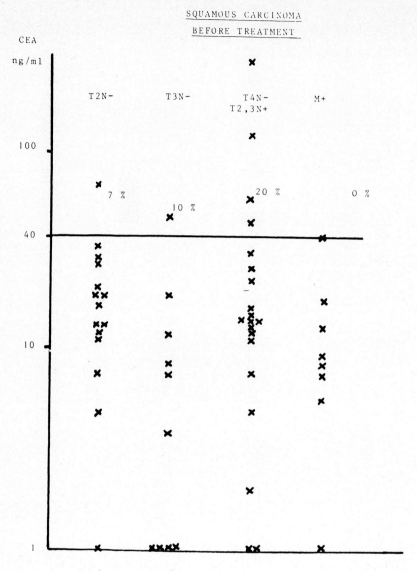

Fig. 2 The distribution of CEA values in epidermoid cancers
(TNM system).

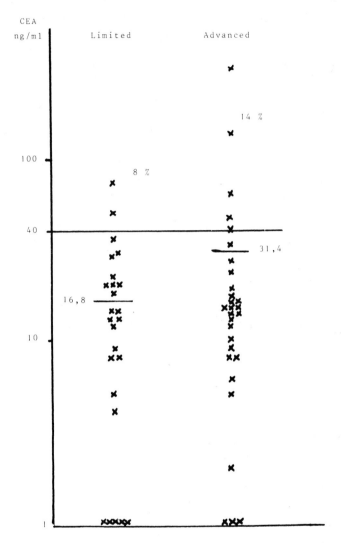

SQUAMOUS CARCINOMA
BEFORE TREATMENT

Fig. 3 The distribution of CEA values in epidermoid cancers

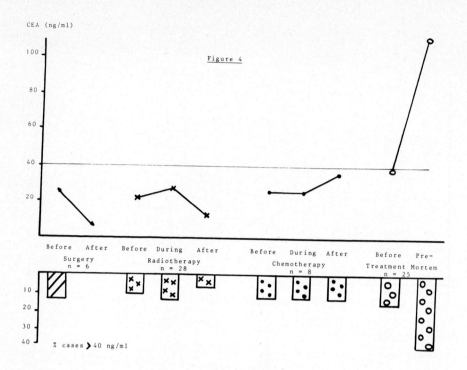

Fig. 4 The follow-up of epidermoid cancer therapy.

202

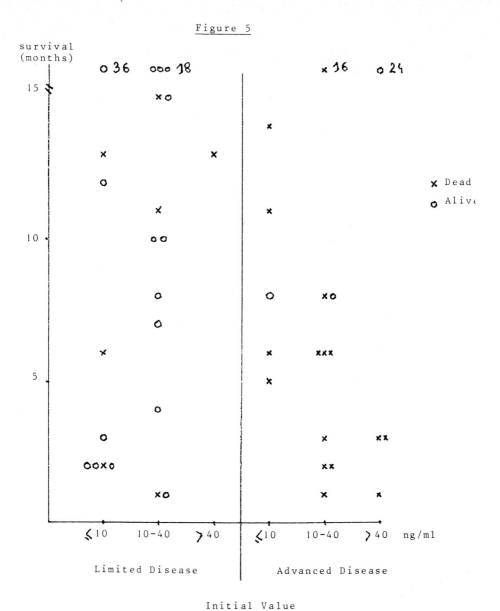

Figure 5

Fig. 5 Relation between survival and initial CEA value in epidermoid carcinoma.

CARCINOEMBRYONIC ANTIGEN AND FERRITIN IN PATIENTS WITH BRONCHIAL CARCINOMA

C. Gropp, F.-G. Lehmann and K. Havemann

Medizinische Universitätsklinik Marburg/Lahn, W. Germany

Carcinoembryonic antigen (CEA) was first described as an antigen specific for colonic cancer by Gold and Freedman in 1965. In the recent years many data have been reported indicating elevated serum CEA levels in non-digestive cancer including bronchogenic carcinoma (1, 2).

Ferritin was found in different molecular forms (isoferritin) in many tissues. In serum, ferritin was detected in patients with liver and Hodgkin's disease. Elevated serum ferritin levels were also described in acute leukemia, in germinal cell tumors of the testis and in breast cancer (3, 4, 5). So far, there were no reports in patients with lung cancer. It was the purpose of this study to define the usefulness of the determination of CEA and ferritin for the detection of lung cancer and especially of recurrence and metastases. Furthermore, serial determinations should show the role of these proteins for the therapeutic monitoring of lung cancer patients.

METHODS

CEA was measured by the commercial radioimmunoassay of Ire-Sorin (Isotopendienst West). The assay was considered positive if the CEA concentration was 10 ng/ml or more.

Serum ferritin levels were determined by the one-dimensional Laurell electrophoresis, using a rabbit antiserum (Behringwerke Marburg) to human placenta ferritin. A human placenta ferritin extract served as a standard. Ferritin levels were expressed in µg/ml.

RESULTS

CEA levels of 10 ng/ml or higher were found in 55 out of 114 (47 %) patients with confirmed lung cancer before treatment. In patients without clinically detectable metastases at the time of diagnosis only four had CEA levels of more than 10 ng/ml. On the contrary elevated CEA values were found in 51 of 60 patients with metastases. 9 patients had CEA values below 10 ng/ml

(Fig. 1).
CEA levels of lung cancer patients in relationship to the histological type of carcinoma showed no difference between small cell, squamous and large cell carcinoma. The highest CEA levels were found in patients with bone and/or liver metastases.

Serial CEA determinations were performed before and after radiotherapy and during chemotherapy with adriamycin, cyclophosphamide, vincristine and DTIC.

Figure 2 shows serial CEA determinations in responders to radiotherapy. CEA levels decreased after therapy or remained undetectable, but increased at the time of recurrence and tumor progression. In figure 3 serial determinations of patients, who did not respond to radiotherapy are shown. They all had tumor progression during therapy and had no further treatment. Figure 4 shows some examples of serial CEA determinations in patients with extended disease treated with chemotherapy. Most patients, who responded to therapy had temporary decreased CEA levels, but at the time of recurrence CEA levels increased. It is of great importance that there were some patients with tumor dissemination, who had normal CEA values at any time (see figure).

Ferritin was detectable by the Laurell electrophoresis in the serum of 58 out of 81 (72 %) patients with confirmed lung cancer at the time of diagnosis. Ferritin levels were significantly higher in patients with metastases (Fig. 5). Ferritin was not detectable in the serum of normal controls, but in some patients with liver cirrhosis and severe pneumonia. Serial ferritin determinations showed decreased or unchanged levels, when patients responded to radio- or chemotherapy (Fig. 6). Non-responders generally showed a rise of ferritin values. But there were also some patients without correlation of ferritin levels and tumor growth (Fig. 7).

CONCLUSION

The results suggests that determination of CEA and ferritin in the serum of lung cancer patients may be useful as an additional method to detect metastases or recurrences and in monitoring the results of treatment. As there are some cases in which CEA and ferritin are not detectable at any time determinations of these proteins should be used only in context with other clinical and laboratory findings.

REFERENCES

(1) Concannon, J. P., Dalbow, M. H., Liebler, G. A., Blake, K. E., Weil, C. S. and Copper, J. W. (1974): Cancer 34, 184

(2) Gropp, C., Lehmann, F.-G. and Havemann, K. (1977): Dtsch. med. Wschr. 102, 1079
(3) Jones, P. A., Miller, F. M., Worwood, M. et al. (1973): Br. J. Cancer 27, 212
(4) White, G. P., Worwood, M., Parry, D. H., et al. (1974): Nature 250, 584
(5) Marcus, D. M., Zinberg, N. (1975): J. Natl. Cancer Inst. 55, 791

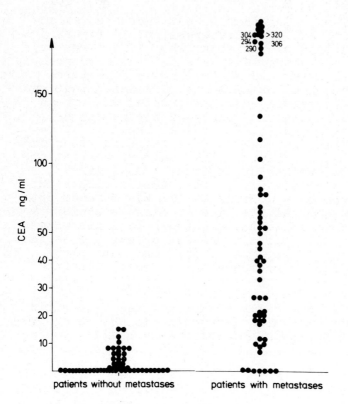

Fig. 1 CEA levels in lung cancer patients with and without metastases.

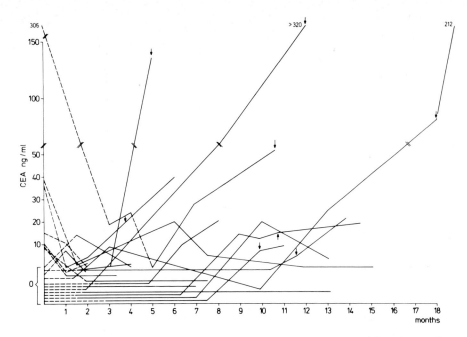

Fig. 2 Serial CEA levels in lung cancer patients, who received complete or partial remission during radiotherapy. The clotted lines mean the time of radiotherapy (↑↓ = time of recurrence).

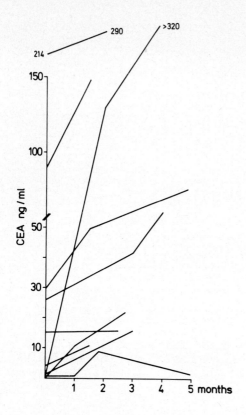

Fig. 3 Serial CEA levels in lung cancer patients with
progressive tumor growth during radiotherapy.

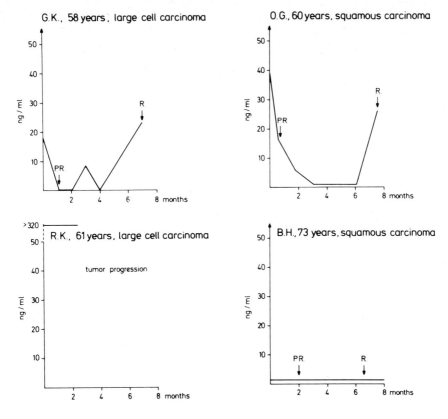

Fig. 4 Serial CEA levels in patients with metastatic lung cancer during chemotherapy. P. R. = partial remission, R. = recurrence.

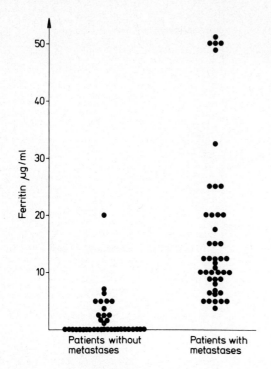

Fig. 5 Ferritin levels in lung cancer patients with and
without metastases.

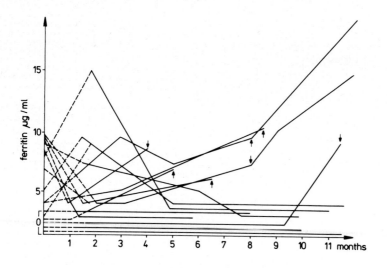

Fig. 6 Serial ferritin levels in lung cancer patients,
who received complete or partial remission during radiotherapy. The clotted lines mean the time of radiotherapy
(↑↓ = time of recurrence).

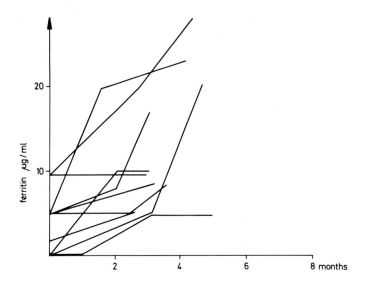

Fig. 7 Serial ferritin levels in patients with progressive tumor growth during radiotherapy.

LEUKOCYTE MIGRATION REACTIVITY IN PATIENTS WITH LUNG CANCER OF THREE DIFFERENT HISTOLOGICAL TYPES

M.Zöller, S.Matzku, P.Georgi and D.Zeidler

Institut für Nuklearmedizin, Deutsches Krebsforschungszentrum and Thoraxchirurgische Spezialklinik, Rohrbach,
Heidelberg

The leukocyte migration reactivity of cancer patients is mostly tested by exposing leukocytes to one single extract, which is usually selected for the absence of non-specific interferences and for a high specific response. This may of course generate some bias, since negative responses could result from lack of sensitization of lymphocytes as well as from an incomplete spectrum of antigens contained in the particular extract.

When we sought to overcome this difficulty by proceeding to a panel of extracts, we observed a surprisingly high degree of cumulative positivity in patients bearing tumours of the gastrointestinal tract. However, the success of the panel test mode with these tumours could have stemmed from the fact, that most of the tumours of the gastrointestinal tract are adenocarcinomas.

The situation is quite different in the lung, where very different histological types of tumours arise within the same organ. Hence, testing of LM reactivity against panels of extracts of different lung tumours probably could answer the following questions: 1.) How is the performance of LMT with tumours differing in histology but arising in the same organ. 2.) Can we, by using multiple extracts, get insight into the expression of antigen specificities on tumours of differing histological type?

PATIENTS

Patients hospitalized in the clinical center for thoracic surgery, Heidelberg-Rohrbach, (benign and malignant pulmonary disease) and outdoor patients of the Institute of Nuclear Medicine were comprised in the study. Healthy volunteers were recruited from the institute's staff.

METHODS

The details of LMT are described elsewhere (1). Patients' leukocytes were tested against 3 media controls and against one of two panels of tumour extracts (5 squamous cell carcinoma extracts and 5 adenocarcinoma ex-

tracts). Positive response was defined as the occurance
of abnormal MI's with ≥3 out of 5 extracts.

RESULTS

Table 1 summarizes the results for different groups
of patients with malignant and nonmalignant diseases and
it shows patient's reactivity against normal lung extracts.

TABLE 1   Leukocyte migration reactiviy with 3M KCl extracts of normal lung, squamous cell carcinomas (SCC) and
adenocarcinomas (AC).

Leukocyte donor	abnormal MI[+] with normal lung extr.	pos.react.[++] with SCC extr.	pos.react.with AC extracts
Malignant disease:			
lung cancer	11/33 (33%)	113/159 (71%)	27/33 (82%)
other tumours	-	21/110 (19%)	-
Nonmalignant disease:			
lung, various	6/33 (18%)	10/81 (12%)	6/33 (18%)
other organs	0/4 -	14/257 (5%)	0/4 -
Healthy donors	0/17 -	0/16 (0%)	0/17 -

[+]   relative migration area ≤0.8 and ≥1.2
[++]   abnormal MI with ≥3 out of 5 extracts

Patients with non-pulmonary disease and healthy donors did not react with a normal lung tissue extract, while
an abnormal MI was observed with some of the lung cancer
patients. It is interesting to note, that all patients with
benign pulmonary disease (especially M.Boeck), who reacted
with the normal extract, concomitantly showed positive
reactivity with tumour extracts.
Healthy individuals and patients with nonmalignant,
non-pulmonary disease reacted very rarely with either type
of tumour extracts.
Nineteen percent of patients with extra pulmonary
cancer showed crossreactivity with squamous cell carcinoma
(SCC) extracts. The panel reactivity of lung cancer patients with both extract types was 71% and 82%; this
difference was not significant (p 0.05) by the chi-
square test.

Evaluating the reactivity of leukocytes with respect
to the histological type of the patient's tumours
(Table 2), it turned out that the lower level of reactivity against SCC extracts was due to a "hyporeactivity" of
SCC bearer's leukocytes.

TABLE 2 LM reactivities of leukocytes from patients
bearing different types of tumours (homologous combinations and cross combinations).

Leukocyte donor	pos.reactivity[+] with SCC extracts	pos.reactivity with AC extracts
squamous cell Ca	28/46 (61%)	9/13 (69%)
adeno Ca	7/8 (88%)	2/2 (100%)
Oat cell Ca	22/27 (81%)	6/7 (86%)
tumours not classi- fied/not classifiable	56/78 (72%)	10/11 (91%)

[+] see above

This resulted from a comparison of leukocyte reactivities, with SCC and AC extracts. SCC bearer's leukocytes
showed the lowest frequency of positive reactivity with
the matching panel of extracts, but a low percentage of
reactivity was also observed with AC extracts. AC bearers'
leukocytes on the contrary were highly reactive with AC
extracts (note however the small number of cases) as well
as with SCC extracts. Oat cell carcinoma bearers' leukocytes and leukocytes from patients with unclassified or
unclassifiable tumours (all patients in this group were
inoperable) ranged in between. The data concerning this
latter group of patients demonstrates, that the high incidence of positive LMT reactivities reported here is in
no way due to some bias in the selection of patients or
in the establishment of histological diagnosis.
In addition, Table 2 substantiates a trend that
emerged already from data in Table 1: AC extracts seem to
induce a higher frequency of positive reactivities with
leukocytes from patientsbearing any kind of lung cancer
than do SCC extracts. Now the question arises, whether AC
extracts also induce stronger reactions than do SCC extracts. Reaction strength in our LMT system sofar could
only be analysed by taking advantage of an observation
based on extract titration studies: We have shown (1),
that LM inhibition is generally induced by high extract
concentrations, whereas dilute solutions of the same extract lead to LM enhancement. Hence LM inhibition to us
indicates strong reactivity and LM enhancement indicates

weak reactivity. In Fig.1, LM reactivities in the various combinations of leukocytes and extracts were analysed with respect to both types of migration. Again it became clear, that AC leukocytes showed strongest reactions (highest proportion of LM inhibition) with AC extracts, whereas SCC leukocytes tested with SCC extracts ranged at the other end of the scale (highest proportion of LM enhancement).

Finally we wanted to find out, whether the low levels of reactivity observed in SCC patients might be ascribed to a subgroup of patients being unreactive with any extract or whether this might rather be caused by single extracts which did not react with any patients' leukocytes.

In Fig.2 panel reactivities are depicted for AC and SCC extracts. We realize that unreactivity of single SCC extracts could not have taken place, since we found a definite frequency of 5/5 reactivities in every group of patients tested with the SCC panel. Furthermore we can state that complete unreactivity (0/5) takes place indeed, but it is by no means confined to any particular tumour type.

DISCUSSION

In various reports on the validity of the LMT in lung cancer monitoring an overall test sensitivity of about 60% was described (3,4,5). This figure is in accordance with our findings, since we observed 52% and 68% reactivity when calculating our data on the basis of single extracts of SCC and AC (fig.2). By the panel modification, test sensitivity could be increased with SCC extracts up to 71% and with AC extracts up to 82% (Table 1). Thus, the panel modification of LMT again proved to be effective from a diagnostic point of view.

However, there are two points which require detailed discussion: 1) What information do we get from LM reactivity data with respect to antigen expression, and 2) what is the interpretation of different reactivity profiles observed in patients bearing lung tumours of different histological type?

The following findings are related to the question of antigen expression: No extract of any kind of tumour did induce reactivity in none of the patients. This can be judged from the consistent frequency of 5/5 reactions in every lung cancer patients' group. Patients bearing lung tumours of any histological type did react more frequently with AC than with SCC extracts. Accordingly, AC extracts induced strong reactivity (LM inhibition) more frequently than did SCC extracts. Cross reactivity between the different histological types of lung cancer was hardly lower than reactivity in homologous combinations (Table 2). Reactivity in patients bearing tumours localized outside the lung was much less frequently observed (Table 1). The

high degree of crossreactivity between the different
histological types of lung cancer and the rather low degree of crossreactivity with tumours of other localizations forces the hypothesis, that the antigenic pattern
of tumours is not essentially dependent on the histological type of the tumour but rather shows some degree of
organ specificity. The higher frequency and strength of
reactivity with AC extracts may be interpreted in the
sense, that antigen expression on this tumour is more
dense or more comprehensive than e.g. on squamous cell
type tumours.

When looking at patients leukocytes' sensitization,
the following findings seem to be important: Patients
bearing any type of lung cancer can (in a few cases) be
unreactive to both types of extracts tested. Patients with
AC and with oat cell carcinomas react more frequently and
in a "stronger manner" than patients with SCC, irrespective of the type of extract used. Hence we postulate, that
AC provokes a higher degree of sensitization than SCC.
Furthermore, since AC bearers' leukocytes react more often
and in a stronger way with SCC extracts than do SCC bearers' leukkocytes with homologous SCC extracts, we conclude
that LM reactivity rather refelcts patients' leukocytes
sensitization than the variability of antigen concentrations in tumour extracts.

REFERENCES

(1)   Zöller,M., Matzku,S. and Schulz.U. (1977): J.Nat.Canc.
      Inst.58, 897.
(2)   Zöller,M., Matzku,S., Schulz,U. and Rapp,W. (1977):
      Digestion 15, 373.
(3)   Oldham,R.K. et al. (1976): Int.J.Cancer18, 739.
(4)   Boddie,A.W. et al. (1975): Int.J.Cancer 15, 823.
(5)   Vose,B.M., Kimber,I. and Moore,M. (1977): J.Natl.Can-
      cer Inst.58, 483.

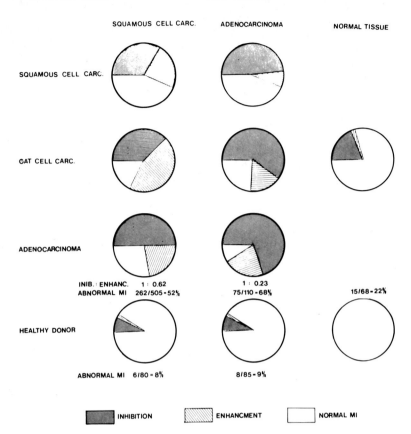

Fig.1: Comparison of frequency and strength of reactivity of patients' lymphocytes bearing different histological types of lung tumours against either SCC or AC extracts.

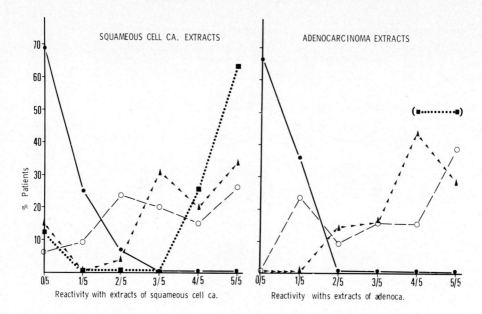

Fig.2: Panel reactivities of SCC, AC and oat cell carcinoma patients' leukocytes against SCC and AC extracts.

PROGNOSTIC VALUE OF CEA[+] IN PATIENTS WITH SQUAMOUS CELL CARCINOMA OF THE LUNG

H. GAUTIER, P. BARON, P. HUGUENIN, P. MORIN, A. BARON, R. PARROT*
H. MAGDELENAT, R. GONGORA, M. JOUVE, P. POUILLART**
T. PALANGIE, E. GARCIA GIRALT***

*   CMC BLIGNY 91640 BRIIS SOUS FORGES
** FONDATION CURIE PARIS
***VILLEJUIF

Some previous trials have demonstrated the poor interest of CEA level for the diagnostic of bronchial carcinoma. However, in some conditions a good correlation between CEA level and prognosis appears.
The aim of this work is to study the interrelationship in patients with squamous cell lung cancer between CEA level before treatment and clinical or immunological variable, in order to specify the prognostic significance of CEA assay.

PATIENTS AND METHODS

Since May 1975, CEA level was systematically measured in all patients with proven squamous cell bronchus carcinoma. 94 patients ranged from 48 to 76 years of age were included in this trial. 12 of them had been surgically treated 4 to 6 weeks before, 35 patients had a stage III or limited disease, 47 patients presented a stage IV or extensive disease.
The immunological status of all these patients was defined according to the skin responses to 3 different recall antigens, LIF activity of the serum and the mean peripheral lymphocytes count.
With the serum CEA determination's technique - CIS - we used, a level of 10 ng/ml was considered as upper value in normal subjects ; a level of 25 ng/ml was considered as the superior limit which correspond to inflammatory non malignant bronchus or lung diseases.
Clinical evolution, survival time, response to treatment and immunological status, were studied according to CEA level.

RESULTS

After analysis of the data, no good correlation was found between initial CEA level and clinical staging of disease (table 1). Although 11 adequate resected patients

[+] CarcinoEmbryonic Antigen

out of 12 had a normal level of CEA and so presented
a good relationship between CEA level and a good surgical resection, a great dispersion of results was
obtained in stage III and IV patients. Furthermore,
29 out of 47 patients with extensive disease presented
CEA level lower than 25 ng/ml.

TABLE 1 Initial CEA level according to staging of
disease. 94 squamous cell lung cancer

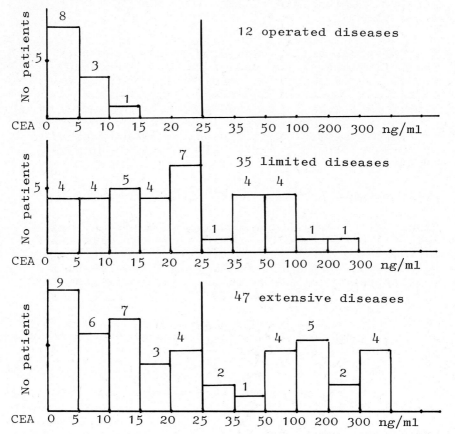

All patients who entered into this trial were submitted
either to immunorestoration protocol if they were initially non immunocompetent or to chemotherapy program
if they were immunocompetent. The study of survival in
these patients showed a good correlation between CEA
level prior initiation of treatment and median survival
time. Survival median was significantly higher for population of patients with CEA level under 25 ng/ml (Figure 1)

FIGURE 1 Survival of 82 patients according to initial
CEA level. Squamous cell lung carcinoma

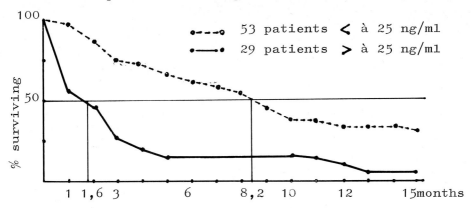

However, this survival prolongation was not related to
an improvement of tumor response rate to treatment
(table 2). The response rate was approximately the
same for the patients with CEA level upper than
25 ng/ml and for those with CEA level under 25 ng/ml.

TABLE 2 Responses to treatment for 80 patients with
inoperable squamous cell lung cancer

	Responses	Failures	Number of patients
CEA < 25 ng/ml	17 (33 %)	35 (66 %)	52
CEA > 25 ng/ml	6 (26 %)	22 (74 %)	28

In a previous trial it was demonstrated that prognosis is
directly related to immunological status of patients.
In this present trial we observed CEA level's medians of
23 ng/ml for immunocompetent patients and 76 ng/ml for
immunodeficient patients. In fact, 81 % of patients with
positive reaction to recall antigens opposed to only 50%
with negative reaction had CEA level lower than 25 ng/ml
(table 3). This difference is significant.
In the group of immunodeficient patients, the application of BCG on a scratched area every 2 days for 3
weeks induced immunorestoration only in patients whom
CEA level was lower than 25 ng/ml.

TABLE 3. ACE level according to immunological status.
83 squamous cell lung carcinoma

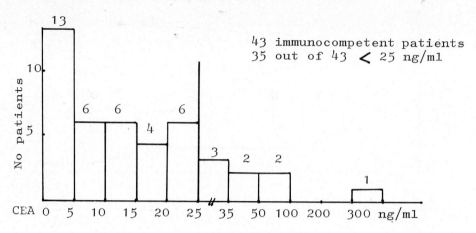

43 immunocompetent patients
35 out of 43 < 25 ng/ml

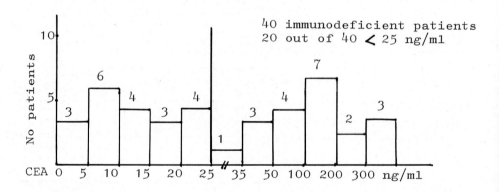

40 immunodeficient patients
20 out of 40 < 25 ng/ml

CONCLUSION

In this trial, CEA level was not related with tumor volume defined by clinical staging. It was also impossible to establish a relationship between CEA level and sensitivity to chemotherapy.
However, we found that immunological status of patients and CEA level were strongly correlated. As well, we obtained a good relationship between CEA level prior to medical treatment and median survival time. CEA level predicted likewise the immunorestoration possibility for immunodeficient patients.
These data suggest that CEA level is a factor which can be used in the pretherapeutic assessment of patients with squamous cell lung carcinoma.

REFERENCES

(1) Lanzotti Victor J., Thomas David R., Boyle Liam E., Smith Terry L., Gehan Edmund A., and Samuels Melvin L. Cancer 39, 303-313 1977.

(2) Lo Gerfo P.L., Herter F.P., Braun J., Hansen H.J. Tumor associated antigen with pulmonary neoplasms. Ann. Surg. 175, 495-500, 1972.

(3) Mach J.P., Pusztazseri G., Dysli M., Kapp F., Bierens de Haan B., Loosli R.M., Grob D. et Isliker H. Dosage radioimmunologique de l'antigène carcino-embryonnaire dans le plasma de malades atteints de carcinomes. Schweiz. Med. Wschr. 103, 365-371, 1973.

(4) Mac Sween J.M. and Andersen G.H. The quantitative relationship of carcinoembryonic Antigen to tumor cells of different organs. Cancer 40, 808-812, 1977.

(5) Morin P., Baron A., Gautier H., Gongora R., Jammet H. Evolution du taux d'ACE au cours du traitement des cancers bronchiques par chimiothérapie. Bull. du cancer 63, 525-530, 1976.

(6) Vincent R.G., Chu T.M. Carcinoembryonic antigen in patients with carcinoma of the lung. J. Thorac. Cardiovasc. sug. 66, 320-328, 1973.

IMMUNORESTORATION AND CEA$^+$ LEVEL IN NON-RESECTABLE SQUAMOUS CELL CARCINOMA OF THE LUNG

H. GAUTIER, P. BARON, P. HUGUENIN, P. MORIN, A. BARON,
R. PARROT*
H. MAGDELENAT, R. GONGORA, M. JOUVE, P. POUILLART**
T. PALANGIE, E. GARCIA GIRALT***

* CMC BLIGNY 91640 BRIIS SOUS FORGES
**FONDATION CURIE PARIS
***VILLEJUIF

The prognosis of patients with no resectable squamous cell carcinoma of the lung is very poor. In a previous work it was demonstrated a good correlation between survival and immune status of the patients before application of the treatment (Pouillart and all 1976) in a same trial a high level of CEA appears as one of the most significant marker of immune deficiency : later an other trial was began in order to test the prognostic signification of immune manipulations before application of other treatments.
The aim of this work is to test the signification of CEA level in patients submitted to immunorestoration.

PATIENTS AND METHOD

40 patients from 47 to 78 years old with non-resectable squamous cell carcinoma of the lung were considered as not immunologically competent on study of delayed hypersensitivity skin reactions and entered into an immunorestoration protocol using BCG. BCG was applied on a scratched area at the dose of 75 mg of living bacilli three times a week for 3 weeks. 15 days later, the patients were submitted to a new immunological control comprising skin tests to recall antigens, circulating lymphocytes count. The CEA level was measured in all the patients before BCG treatment and was controlled 5 weeks later at time of the new study of immune competence.
We have considered two groups of patients according to the level of CEA before the immunorestoration start. The limit was determined at 25 ng/ml corresponding to the highest value observed in patients with inflammatory non malignant diseases of the bronchus or the lung which have been considered as a control group.
In the other part in commune therapeutical conditions level of CEA more than 25 ng/ml was previously demonstrated as significant factor of poor prognosis for
+ Carcinoembryonic Antigen.

224

patients with squamous cell carcinoma of bronchus.
The serum CEA level was determined with CIS method : the
upper value was 10 ng/ml in healthy individuals.

RESULTS

5 weeks after initiation of immunorestoration with
BCG, 20 patients presented with positive skin tests to
recall antigens, 20 others patients fail to respond to
BCG stimulation. The distribution of the patient according to the level of CEA in each of these 2 groups was
quite different : the patients who become "immunocompetent" after this phase of treatment presented initially a level of CEA lower than 25 ng/ml (table 1)

TABLE 1   40 squamous cell carcinoma of bronchus submitted to immunotherapy

Initial CEA level	Non respon-ders to immuno therapy - → -	Responders to immuno therapy - → +	% Repositivation	Median survival time
CEA < 25ng/ml	8	19	70,5%	8 months
CEA > 25ng/ml	12	1	8,3%	1,6 months

The mean level of CEA was 15 ng/ml in this group of
patients which respond to BCG and 70,7 ng/ml in the group
of patients which fails to respond (table 2)

TABLE 2   CEA level before and after immunostimulation for
33 squamous cel carcinoma of bronchus

	CEA level before immunostimulation	CEA level after immunostimulation
Non responders to immunotherapy - → -	70,7 ng/ml	73,5 ng/ml
Responders to immunotherapy - → +	15 ng/ml	7 ng/ml

In 12 patients out of 20 whom skin tests to recall antigens became positive after BCG treatment a significant
reduction of CEA level was observed. Inversely in the
patients who do not respond to BCG a slight increase of
CEA is observed (table 3).

TABLE 3 Variations of CEA level according to response to
immunotherapy for 33 squamous cell carcinoma of bronchus

	Non responders to immunotherapy - ⟶ -	Responders to immunotherapy - ⟶ +
CEA level ↘	3	12
CEA level ↗	7	3
stable CEA level	3	5
TOTAL	13	20

In all the cases studied no significant variations of the
tumor mass was measured.
The median survival time of all the group of patients
is 5 months but the shape of the curve of median survival was different according to response we observed with
BCG treatment (fig 1).

Fig 1 Survival curves according to response to immuno-
therapie
    ----20 non responder patients (median CEA level 70,7ng/ml)
    ——20 responder patients (median CEA level 15ng/ml)

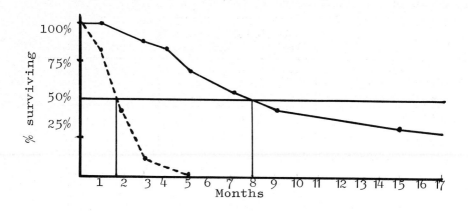

The median of survival of the patients who respond to immunostimulation is 8 months and the median of survival of the patients who fail to respond was of 1,6months.

DISCUSSION

Althrough the serum CEA level in patients with bronchus carcinoma has no diagnostic interest, some previous works have noted the prognostic signification of levels higher than 25 ng/ml. The aim of this trial was to study the prognostic signification of a manifestation of immuno status for non immuno competent patients (Pouillart and all, to be published) before any attempt of reduction of tumoral volume.

3 points can resume the results of this work :

1) the immune status of patients with non resectable squamous cell carcinoma of the lung appears as one of the most significant factor of prognosis.
2) the stimulation of immunological reactivity of these patients with BCG given for 3 weeks is able to transform the poor prognosis of 50 % of the patients.
3) the benefical effect of the stimulation with BCG can be obtained only when the level of CEA is lower than 25 ng/ml. In this group of patients the level of CEA decreased during the BCG treatment.

REFERENCES

(1) Concannon J.P., Dalbow M.H, Liebler G.A. The carcino embryonic antigen assay in bronchogenir carcinoma. Cancer 34, 184-192, 1974
(2) Gautier H, Botto H.G., Pouillart P, Magdelenat H, Huguenin P, Parrot R. Etude comparative entre le taux d'inhibition de la migration des leucocytes dans les cancers bronchiques. Bull. du cancer 63, 633-638, 1976
(3) Pouillart P., Botto H.G., Gautier H., Huguenin P., Baron A., Lappare C, Hoang thy, H.T., Parrot R., Mathé G. : Relation entre l'état immunitaire et la réponse à la chimiothérapie. Résultats chez 64 malades avec cancers bronchiques épidermoïdes inopérables. Nouv. Presse Med 5, 1037 (1976)
(4) Vincent R.G., Chu T.M. Carcinoembryonic antigen in patients with carcinoma of the lung. J. Thorac. Cardiovasc. sug. 66, 320-328, 1973.
(5) Steward A.M., Kupchik H.Z., Zamcheck N. Circulating carcinoembryonic Antigen levels and serum suppression of phytohemagglutinin-stimulated lymphocyte DNA synthesis : an inverse correlation in the cancer patient. Journal of the Nat. Cancer Inst. 53, 1, 3-9, 1974

DISCUSSION

NAMER M. (Nice) : In lung cancer, are high levels of CEA a worse
prognosis than widespread of disease.

GAUTIER H. (Briis-sous-Forges) : Our patients were inoperable,
so the TNM classification was not used. Nevertheless, we found that
the tumour is not so important than the immune status concerning
prognosis.

GROPP C. (Marburg) : I think the immuno-competence of these patients
depends on the extent of disease. If you have a widespread tumour,
you have also a bad immunocompetence and, if you had an extended
tumour, you have also a high CEA level. I think the immunocompetence
does not depend on the CEA level but depends on the tumour extent.

GAUTIER H. (Briis-sous-Forges) : I am speaking about immunocompetence
but in response to immunostimulation . This immunostimulation is
impossible if CEA is higher than 25 ng/ml. In contrast, we found
patients with high levels of CEA with positive immunocompetence.

CLINICAL INTEREST OF CEA DETERMINATION IN BRONCHIAL SECRETIONS.
COMPARISON WITH PLASMA LEVELS.

J.M.Aubanel, G.Milano, M.Schneider, B.Blaive, M.Namer, C.Bonet,
B.P.Krebs, E.A.MacDonald, C.M.Lalanne

Centre Antoine Lacassagne, 36 Voie Romaine, 06054 Nice Cedex,France

INTRODUCTION

Following the work of BLAIR and GOLDENBERG (1) we wanted to
find out if CEA levels in bronchial secretions would reflect the
"clinical status" in neoplastic conditions compared with benign
bronchial affections.

METHODS AND PATIENTS

1. Endoscopic exploration was performed under local anesthesia
with 1% adrenalin free xylocaïn. Bronchial secretions were obtained
by bronchial washing with 10 ml of normal saline before biopsy to
avoid blood contamination. CEA determination is done by the radioimmunoassay of Roche indirect method using AMICON ultrafiltration
system instead dialysis.
Protein levels are simultaneously assessed on a separate aliquot
by the Lowry method , and subsequently the CEA level is given in
terms of the protein content, the unit being ng CEA/mg protein.
Plasma measurements of CEA obtained by radioimmunoassay using the CIS
method commercialised by the Commissariat à l'Energie Atomique.
Since the work of CONCANNON et al.(2) the reference value of
serum CEA in bronchial disease has been placed at 5ng/ml.

2. Patient classification :
A) The population of 68 patients presenting squamous cell carcinoma
of the bronchus was divided into the following groups :
. 29 cases of carcinoma before treatment classified according
to the TNM of the U.I.C.C.; 16 T1-T2, 13 T3 (where the tumour lies
at less than two centimeters from the carena).
. And 49 bronchial tumours after treatment during endoscopic
surveillance. This group of patients is divided into 23 patients
with progressing disease (biopsy positive) and 16 patients without
recurrence (biopsy negative at fibroscopy).

B) Benign bronchial disease (18 patients) :
. in 12 cases fibroscopy showed macroscopic and histological
evidence of inflammation.
. In 6 cases, fibroscopy was normal.

RESULTS

TABLE 1 Population submitted to fibroscopy : 86 patients

Benign bronchial affection	Inflammatory	12
	Normal	6
Bronchial carcinoma before treatment	T1-T2	16
	T3	13
Bronchial carcinoma in follow-up	Fibroscopy negative	16
	Fibroscopy positive	23

Results of CEA determination in bronchial secretions are shown in figures 1 and 2.

a) In benign bronchial conditions without inflammation, measurements on bronchial aspirates are alwalys below 10 ng/mg of protein, the median being below 5 ng/mg protein. In our estimation the maximum normal level of CEA in bronchial secretions at normal bronchoscopy is 15 ng/mg protein.

In benign bronchial inflammatory conditions the median level is found at 10 ng/mg protein. The one mesaurement of 50 ng/mg protein was found in a formarly tuberculous patient with mechanical irritation of the bronchial mucosa by a broncholithe. The results at 27 and 32 ng/mg protein were seen in a patient presenting middle lobe syndrome with diffuse bronchiectasis and chronic expectoration, who also presented bronchial dilatation.

b) In malignant conditions before treatment :
T1-T2 lesions give highly variable results with a median at 11 ng/mg protein, not far removed from results in benign inflammatory conditions. T3 lesions on the other hand have a median of 42 ng/mg protein - 6 cases presenting results of 50 ng and above.

c) Follow-up of treated bronchial tumours reveals two distinct groups:
1- one where biopsy is negative and the median CEA level is below 10 ng/mg protein. In each of the four cases where the results reached 50 ng the patients subsequently developped recurrent disease.
2- The second group with positive bronchial biopsies produce a median CEA level of 50 ng/mg protein.
In addition we wanted to establish whether the serum CEA level taken 10 minutes before bronchoscopy in combination with the CEA measurement in bronchial secretions could in combination prove diagnostic of cancer.

The histogram (fig.3) demonstrates the percentage of patients with abnormal serum CEA plasma levels (upper limit of normal 5 ng/ml) (column P) and the incidence of positive levels in bronchial aspirates (upper limit of normal 15 ng/mg of protein) (column A).

The column PA represents the percentage of positive results obtained by either method . It is evident that in benign conditions with normal or inflammatory findings at biopsy there are fewer false positive results when one considers the bronchial aspirate results alone. In untreated malignant conditions the two methods together give positive results in 80% of cases.

By chance it came to our attention that CEA levels measured on blood samples taken 10 minutes after the trauma of bronchoscopy and biopsy revealed an elevation of serum levels of circulating CEA.

Figure 4 represents 56 samples taken before and after fibroscopy and shows that the level of CEA rises sometimes quite markedly : in one case the plasma level increased 20 fold after bronchoscopy.

The deduction that can be proposed from this observation is that trauma to the bronchial epithelium stimulates the release of CEA into the circulation.

CONCLUSION

This new method of obtaining tumour markers from their very site of production in the respiratory tree produces some interesting results.
A) A signigicant difference (P = 0,01) exists between benign normal and inflammatory conditions and malignant disease before treatment.

B) The results of CEA bronchial estimations in patients during follow-up after treatment of bronchial carcinoma show a significant difference between aspirations from biopsy positive and biopsy negative cases (P = 0,025). These aspirations can be predictive of recurrent disease.

On the other hand there appears no significant difference between benign inflammatory conditions and early untreated tumours (T1-T2). Results in this category do not reflect the clinical situation.

The fact that one sees a systematic rise in serum CEA levels after bronchoscopy compared with serum levels before this investigation may lead to a possible CEA stimulation test of interest in certain patients with apparently benign bronchial lesions and normal serum CEA levels before fibroscopy but with positive levels after bronchoscopy. These patients may develop in time a malignant condition.

In conclusion, this study demonstrates that CEA levels in the bronchial aspirate reflect with greater fidelity the clinical situation than does the estimation of CEA in the general circulation.

REFERENCES

(1) Blair, O.M., Goldenberg,D.M. (1974) : Acta Cytologica 18, 510.

(2) Concannon, J.P., Dalbow,M.H. , Liebler, G.A., Blake,K.E., Weil, C.S., Cooper, J.W. (1974) : Cancer 34, 184.

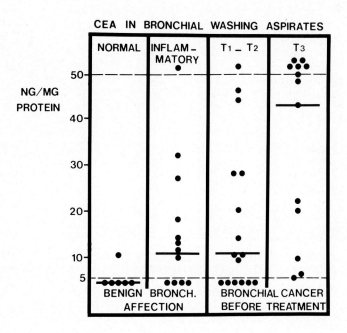

Fig.1 CEA in bronchial washing aspirates. Comparison between benign and malignant diseases.

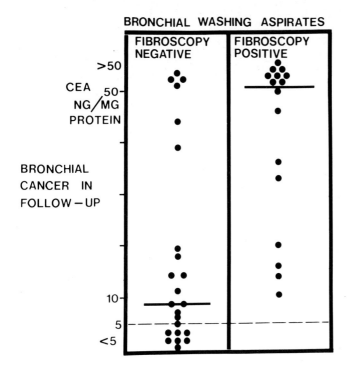

Fig.2 Bronchoscopy in follow-up.

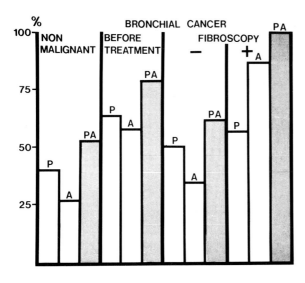

Fig.3 Histogram. Comparison between results in plasma levels and aspiration .

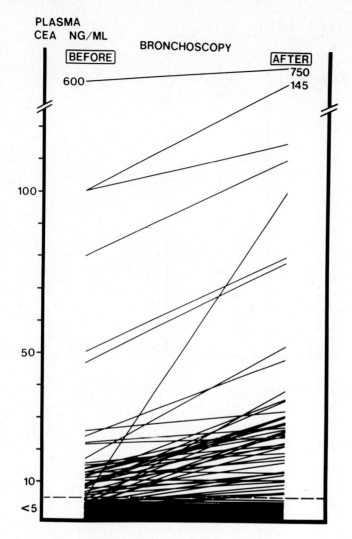

Fig.4 Modification of CEA levels in plasma before and after bronchoscopy.

234

TUMOR MARKERS IN RELATION TO CANCER OF THE BREAST

J.C. Hendrick, P.F. Zangerlé, A. Thirion and
P. Franchimont

Belgian National Scientific Research Fund, Radioimmunoassay Laboratory, University of Liège, Liège

INTRODUCTION

Cancer antigens belong to several categories. The
first includes fetal and embryonic antigen, carcinoembryonic antigen (CEA and α-fetoprotein (AFP) are representative of the first group. Other substances which are
synthesized by the cancer cells are placental antigens.
Among those placental antigens are found human chorionic
gonadotropin (HCG) and its α- and β-subunits. A third
group of antigens produced by tumors is made up of the
polypeptide hormones. Finally, certain tumor cells recover
the property of synthesizing exocrine products such as
casein, a phosphoprotein present in milk.
Having established methods for measuring these
antigens, we have first investigated the production of
these substances in normal conditions. Then, we have
determined the frequency with which at least one of these
antigens, which can be produced by malignancies, is present in a population of normal non pregnant and non
lactating subjects, in patients with benign mastopathy
and in patients with breast cancer at the beginning of
their clinical course in order to determine the specificity and practicability of these biochemical parameters
as a diagnostic tool in this neoplastic disease. We
have also investigated the effect of metastatic spread
on the frequency with which these tumor markers can be
detected. Finally, the effect of breast tumor removal
of chemotherapy or radiotherapy on tumors in situ has
been defined.

MATERIAL AND METHODS

Methods of assay

The methods of assays for CEA (1,2), AFP (3), HCG (4,
5), α-HCG (4,5) are extensively described in original
papers which may be consulted by the readers.
Concerning casein assay the following methods were
used :
Preparation of human casein. The different fractions
of casein were isolated from human milk using the method

of Groves and Gordon (6). Human milk was defatted, dialyzed overnight against distilled water at 4°C. Casein was precipitated at room temperature by additions of acid at ph 4.6., centrifuged, washed and lyophilized Separation of the casein component was performed by stepwise chromatography at 4°C on DEAE-cellulose. All the different protein peaks were dialyzed against water and lypholized.

Labelling of casein. Casein was labelled with ^{125}I by the classical CT method (7).

Radioimmunoassay. Radioimmunoassay was performed using the double antibody method with incubation at ordinary temperature (8). Antiserum was obtained in rabbit by intradermal injection of whole casein (8).

Serum Studied

Normal serum. Cancer-related antigens were measured in the serum of 350 pregnant women, of 19 lactating women during the 6 days following delivery and of 935 blood donors of different ages (20-60 years) in whom clinical and biochemical investigation led to the exclusion of any renal or hepatic disorder.

Patients with benign mastopathy. Serum from 55 women with benign breast diseases were assayed : 7 with polycistic disease, 30 with single cyst and 18 with fibroadenoma. All the benign breast diseases were investigated by histological examination. Furthermore, casein and prolactin were assayed in 12 cases of functional galactorrhea with or without menstrual disturbances but without any evidence of pituitary adenoma. Some of these have shown galactorrhea appearing after hormonal contraceptive treatment.

Women with breast cancer. The investigation of the cancer antigens included 145 sera from patients with breast cancer. Histological confirmation of neoplastic disease was available in each case. Breast cancers were classified into 4 groups on the basis of their clinical progress and the treatment which had been given : (1) onset of the disease before any treatment in absence of metastases; (2) metastatic spread of the tumor. Presence or absence of metastases was established by clinical examination. X-rays of chest, lung, skull, pelvis and liver scintigraphy; (3) following ablation of the tumor without any clinical, biological, radiological and isotopical signs of recurrence or of metastasis. The samples were obtained 2 months to 3 years after primary surgical therapy; (4) following chemotherapy or radiotherapy, the tumor not having been removed. This small groups was investigated to compare the incidence of positivity with the preceding groups but not to assess the follow-up of these patients under therapy.

236

RESULTS

Normal Subjects

Serum of pregnant women. In normal pregnancy, the concentration of AFP increases from the 8th week of gestation to the 32nd, then stabilizes or gradually decreases (3). CEA levels range from 0 to 10 without any systematic variations. -Subunit increases progressively whereas native HCG and β-HCG subunit is maximum at the beginning of gestation with a maximum between the 10th to the 12th week and decreases afterwards (4). The ratio λ-HCG to β-HCG will increase; during the three first months of gestation the ratio is less than 2 whereas during the last trimester it is higher than 5. κ-Casein progressively increases during the pregnancy (9). There exists a statistically significant difference between the mean values of κ-casein between the 4th and the 10th week of pregnancy on one hand and between the 30th and 40th week on the other.

Serum of lactating women. Only κ-casein was assayed simultaneously with prolactin. In these conditions, mean prolactin levels increased to reach their maximum the 2nd day of postpartum. These progressively decreased and on the 5th day the level reached was significantly less than the mean value determined at the delivery (9). The mean casein level progressively increases during the lactation and is found to reach its maximum on the 4th day after delivery, i.e. when the milk is in full flow.

Serum of blood donors. In the sera of 935 normal non pregnant and non lactating subjects, the levels of CEA, AFP, native HCG, °-subunit of HCG and casein were often undetectable and never greater than 10, 20, 1, 1.5 and 25 ng/ml, respectively. We would regard as abnormal any value greater than these.

Patients with benign breast diseases.

In the serum of 55 women with benign mastopathy, κ-casein, native HCG and β-HCG subunit were found higher than the normal limit, each in one case. Thus, the incidence of positivity of one cancer-related antigen was 5,5 %. Pathological values (i.e. higher than 25 ng/ml) of κ-casein were found in 8 out of 12 cases of galactorrhea. The other cancer-related antigens were not detectable in the sera of these patients.

Patients with breast cancer.

As shown in table I the incidence of finding at least one antigen was 69 % at the beginning of the clinical course, 88 % in the presence of metastases, 34 % following removal of the tumor and 83 % when the tumor was left in place and chemotherapy and/or radiotherapy administered. Individual incidence for each antigen shows that CEA and casein were found most frequently in the sera of patients with breast cancer.

TABLE I Breast cancer : incidence of positivity of cancer-associated antigens

Circumstances	Total	Incidence of at least one positive antigen		Incidence of				
		n	%	CEA	α-FP	HCG	κ	casein
						β-HCG		
Onset of clinical course	39	27	69	20	0	6	1	6
In the presence of metastases	25	22	88	14	0	0	0	11
Following removal of the tumor	69	24	34	15	1	4	3	6
Following chemotherapy or radiotherapy	12	10	83	9	0	0	0	2

Among the patients who had been operated on, 30 patients had no evidence of lymph node involvement or of distant metastases. HCG, β-HCG and casein were each found in one case. The incidence of positivity of at least one antigen was therefore 3 out of 30, i.e. 10 %. In contrast, 39 patients who had been treated surgically had at least one lymph node metastasis in the draining glands. The frequency of appearance of at least one antigen was 21/39 i.e. 54 %.

12 patients were treated by radiotherapy and/or chemotherapy, the tumor not having been removed. The incidence of positive findings of at least one cancer-associated antigen was 83 %.

DISCUSSION

Measurement of cancer-associated antigens is a useful diagnostic procedure, which, however, is neither absolute nor specific. In considering as abnormal levels, values higher than the concentration observed in normal subjects, i.e. CEA greater than 10 ng/ml, HCG greater than 1 ng/ml, β-HCG greater than 1.5 ng/ml, casein greater than 25 ng/ml and AFP greater than 20 ng/ml we confirm the fact that the incidence of positive findings for one of these antigens is 5.5 % in benign breast diseases and 14.7 % in all the non-neoplastic disorders (10). When galactorrhea exists, the κ-casein levels are elevated in a high percentage of cases (8/12).

This high incidence was observed by the simultaneous measurement of 5 cancer antigens. In fact, CEA alone displays the highest incidence in breast cancer at the onset

of the clinical course and when complicated with metastases; the other markers allow an increase of incidence of
18 % at the onset of clinical symptoms and of 28 % when the
cancer is complicated by metastases (table II).

TABLE II Incidence of positivity of one cancer-related
antigen compared with CEA incidence

	Benign diseases	Breast cancer	
		initial	metastases
CEA			
n	0/55	20/39	14/25
%	0	51	60
All CRA			
n	3/55	27/39	22/25
%	5.5	69	88

It shoud be noted that AFP was found in one case of
breast cancer after removal of the tumor. Thus, AFP would
not appear to be an essential tumor marker in the screening of patients suspected to be suffering from breast
cancer if the other antigens investigated in this paper
are measured. The incidence of positive findings should,
on the other hand, increase if the number of tumor markers
is increased by the assay of new cancer-associated antigens.
No correlation was found between the histological
type of tumor and the incidence of one particular antigen,
which confirms the experience of other authors with HCG,
β-HCG and CEA (11-16).
Spread of neoplasm leads to an increase in the incidence of positivity for cancer-associated antigens and an
increase in their levels. In fact, the incidence of positivity of at least one cancer antigen is 88 % in the presence of metastases while it is 69 % at the onset of the
disease. Further, the mean level of CEA and of casein is
statistically significantly higher in the presence of metastases as compared with mean level present at the onset
of the disease (table III).

TABLE III

	Presence of metastases	Undetectable levels		Mean (ng/ml) $\pm$ SEM
		n	%	
CEA	M_O	9/39	23	14.1 ± 3.8
	M_+	5/25	20	75.8 ± 21.7
κ-Casein	M_O	19/39	48.7	22.6 ± 6.5
	M_+	5/39	12	60.1 ± 21

Currently, clinicians have few reliable criteria for
the study of the progress of cancer therapy.

In our experience the value of this biochemical method is shown particularly in patients who have been operated on. In these the incidence of positive findings drops to 34 %. The persistence of antigens in pathological concentrations appears to be correlated with the likelihood of recurrence; thus when the tumor has been removed at stage N- the incidence of positivity of at least one antigen is only 10 % while it reaches 54 % when the tumor has been removed when there had already been invasion of the regional lymph gland (N+). Further follow-up of the involved patients will be necessary to assess the values of the positivity as a precocious index of recurrence and/or metastases.

In the group of patients treated by chemotherapy and radiotherapy the incidence of positivity of at least one cancer-related antigen is between those in patients at the onset of the clinical course and those complicated with metastases.

SUMMARY

Five tumor markers can be simultaneously determined in the serum by radioimmunoassay : carcinoembryonal antigen (CEA), λ-fetoprotein (λ-FP), human chorionic gonadotropin (HCG), β-subunit of HCG (β-HCG) and κ-casein. In a series of 935 healthy subjects, these antigens remain detectable or are detected within very precise limits. At the start of the clinical evolution of breast cancer, the incidence of pathological concentrations is increased as compared with the highest level observed in normal subjects. This high incidence is mainly due to a concomitant determination of CEA, κ-casein, HCG and β-HCG. The λ-FP test is never positive, while the κ-casein concentration is particularly high in the first clinical stages of breast cancer and with metastases. The concomitant determination of these tumor markers may be a biological element contributing to the diagnosis of neoplasia, although it is neither an absolute nor a specific criterium. Indeed, a pathological concentration of at least one antigen was observed in 5.5 % of the subjects presenting with benign mastopathy. When metastases occur (25 patients), the incidence of pathological conditions of at least one antigen increases : 88 %, the absolute values of these levels increasing simultaneously. The determination of the antigen concentration therefore allows an evaluation of the extension of the disease.

Surgical removal reduces the incidence of positivity of these antigens to 34 %. Persistence of pathological levels seems to be related to a possibility of relapse or metastatic spreading. Finally, chemotherapy and radiotherapy applied on a tumor which is not excised, does not decrease the incidence of positivity of the tumoral markers, although their levels seem to fluctuate with the clinical evolution.

REFERENCES

(1) Franchimont, P., Debruche, M.L., Zangerlé, P.F. and
    Proyard, J. (1973) : Ann. Immunol., 124, 619-630
(2) Franchimont, P., Debruche, M.L., Zangerlé, P.F. and
    Proyard, J. (1974) : in Radioimmunoassay and related
    procedures in medicine, Istanbul, September 1973.
    International Atomic Energy Agency, 2, 267-274
(3) Franchimont, P., Zangerlé, P.F., Debruche, M.L.,
    Proyard, J., Simon, M. and Gaspard, U. (1975) : Anns.
    Biol. Clin., 33, 139-148
(4) Franchimont, P., Hendrick, J.C., Reuter, A. and
    Zangerlé, P.F. (1977) : Proceedings of International
    Congress of Endocrinology Hamburg, July 1976 (Excerpta
    Medica, Amsterdam, in press)
(5) Reuter, A., Roulier, R., Ulama-Dubois, N., Gaspard, U.
    and Franchimont, P. (1977) : Path. Biol. Paris (in
    press)
(6) Groves, M.L. and Gordon, W.G. (1970) : Archs. Biochem.
    Biophys., 140, 47-51
(7) Greenwood, F., Hunter, W. and Glover, S. (1963) :
    Biochem. J., 89, 114
(8) Hendrick, J.C. and Franchimont, P. (1974) : Eur. J.
    Cancer, 10, 725-730
(9) Zangerlé, P.F. (1976) : in Franchimont, Proceedings of
    the Symposium on Cancer Related Antigens (Excerpta
    Medica, Amsterdam), 61
(10) Franchimont, P., Zangerlé, P.F., Nogarede, J., Bury, J.,
    Molter, F., Reuter, A. Hendrick, J.C. and Collette, J.
    (1976) : Cancer (in press)
(11) Braustein, G.D., Bridson, W.E., Glass, A., Hull, W.H.
    and McIntire, K.R. (1972) : J. Clin. Endocr. Metab.,
    35, 857-862
(12) Fuks, A., Banjo, C., Shuster, J., Freedman, S.O. and
    Gold, P. (1974) : Biochem. Biophys. Acta, 417, 123-152
(13) Laurence, D.J.R., Stevens, U., Bettelheim, R.,
    Darcy, D., Lesse, C., Turberville, C., Alexander, P.,
    Hohns, E.W. and Neville, A. Munro (1972) : Br. Med. J.,
    iii, 605-609
(14) Laurence, D.J.R. and Neville, A.M. (1972) : Br. J.
    Cancer, 26, 335-355
(15) Vaitukaitis, J.L. (1975) : Ann. Intern. Med., 82,
    71-83
(16) Weintraub, B.D. and Rosen, S.W. (1971) : J. Clin.
    Endocr. Metab., 32, 94-101

DISCUSSION

MACH J.P. (Lausanne): You have been discrete on the importance of casein in your panel of five markers.

HENDRICK J.C. (Liège): Casein increases true positive incidence.

ROCHMAN H.(Chicago): You spoke about the instability as a reason for differences in casein estimations from different laboratories; instability in term of storage of sera samples. What would you suggest as the most appropriate means of storing samples for assay. It does become difficult to be able to measure them on the same day.

HENDRICK J.C. (Liège): In fact, we have not made a lot of investigations in this field. We said only that it could be a problem, but we have not solved the problem. It is practically impossible with clinicians to get samples in good condition. In bad conditions, you have false results, the assay being so difficult to perform, it might be better not to do it.

HERBERMAN R.(Bethesda): I have a question related to your comments on the use of five markers. It seems that CEA and casein must be sufficient. It is hard for me to see why you use 5 tests. In your published data, almost all cases were detected by CEA and casein, AFP, HCG and βHCG seem to contribute very little.

HENDRICK J.C. (Liège): Yes, but you see our results are coming from a study on different cancers and not only breast cancer and the five markers were measured for a prospective purpose. But you are right: CEA and casein should be sufficient in breast cancer.

HERBERMAN R. (Bethesda): Concerning the controversy about casein, did you perform parallel assays with the Kappa casein specific assay and with an assay for the other caseins.

HENDRICK J.C. (Liège):There is a difference: one serum sample could be positive in one assay and negative in the other.

BOHUON C. (Villejuif): What is your methodology for CEA assay? In fact, we never found 51% of positivity in loco-regional breast cancer, but 10%,using the kit from Saclay.

HENDRICK J.C. (Liège): We use our own method, this may explain differences of incidence.

BRIERE M.(Saint-Cloud): Is your own antigen extracted from breast cancer?

HENDRICK J.C. (Liège): I do not think so. We use the well-known method from liver metastases of colonic cancer.

DIAGNOSTIC AND PRONOSTIC USE OF CARCINOEMBRYONIC
ANTIGEN IN HUMAN MAMMARY CARCINOMA

P.HAEGELE, J.C.PETIT , J. HERDLY, P.PILLEMENT,M.EBER

Centre Regional de Lutte contre le cancer Paul Strauss
Strasbourg.

SUMMARY

   Carcinoembryonic antigen (CEA) assays performed on 124 patients
with primary breast cancer and on 84 patients with recurrences after
adequate primary treatment of breast cancer. Serum CEA determinations
were accomplished by radioimmunoassay using the method CIS of Saclay
(France). The percentage of elevated (above 15 mg/ml) CEA levels
increased from earlier stages (TI-TII : 17 %) to later stages (TIII :
37 %) and to advanced malignant diseases (TIV : 60 % and especially
recurrences : 75 %). In the group of metastases the frequency and
magnitude of elevation were related to the sites of tumor metastases,
with an increasing order from soft-tissue and pulmonary to osseous
metastases. In most patients elevated values dropped to normal ranges
after primary treatment; persistent elevation, partial decrease or a
rise in CEA titer were associated with demonstrable metastases during
follow-up; however a limited number of patients had elevated levels
without apparent disease at time of the follow-up. It appears that the
greatest value of the CEA assay lies in detection of distant metastases
when these are still undetectable by the usual diagnostic aids in the
early recognition of recurrence during longterm management of cancer.

   In this study 208 patients with breast cancer were
investigated in order to evaluate the diagnostic and pronostic use of serum CEA levels, before surgical resection
or radiotherapy of primary cancer and during the course
following this treatment. The follow-up of patients with
recurrences was excluded.

I.   PATIENTS AND METHODS

   A. Patients Selection and Classification

   Patients admitted to hospital with primary breast cancer histologically confirmed were evaluated by clinical history, by physical examination and by roentgenogram and
radioisotope scan of liver and bone. Patients were staged
according to the TNM classification (UICC, 1972). In tumor I
and II, the tumor does not exceed 5 cm diameter.In tumor III
the tumor is larger than 5 cm diameter.Tumor IV patients in
addition had chest well fixation, skin edema or ulceration.

Stage I-II formed with tumor I-II patients without axillary node fixation (N2), subclavian node or arm edema (N3).
Stage III are formed with tumor I-II patients when preceding signs (N2-N3) are present and with tumor III-IV patients. All patients with metastases are in stage IV. Patients with distant recurrences were considered to have
had adequate primary treatment and metastases were confirmed by the usual methods at time of first view.

B. Serial CEA Measurements

Blood specimens were drawn for CEA evaluation before
treatment (tumor resection or irradiation, hormonal or
chemotherapy),at the end of the radiotherapy or 7 days
after surgery, and 3 months to 24 months afterwards in
many cases.

C. Method of CEA determination

Serum CEA estimation were carried out by the double
antibody solid phase radioimmunoassay, without perchloric
extraction (Method CIS Saclay, France). A CEA level of
10 ng/ml or greater was considered as "positive" but
15 ng/ml may be more realistic and above this cut-off point
the values are considered as "elevated".

II. RESULTS

A. CEA Levels and Disease Stage

The serum CEA values of breast cancer patients in later
stages of disease were higher than those in earlier stages.

TABLE I : Carcinoembryonic Antigen Values in 208 Patients
with Mammary Carcinoma in Relation to the Clinical Stage.

Stage*	Number	Serum CEA (ng/ml) 0 - 4	5 - 9	10 - 14	>15
T I - T II	59	29(49%)	15(25,5%)	5(8,5%)	10(17%)
T III	27	10(37%)	6(22 %)	1(4 %)	10(37%)
T IV	38	6(16%)	4(10 %)	5(14 %)	23(60%)
Stage I-II	55	28(51%)	15(27 %)	5(9 %)	7(13%)
Stage III	45	16(36%)	10(22 %)	4(9 %)	15(33%)
Stage IV	24	1(4%)	/	2(8,5%)	21(87,5%)'
Recurrences	84	5(6%)	10(12 %)	6(7 %)	63(75%)

✹ TNM Classification (UICC,1972).

With increasing spread of tumor , CEA values of the
patient group increased : the mean values of all patients
were 6,5 ng/ml in stage I-II, 14,8 ng/ml in stage III and
170 ng/ml in stage IV. The percentage of elevated CEA
levels increased from stage I-II to stage IV,respectively

244

13%, 33% and 87%. Inversely the percentage of very low
(below 5 ng/ml) values decreased from 51% to 36% and to
4 % respectively. In the group of recurrences the mean
value was 87 ng/ml, the percentage of elevated levels was
75% and the percentage of very low levels was 6%. When the
patients with recurrences, the stage IV patients and those
with metastases at any time of their course, were considered as a single group (Metastases group,Table II). 76%
had elevated values, 86 % had values above 10 ng/ml and
6% had very low values. The percentage of elevated values
was high (96%) in group of isolated osseous metastases
whereas this percentage was 33% in group of isolated pulmonary metastases and 31% in group of isolated soft-tissue.
No isolated hepatic metastasis was found.

TABLE II : Carcinoembryonic Antigen values in 118 patients
with metastases of mammary carcinoma in relation to the
site.

Site	Number	Serum CEA (ng/ml)			
		0 - 4	5 - 9	10-14	>15
Multiple	48	/	2	3	43
Osseous	45	/	2	4	39
Pulmonary	9	2	2	2	3
Soft-times	16	5	4	2	5
Total	118	7(6%)	10(8%)	11(9%)	90(76%)

B. CEA levels Following Primary Tumor treatment

Following CEA values were taken once or more in most
patients between the end of radiotherapy or the 7th day
after resection and the 24th month after treatment.

1. Tumor I-II patients :
In 34 out of 36 patients with initial values below 15 ng/ml, the level did not change during the first year
of follow-up;in one patient appeared pulmonary metastasis
and in another soft-tissue metastasis without any rise in
CEA level ; in 2 patients of these 36 the level increased
at 6 months and at a year and one developed pulmonary metastasis.
For the 10 patients with initial CEA values
above 15 ng/ml, one had stable value for over 2 years without recurrence but with cirrhosis of liver, two had metastases at time of diagnosis and died within first year,
three had repeated borderline values, three had decreasing
values and one had rising serial values and developed
osseous metastases several months later.

2. Tumor III patients :

For 16 out of 17 patients with initial va-
lues below 15 ng/ml the level remained low after treatment;
one of those had rising values 18 months later and developed
osseous metastases after 3 months and 4 out of those had
borderline values : in two cases pulmonary metastases
appeared later. One patient out of these 17 had persistent
borderline values at a year without clinical disease.
In 8 out of 10 patients with CEA values
above 15 ng/ml before treatment the level decreased to low
range and 2 out of 10 patients it decreased to borderline
range. In this series 3 patients died before 6 months.

3. Tumor IV patients :

In the group of 15 patients with CEA values
below 15 ng/ml before treatment were noted persistent low
levels in 11 patients, borderline levels in 2 patients without measurable disease and increasing levels in 2 patients:
multiple metastases were detected at the 4th month and at
the 12th month respectively.
In the group of 23 patients with elevated
levels before treatment were seen a decrease to low values
in 5 patients, variable elevated levels in the other cases.
Six months after this onset 11 patients were dead. This
mortality rate was much greater than that noted with the
former group in which only 1 patient died before one year.

DISCUSSION

Earlier reports have shown a correlation between the
amount of tumor or the extent of dissemination in breast
cancer and the incidence of elevated serum levels of CEA
(1,2,3,4,5,6). Besides it was reported (3) that frequency
and degree of CEA elevation were related to the sites of
metastases, with an increasing order from soft-tissue to
osseous, pulmonary and hepatic metastases. The findings
reported here thus confirm these previous observations
except for the percentage of elevated levels in pulmonary
metastases who was similar in our study to that seen in the
soft-tissue metastases. In this view no differences in CEA
levels were seen between the 21 tumor I-II patients with
histologically negative axillary nodes and the 19 tumor I-
II patients with histologically positive axillary nodes.
It was also suggested (4) that serial CEA assays may
be of use for the response to treatment in breast carcinoma
as in patients with gastrointestinal tumors. But several
patients with soft-tissue and pulmonary metastases had low
CEA levels and this would appear to be a limiting factor
in the use of CEA as an indicator of emerging metastasis
after primary treatment. However in case of osseous metastases sequential determination after treatment of primary
tumor showed a rise in CEA levels prior to clinically

manifest recurrence in a high percentage of patients.Besides, the findings reported here tend to confirm other observations (7,8) about the pronostic use of the CEA value before treatment: the mortality rate was higher when patients had elevated levels prior to the treatment.

ACKNOWLEDGMENT : The authors are grateful to Mrs.C.AZULAY and Mrs.S.MAIRIE for technical help.

REFERENCES

(1) LAURENCE D.J., STEVENS U., BETTELHEIM R. et al.(1972)
    Br. Med. J. 3 , 605
(2) REYNOSO G., CHU T.M., HOLYOKE D. et al:(1972)
    JAMA 220, 361
(3) CHU T.M., NEMOTO T. (1973)
    J.Nat. Cancer Inst. 51, 1119
(4) STEWARD A.M., NIXON D., ZAMCHECK N. et al. (1974)
    Cancer 33, 1246
(5) BOENISCH T., RAHM S., (1975)
    Clinica Chimica Acta 58, 195
(6) PICO J.L., HENRY R., MERIADEC B. et al. (1976)
    Bull. du Cancer 63, 595
(7) BOOTH S.N., JAMJESON G.C., KING J.P. et al. (1974)
    Br. Med. J. 4, 183
(8) CHU T.M., HOLYOKE E.D. , MURPHY G.P. (1974)
    N.Y.State J. Med. 74, 1388

Tumours of the breast: clinical, histological and developmental characteristics related to determination of carcinoembryonic antigen.

M. Brière, G. Moulin, M. Brunet, J. Gest in collaboration with F. King, J. Delaunay and A.M. Hersant.

Centre René Huguenin de Lutte Contre le Cancer,
Saint-Cloud, France.

A study was made on homogeneous populations of tumours of
the breast (225 cases including 63 benign and 162
malignant tumours) with respect to the clinical
characteristics (T.N.M. classification of the International Union against Cancer), histological aspects
(histopathological code of human tumours - Inserm 1971)
and evolution as related to measurements of serum
carcinoembryonic antigen (CEA).

MEASUREMENT TECHNIQUE

Radioimmunological assay of CEA was carried out directly
on the serum; the standard range used was from 5 to
320 ng/ml, with a sensitivity limit corresponding to
2 ng/ml. The levels were defined as follows: normal
(0 to 5 ng/ml), dubious (6 to 10 ng/ml), high (over
10 ng/ml).

False-positive results have been found in patients with
serious hepatic insufficiency and heavy smokers without
cancer. These elements were taken into consideration in
the statistical analysis.

Within a short time and without clinical changes in the
cancer, repeated determinations of the same patient were
made: in 22 cases of malignant tumours CEA level was
always zero; in 7 cases CEA levels were between 2 and
10 ng/ml with constant values; in 12 cases CEA levels
were always over 10 ng/ml and the standard deviation was
always smaller than a third of the mean. From this, the
conclusion can be drawn that variations in concentration
for an individual case are small.

CEA ACCORDING TO THE TYPE OF LESION

The study concerned 225 women with tumours of the breast.
Of the 162 cases of malignant tumours only 125 were
treated from the onset of the disease in the Centre René
Huguenin. For these, therefore, a clinical description
of the tumour was available. Table 1 gives the distribution of T and of N for these 125 cases.

Table 1. T and N of the TNM classification for cancer of the breast in women

		Total	N0	N1	N2	N3
Total	N	125	56	49	12	8
	%	100	100	100	100	100
T0	N	2	2	0	0	0
	%	1.6	3.7	0	0	0
T1	N	13	10	3	0	0
	%	10.4	17.8	6.1	0	0
T2	N	46	29	16	0	0
	%	36.8	51.8	32.7	0	12.5
T3	N	37	10	20	3	4
	%	29.6	17.8	40.8	25	50
T4	N	27	5	10	9	3
	%	21.6	8.9	20.4	75	37.5

It may be pointed out that most patients belonged to T2 N0 and T3 N1.

Table 2 shows the distribution of the levels of CEA according to the type of lesion.

Table 2. Distribution of tumours by CEA level and type of lesion

Overall category of lesion

Distribution of CEA levels in 3 classes	Total	Suggestive of benign lesion	Suggestive of malig- nant lesion	Rejects[1]
Total	235	63	162	10
Normal	187	61	117	9
Dubious	25	2	23	0
High	23	0	22	1

1) rejects: rejected histories, incomplete for this contingency table.

Division of the results into three classes appeared to be of value since the intermediate class of dubious results (5-10 ng/ml) has been found to be significant for certain subjects.

Of the total of 235 subjects, 48 (20.4%) had an abnormal CEA level. Of the 63 patients with benign tumours, only 2 (3%) had abnormal levels. In contrast, 45 patients (27.8%) with malignant tumours had abnormal levels. The statistical tests are highly significant (P < 0.001).

Despite this, the percentage of abnormal CEA levels is low. It is certainly not a screening test, but a study was made of the "prognostic" value of this test and its value for monitoring the result of treatment. Possibly, in the near future, CEA measurements more specific for cancer of the breast can be obtained (with an antigen from mammary tumour, not from colon tumour).

CEA AND CLINICAL CHARACTERISTICS OF THE MALIGNANT LESION

We looked for a possible relationship between the levels of CEA and the various characteristics of the malignant tumour. No statistically significant relationship was found between a high CEA level and the classes of T and clinical N, except for the metastasis class (M), for which very high antigen levels often corresponded principally to hepatic metastases, followed by bone metastases. We also examined the relationship between developmental flare-up and CEA levels.

Table 3. Initial level of CEA (ng/ml) prior to treatment in malignant tumours of the breast according to clinical characteristics and age

Developmental flare-up for malignant tumours of the breast	Age of the patient on first examination in the centre (years)				
	Total	0-34	35-49	50-65	65 and over
Total					
average	94.8	57.1	198.4	45.7	36.1
S.D.	794.5	140.0	1346.9	205.7	129.1
no. of cases	162	7	54	63	38
No flare-up					
average	51.8	133.3	2.4	74.4	62.9
S.D.	215.6	188.6	4.9	301.5	178.3
no. of cases	72	3	22	28	19

Table 3 Continued

	Total	0-34	35-49	50-65	65 and over
Flare-up 1					
average	12.8	0	0.9	28.3	6.4
S.D.	46.5	0	1.5	72.8	8.0
no. of cases	24	1	7	9	7
Flare-up 2					
average	27.4		47.3	18.3	10.0
S.D.	27.3		30.1	12.5	14.1
no. of cases	10	0	4	3	3
Flare-up 3					
average	4.7	0	0		14
S.D.	6.6	0	0		0
no. of cases	3	1	1	0	1
Undefined flare-up					
average	208.3	0	523.3	21.2	10.6
S.D.	1358.5	0	2174.8	36.0	10.4
no. of cases	53	2	20	23	8

It seems that the antigen levels were higher in flare-up
2. For these various distributions of the antigen
determinations attempts were made at statistical
evaluation for various characteristics of the malignant
lesions, by calculating the averages of the determinations and the standard deviations per category of lesion.
Very high standard deviations indicated the very marked
variability of this determination in different populations. Therefore, comparison tests of these averages
were not used since this is not a case of normal
distribution, the antigen being absent in principle.
Use was made of a Chi-squared test permitting a
comparison of two populations with or without the
qualitative characteristic "presence of CEA at a level
above or below a threshold" and if necessary a
distribution-free test eliminating the normality
hypothesis (the Wilcoxon test).

CEA AND HISTOLOGICAL CHARACTERISTICS OF THE LESION

A histological study of the tumours revealed the following points.

The number of histologically invaded lymph nodes (Table 4)

Table 4. CEA levels in malignant lesions of the breast as a function of the number of histologically invaded lymph nodes

	number of histologically invaded lymph nodes			
	none	1-2	3-4	5 and over
Negative	22	7	3	3
Dubious (<10 ng/ml)	7	1	3	1
High (>10 ng/ml)	2	1	4	0

	0-2	3 and over
Negative	29	6
Positive	11	8

$$\chi^2 = 4 \qquad P = 0.046$$

The statistical test was very significant (P = 0.046) and permitted the conclusion that there is an important relationship between a high CEA level and the presence of at least three histologically invaded lymph nodes.

Distribution of the CEA levels according to the histology of the lesion: this was not statistically significant (P > 0.10) (Table 5).

Table 5. Distribution of tumours by CEA level and histological type of lesion

CEA levels

Histological type	Total	Normal	Dubious	High
Total	235	187	25	23
Differentiated glandular carcinoma	20	15	4	1
Polymorphic adenocarcinoma	39	31	3	5
Undifferentiated adenocarcinoma	18	14	1	3
Fibrocystic disease of the breast	19	19	0	0
Adenofibroma	22	22	0	0
Sclerosing adenosis	10	9	1	0
Atypical adenocarcinoma	10	10	0	0
Intracanalicular dendritic adenoma	3	3	0	0
Intracanalicular dendritic carcinoma in situ	3	3	0	0
Comedocarcinoma	5	5	0	0
Undefined	88	56	16	14

This study will be continued in a larger population.

Study of grading

The increase in CEA levels in grades II and III in comparison to grade I has little significance ($P = 0.11$).

CEA AND AGE

Two populations of malignant tumours of the same grade (II) in patients below and over 60 were studied as regards the CEA levels.

Table 6. Grade II malignant lesions related to patient's age and CEA level

CEA level	Age of patient (years)	
	<60	>60
Negative	14	6
Positive	6	9

$x^2 = 3.15$, $P = 0.076$

In patients younger than 60, 30% of the tests were high, but in patients over 60 this figure was 60%. This probability is lower than the normal limit (5% confidence) but this raises the question: with equal grading, can older age lead to a higher CEA level?

CEA AND DEVELOPMENTAL ASPECTS OF THE TUMOUR

As regards the evolution of treated tumours (surgery, radiotherapy, hormonal treatment, chemotherapy), statistical relationships could not be determined since many patients were not followed up. From a descriptive point of view several observations may be presented which are interesting as regards the chronology of these various events and the subsequent levels of CEA.

In several patients of T1 NO MO, N-, the zero levels of CEA at the onset of the disease became positive before the clinical appearance of the worsening of the disease. In contrast, the high CEA levels at the onset in patients of T2, T3 NO MO without flare-up became negative after surgery and radiotherapy or after chemotherapy. A study over a longer period of these samples will permit better definition of the prognostic value of this test from a statistical point of view.

254

INTEREST OF CARCINO-EMBRYONIC ANTIGEN IN THE FOLLOW-UP AND TREATMENT OF BREAST CANCER

M.Namer, M.Hery, C.Bonet, M.Abbes, B.P.Krebs, J.L.Boublil,E.A.MacDonald
C.M.Lalanne, A.Ramaioli

Centre Antoine Lacassagne, 36 Voie Romaine, 06054 Nice Cedex,France

INTRODUCTION

Carcino-embryonic antigen has been demonstrated to be a good marker for the evolution of disease and eventually in the monitoring of treatment. The general agreement is that breast cancer is not the most interesting tumour for CEA measurement. Breast cancer does not come from entodermal origin; nevertheless the production of CEA occurs frequently when disease is disseminated.

MATERIAL AND METHODS

Carcino-embryonic antigen was measured with CIS reagents in 194 women with breast cancer, 62 of whom presented localised disease and 132 with widespread cancer. The results were analysed with respect to four points :
- correlation of CEA with clinical status
- prognostic value of pre-operative levels
- CEA variation in follow-up of patients with clinical evidence of disease
- and use of CEA in monitoring of treatment.

RESULTS

Correlation of CEA with clinical status

In agreement with the literature, pre-treatment levels of CEA (fig.1) show that incidence, mean and median levels are greatly increased in women with disseminated breast cancer compared with those who have a tumour confined to the breast. On the other hand, published data is contradictory when one subdivides this last group of patients, according to the characteristics of primary tumour (T) ;node status (N) or according to Columbia Staging A, B, C and D.

For Pico and co-workers(1), there exists a close relationship between tumour size and the frequency of positive CEA level. They also found a correlation between T and the actual CEA level. Once more they described an increase of CEA when involvement of lymphnodes was clinically noticed. Although Steward, Nixon, Zamcheck (2) confirm this finding, the difference appears less evident in their work. On the other hand, Douglas, Tormey et al.(3) from the National Carcer Institute, Borthwick et al. (4) in Cardiff, Wang et al. (5) in London and Franchimont (6) in Liège, failed to demonstrate any significant correlation of CEA plasma level and local extension.

Coombes et al.(7) using seven different parameters were unable to find a relationship with the clinical status in loco-regional cancers.

In our 26 pretherapeutic estimations in loco-regional disease, no correlation was found with either tumour characteristics or with clinically or histologically proven lymphnode involvement .

Table 1 : Relationship between plasma CEA level and TNM (mean)

T1	1.4	N0	4.1	N+	1.8
T2	3.8	N1	2.3		
T3	1.4	N2	2.1	N-	1.6
T4	2.9	N3	4.0		

Prognostic value of pre-operative serum CEA

In contrast to the results obtained in colonic cancer, it is generally agreed that pre-operative CEA level has little prognostic significance in breast cancer patients (5). Our cases are in agreement with this finding.

Follow-up of breast cancer patients without demonstrable disease

After initial treatment (radiotherapy or surgery), there exists a period when clinical assessment is unreliable. In fact it would be highly useful for the clinician to be able to appreciate occult residual disease at that moment. In an effort to increase the percentage of cure or in order to delay the appearance of metastases it is now accepted to give adjuvant chemotherapy for those at high risk, especially the premenopausal patients .

However, this treatment is not harmless and through lack of information, needs to be systematic. In various other cancers, post-therapeutic CEA levels do give supplementary information on the necessity for complementary treatment. In breast cancer, pre-therapeutic values rarely reached significantly positive levels. In addition, the operative procedure is almost always satisfactory. The measurement of CEA immediately after surgery is thus of little value. In breast cancer, some authors (5, 7) use CEA determination to define a group with a high probability of recurrence or spread. In order to screen this sub-population with a high risk of relapse we perform a CEA assay in blood every month. On the other hand, it would be of the highest importance to predict several months in advance the occurence of metastases. Thus, the clinician could institute early the relevant treatment.

In the series of 62 women with disease confined to the breast who underwent localised treatment, we tried to estimate monthly serum CEA during a mean of 22.7 months:

-37 patients had a level always below 10 ng/ml. In three of these women recurrence appeared, one of the three cases did not have any CEA measurement during the 6 months preceding appearance of metastases which may conceal a possible rise of CEA during this period.

-25 women had at least on one occasion, an estimation more than 10 ng/ml. 13 of these cases presented recurrence. In two cases, only the last estimation is elevated and we have not therefore enough follow-up for diagnosis of recurrence. The difference between the groups is significant and thus confirms that repeated CEA measurements can be prognostic of recurrence. The average latent period between the first estimation above 10 ng/ml and clinical appearance of recurrence (lead time) is 6.8 months.

MONITORING OF TREATMENT

When recurrent disease or metastases are clinically obvious, CEA is a good marker of treatment. Published data are in this line, much more homogeneous (8, 9, 10, 11, 12, 13). In our series , we find also a correlation between CEA variations and therapeutic effectiveness.

A) When the treatment is effective with clinical improvement, CEA levels are steady or decrease (fig.2). On the contrary, when the treatment is ineffective with clinical deterioration CEA levels rise (fig.3) . Usually it is also increasing when the patient is in the terminal phase (fig.4). However, in a few cases the level could fall to base line just before death, as in these two examples (fig.5).

B) If one compares the general trend of CEA from the first determination through the last one, three groups become clear : those with falling levels, those with stable levels and those with rising levels, the actuarial survival in these three populations is clearly different with disadvantage for the group with increasing levels.

In order to determine if the follow-up of therapeutic results in using CEA assay is more or less reliable according to the treatment, we have divided our population of 67 patients in three groups, one treated by hormonotherapy, the other by chemotherapy and another by hormonochemotherapy (8). The results are shown in Table 2.
Table 2 : Percentage of concordant results according to the treatment.

	Concordant		Discordant		Inevaluable
HORMONO	17	80%	4	16%	4%
CHEMO	9	90%	0	0%	10%
HORMONCHEMO	22	68%	7	21.9%	9.5%

CONCLUSION

In order to appreciate the usefulness of CEA in breast cancer, we have studied 194 patients in measuring this glycoprotein several times during their evolution. We have noticed three positive points and one negative .

1) During post-operative or post-irradiation follow-up, when CEA level is higher than 10 ng, there exists a strong probability of recurrent disease in the next 6-8 months.
2) CEA assay during the chemical treatment is a good parameter to appreciate the effectiveness of the treatment .
3) In general, an increase in CEA level during clinical evolution is of bad prognosis and survival will be shorter than when CEA levels decrease.
The negative point is that the absolute levels of CEA in breast cancer have no significant prognostic value either in the pre or post-therapeutic phase of the primary, or at the time of recurrent disease or in the pre-mortem period.

REFERENCES

(1) Pico,J.L., Henry,R., Meriadec,B., Salard,J.L. (1976): Paper read at the Second Congress of the Medical Oncology Society, Nice, France

(2) Steward,A.M., Nixon,D., Zamcheck, N., Aisenberg,A. (1974): Cancer 33, 1246.

(3) Douglas, W., Tormey,C., Waalkes,T.P., Ahmann,D., Gehrke,C.W., Zumwatt,R.W., Snyder,J., Hansen,H. (2975): Cancer,35, 1095.

(4) Bortwick,M.N., Douglas,W., Philip,A.B.(1977): Europ.J.Cancer,13, 171.

(5) Wang,D.Y., Bulbrook,R.D., Hayward,J.L.,Hendrick,J.C., Franchimont, P. (1975): Europ.J.Cancer, 11, 615.

(6) Hendrick,J.C., Reuter,A., Franchimont,P. (1975): Proceedings, Hormones and Breast Cancer, Inserm,1975,pp.171-180.

(7) Coombes,R.C., Gazet, J.C., Sloane,J.P., Powles,T.J., Ford,H.T., Laurence,D.J.R., Neville,A.M. (1977) : Lancet, 8003,I, 132.

(8) Namer,M., Krebs,P.B.,Lupo,R., Schneider,M.,Lalanne,C.M.(1976): Cancer related antigens , North-Holland, Amsterdam, 1976, pp.189-196.

(9) Krebs,B.P., Turchi,P., Bonet,C., Schneider,M., Lalanne,C.M., Namer,M. (1977): Europ.J.Cancer, 13, 375.

(10)Go,V.L.W.(1976): Cancer, 37, 562.

(11)Neville,A.M., Cooper,E.H. (1976): Ann.Clin.Biomchem.,13, 283.

(12)Zamcheck,N. (1975): Cancer, 36, 2460.

(13)WU,J.T., Bray,P.F.(1974): New Engl.J.Med.,20,1439.

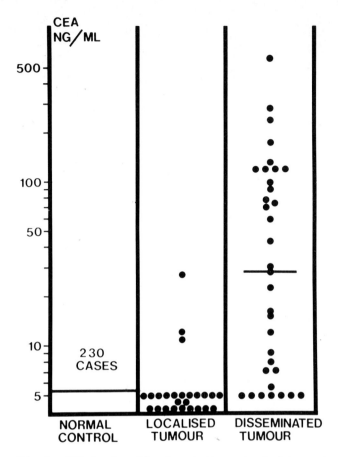

Fig.1 CEA in localized and disseminated breast cancer (on the left, normal non-smoker control group).

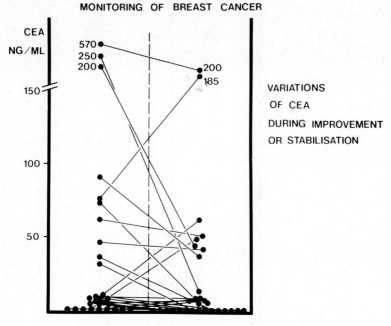

Fig.2   Variations of CEA during improvement or stabilisation.

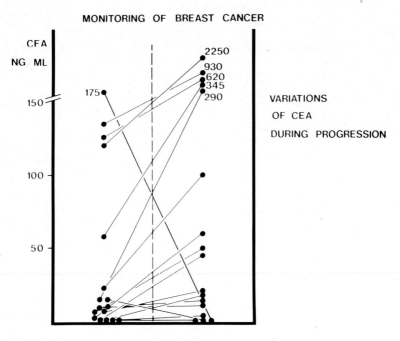

Fig.3   Variations of CEA during progression.

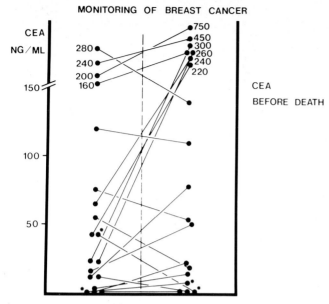

Fig.4   CEA in terminal phase.

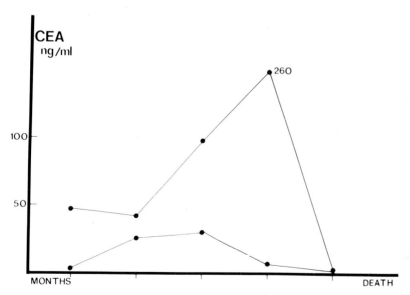

Fig.5   Paradoxal CEA fall during the terminal phase of evolution.

DISCUSSION

CHATAL J.F. (Nantes): In your study, you take care of slightly elevated CEA values. Did you also take care of technological variation
of CEA assay?

NAMER M. (Nice): I agree with you, our initial feeling was that
10 ng/ml could be related to a non-malignant event. But our study
is retrospective and we have been surprised by the great importance
of this slight elevated value.

CHATAL J.F. (Nantes): In the future, will you proceed in the same
manner.

NAMER M. (Nice): In breast cancer, we have very fair results with
post-surgical chemotherapy, So we will take into account these
values for the prescription of this kind of chemotherapy.

THE ROLE OF THE CARCINOEMBRYONIC ANTIGEN IN MONITORING BREAST CANCER PATIENTS UNDERGOING CHEMOTHERAPY

WITH REGARD TO 45 CASES TREATED FOR MORE THAN A YEAR

JF. CHATAL, F. CHUPIN, O. GODIN, A. LE MEVEL-LE POURHIET and
BP. LE MEVEL.
Centre René Gauducheau, Quai Moncousu, 44035 NANTES CEDEX, France.

The encouraging results obtained through polychemotherapy in the treatment of breast cancer suggest that its application, along with other forms of therapy, will appreciably improve prognosis of the disease (1). It is important to have available a sensitive and specific parameter in order to check on the effectiveness of the treatment or to detect recurrences at an early stage. The carcinoembryonic antigen (CEA), despite variable preliminary results (2,3,4,5), may satisfy this need. The purpose of this study is to assess the results of CEA serial assays in the observation of 45 patients undergoing polychemotherapeutic treatment for more than a year's time.

MATERIALS AND METHODS

. With respect to the initial stage of their disease, the patients fall into three groups :

- 19 had node involvement when operated upon (N+)

- 20 had metastatic extension of the disease (M+):
  osseous (9 cases), cutaneous (2 cases), peritoneal
  (1 case) or multiple (7 cases)

- in six cases the cancer showed clinical signs of rapid
  local development so that surgery was out of question
  (PEV+).

. The patients all underwent a chemotherapeutic treatment, according to varying therapeutic schemes, which combined an alkylating agent, an antimetabolite, an antibiotic and a spindle poison. Hormonal therapy was provided for patients with metastases (particularly of the bones).

During the period under study, 304 CEA determinations were performed (an average of seven per patient). Serum CEA estimation was determined directly by analysis of the serum according to the method perfected by the Commissariat à l'Energie Atomique (Marcoule, France). The arbitrary upper limit of normal for this assay was 10 ng/ml.

The progress of the disease, with respect to the treatment, was checked regularly by clinical and biological examination plus, as the case warranted and according to the symptoms detected, a breast check-up, a chest X-ray and bone, liver or brain scans.

A CEA determination was performed for each patient prior to treatment and then regularly at intervals of two or three months on the average.

RESULTS - DISCUSSION

PATIENTS WITH NODE INVOLVEMENT (N+)

Out of the entire 19 patients, considered as a high-risk group and consequently treated by systematic adjuvant chemotherepy after undergoing loco-regional treatment (surgery and/or radiotherapy), 16 are in complete remission and three show loco-regional (two cases) or metastatic (one case) development.

- Before treatment, CEA level was higher than 10 ng/ml in only five cases and no higher than the threshold of 40 ng /ml, except in a single case (48 ng/ml).

- Out of the 16 cases in complete remission more than a year after the beginning of treatment (Fig. 1), CEA level is normal in four cases which had an initial value higher than 10 ng/ml; in the 12 other cases, the level is normal in the vast majority of determinations, and when it is higher than the limit of 10 ng/ml the increase is temporary and not significant (most often less than 15 ng/ml). In a single case, an increase to 30 ng/ml is to be explained as the result of intercurrent intestinal infection.

- Out of the three cases which progressed unfavorably (Fig. 2), there was gradual and moderate increase in CEA level, and fluctuating kinetic activity at the same time as clinical development, in the case of two patients with loco-regional extension of the disease. In the third case, CEA value remained normal despite metastatic development (pulmonary).

On the basis of this study, it is too early to judge the effectiveness of repeated CEA estimations in the detection of recurrences, for the number of patients investigated in whom the disease is in progress is too limited. It is only appropriate to emphasize that when there is no recurrence, CEA level most often remains normal or subnormal, whereas in a study conducted by CHU and NEMOTO (2) raised CEA values were more frequent and higher for a group of patients in complete remission after mammectomy but not undergoing complementary chemotherapy.

Finally, the physiopathological interpretation of the moderate increases in CEA level must be made with caution in view of the relatively high coefficient of variation for the low quantities involved.

PATIENTS WITH METASTATIC EXTENSION OF THE DISEASE (M+)

Among the 20 patients who had metastatic extension before the beginning of treatment, there was partial regression followed by stabilization in 11 cases, and in nine cases persistent progression right away or, secondarily, after initial regression.

- Before treatment, CEA level was higher than 10 ng/ml in 16 cases (80%); it was above the threshold of 50 ng/ml in nine cases and of 100 ng/ml in six cases. Two patients,

264

each with a single occurrence of bone metastasis, had a slightly increased initial CEA value (14 and 20 ng/ml).

- Out of the 11 cases with partial regression followed by stabilization (Fig. 3), CEA value became normal in three instances, decreased significantly without becoming normal in three instances, and remained practically stable in three instances, either at a high level (two cases) or a relatively low level (one case). In two cases CEA level remained normal despite the existence of multiple bone metastases at the beginning of treatment; one of these patients had a temporary increase to 40 ng/ml, without any clinical sign of development of the disease, a circumstance which remains unexplained.

- Out of nine cases in which the disease made progress (Fig. 4), there are three instances of increase at the same time as (two cases) or preceding (one case) clinical development; for these three patients the increase occurred secondarily after a period of stabilization. In three instances CEA value remained stable at a high or very high level; finally, for three patients CEA level remained normal or had a fluctuating pattern of change not in conformity with clinical development. It is important to emphasize that these three patients had local or loco-regional cutaneous metastatic development which corresponded less frequently than for the other metastatic localizations to an increase in CEA level (2).

If all 20 patients initially with metastases are taken into consideration, decrease or increase in CEA level is most often seen to occur simultaneously with favorable or unfavorable clinical development. In one case the increase preceded clinical development. These results do not confirm those of CHU and NEMOTO (2) who frequently found a delay between change in CEA value and clinical development.

PATIENTS INITIALLY SHOWING SIGNS OF RAPID DEVELOPMENT OF THE DISEASE (PEV+)

Among the six patients in this group, the initial CEA level was higher than 10 ng/ml in four cases, but the increase was moderate and did not exceed 50 ng/ml, except in one case (52 ng/ml). The six patients remain in complete remission (Fig. 5). In three cases CEA level is becoming normal, and in three others it is normal or subnormal.

CONCLUSION

Subject to certain precautions in interpretation, it may be said that change in CEA value during chemotherapy seems most often to provide satisfactory indication of the state of the disease. A fall always corresponds to a clinical or paraclinical regression (whether the patients be N+ or PEV+). In the case of a sudden rise, an intercurrent cause must first be sought, and then the rise must be confirmed by the results of a new determination before being interpreted as a sign of unfavorable progress. It appears that local or loco-regional development of the disease less frequently induces an increase in CEA level than does a remote metastatic extension of the disease, a circumstance which places a certain limit on the surveillance value of CEA estimation; but this limit is relatively unimportant to the extent that loco-regional development is often clinically perceptible. The fact that this study is recent and that not enough patients have yet been observed dictates against drawing definitive conclusions, but it would seem that CEA determination provides an interesting means of surveillance in cases of breast cancer.

REFERENCES

(1) SHABEL, F.M. (1977) : Cancer, 39, 2875.

(2) CHU, T.M., NEMOTO T. (1973) : J. Natl. Cancer Inst., 51, 1119.

(3) HENRY, R., MERIADEC, B., PICO, J.L., SALARD, J.L. (1976) : Nouv. Presse Med., 5, 1233.

(4) BORTHWICK, N.M., WILSON, D.W., BELL, P.A. (1977) : Europ. J. Cancer, 13, 171.

(5) STEWARD, A.M., NIXON, D., ZAMCHECK, N., AISENBERG, 1. (1974) : Cancer, 33, 1246.

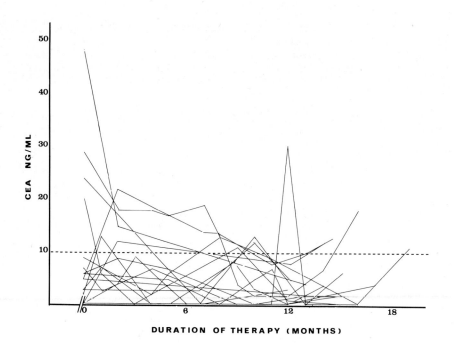

Fig. 1 Patients with node involvement (N+) in complete remission.

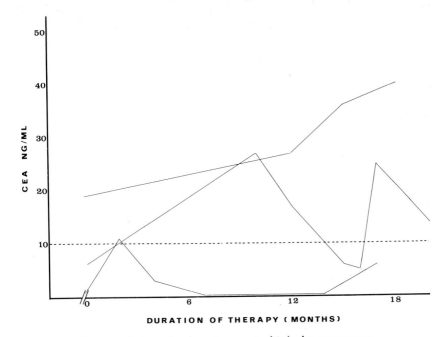

Fig. 2 Patients with node involvement (N+) in progress.

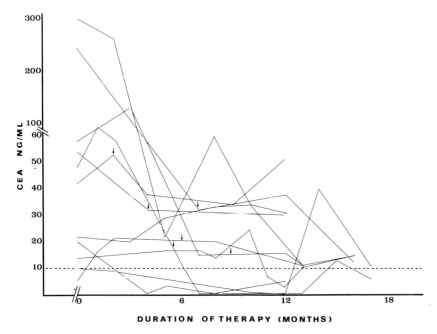

Fig. 3 Patients with metastatic extension (M+) in partial regression.
The arrows indicate the date of clinical regression.

267

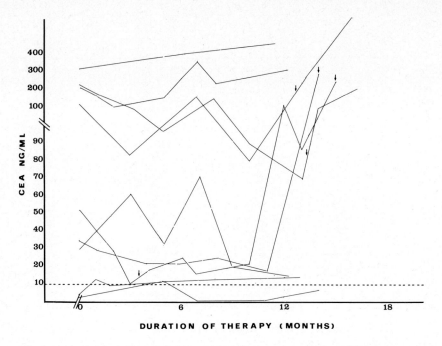

Fig. 4 Patients with metastatic extension (M+) in progress. The arrows indicate the date of clinical progression.

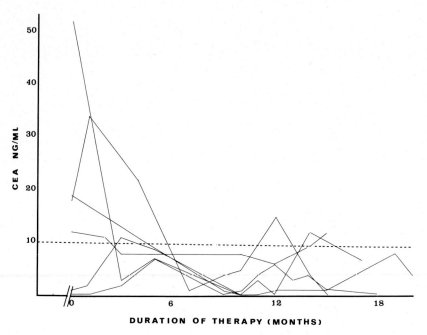

Fig. 5 Patients with clinical signs of rapid development of the disease (PEV+)

DISCUSSION

CALLE R.(Paris): What is the importance in discrepancy between CEA levels and clinical evolution?

CHATAL J.F. (Nantes): Discrepancy exists mainly in cases of local recurrence of disease. But it seems that these discrepancies are few.

LALANNE C.M. (Nice): Do you take into account an elevation of CEA to start of modify chemotherapy?

CHATAL J.F.(Nantes): This must be our conclusion and one of the main interests of follow-up with CEA. At the Nantes Cancer Centre, we modify chemotherapy protocols according to CEA increase even with no clinical change.

THE STUDY OF CEA RATES   BEFORE, DURING AND AFTER TELECOBAL THERAPY

Salabert,M.T.; Romero de Avila,C;Moreno,J.L.;Zaragoza,R; Belloch,V.

Dept.of Radiology & Physiotherapy.Faculty of Medicine. Valencia.Spain.

The scope of our research has been the following:

I) To verify the rate of CEA in persons considered as normal, in order to compare it with those rates consi dered normal in medical literature, since there is no unanimous agreement.

II) To evaluate CEA in neoplasic patients with proven diagnosis of malignant neoplasia and subjected to surgery. Theses patients have been irradiated, later on, with tele cobaltherapy. The rate of CEA has been studied in them, before,during and after telecobaltherapy.

III) To attempt at establishing a correlation between the CEA variations at the end of telecobaltherapy and the later evolution of the process, in order to estimate whe ther that evolution may be unfavourable.

IV) To establish the difference between the serum and the plasma levels of CEA.

In order to estimate normal values we have used 150 people considered as normal. In order to study CEA in neo plasic patients, and under the above mentioned conditions we have screened 60 patients with different localizations.

All the results presented in this research have been carried out by means of CIS method.

RESULTS

I) Our interest in the evaluation of CEA in normal persons is due to the fact that the figures offered as "normal" very greatly according to the methods used.

The results we have obtained in the determination of CEA in normal persons, are shown in Figure. 1.

We have, therefore, considered normal values to be below 5 ng./ml., and pathological all values above, appre ciating the posibilities of high values being obtained by non-neoplasic patients or even by normal people.

II) All patients whose results are included in the re search carried neoplasia, as was ascertained surgically with pathological diagnosis. Thay were later irradiated with telecobaltherapy as above explained.

In these patients CEA was evaluated: 1.- When they first recieved to our treatment of irradiation, and prior to it. 2.-In the middle of their treatment with telecobal therapy (2.000-2.500 rad-t), since we assumed that perhaps the CEA rate could be modified by the radiobiological alterations due to irradiation, both on the tumour cells and on the normal cells. 3.-At the end of treatment with telecobaltherapy.

The table I shows the variations of statistical averages in theses patients before the beginning of the treatment, during it and at the and of it.

TABLE I Variations of average of CEA in neoplasic patients after chirurgical treatment, before, during and at the end of irradiation

Site	No.	Before irradiation	Half irradiation	After irradiation
Breast	27	18.6	27.82	21.46
Uterus	17	22.29	24.46	47.00
Larynx	10	3.00	6.67	5.71
Bladder	6	8.83	23.50	5.33

In all the localizations studied it can be seen that the CEA rate experiences a slight increase in the middle of the treatment and a decrease at the end of it.

III) At the end of the treatment, a detailed study of the patients anabled us to classify them into two groups: firts one was formed by those who had values of CEA below 5 ng./ml.; the second, by those with higher values of CEA, considering 5 ng./ml., as a "compromise" of normal values. According to this guide-line patients are grouped as Table II shows.

TABLE II Values of CEA in neoplasic patients after chirurgical treatment, after irradiation

Site	No.	> 5 ng/ml	$\leqslant 5$ ng/ml
Breast	27	8	19
Uterus	17	5	12
Larynx	10	2	8
Bladder	6	4	2

The follow-up of these patients, once finishing their treatment with telecobaltherapy, has shown that the ones who evolved to methastasis belonged to the group with high rates of CEA after irradiation. Those patients who after irradiation did not have high values of CEA, belonged to patients with nomethastasis during the time of this research (1,5 years).

In this way, out of the 8 cases of breast neoplasic with rates of CEA above 5 ng/ml. at the end of our treatment, 3 showed bone methastasis, 4 lymph nodes methastasis and 1 skin methastasis.

Out of 5 cases of uterus neoplasia, 1 had liver methastasis and 2 rectum invasion. Out of 2 cases of larynx carcinoma, 1 had lymph nodes methastasis. Out of 4 cases of bladder carcinoma, 1 had rectum methastasis and 1 had local recurrence.

IV) We studied 56 cases in which simultaneously we analised the CEA in both plasma obtained with EDTA-k2 and serum, with the intention of establishing some relation between them. In all cases we found that the quantity of CEA detectar was higher when we used serum than when we employed plasma. Figure 2.

CONCLUSIONS

1.- The evaluations of CEA in normal people has offered some results, wich enable us to consider as "normal" values below 5 ng/ml.

2.- In neoplasic patients, we have found a great dispersion of values. Out of the 60 patients studied, the rate of CEA was below 5 ng./ml. in 41. Having considered 5 ng/ml. as the limit of normal values, 68% of these patients showed "normal" values of CEA.

It has to be considered that all theses patients had suffered a surgical treatment, and thus, the above figures have little value, since we do not have values of CEA prior their surgical treatment. Therefore, we cannot draw any conclusion about the validity of CEA for the diagnosis of neoplasia.

3.- In those neoplasic patients, irradiated with tele cobaltherapy after surgical treatment, the rate of CEA shows an increase at the middle of the irradiation, in most cases, and a decrease at the end of treatment.

4.-The follow-up of these patients anables us to establish a strong correlation between high rates of CEA at the end of treatment and the sppearance of methastasis in the short run. In some neoplasic sites this correlation schieves a 100% as observed in our patients with breast neoplasia.

5.- And last, but by no mens least, we have determined that the use of serum in these tests, is more to be prefered than the use of plasma.

REFERENCES

Gold,P.;Freedman,S.O. (1965):J.Exp.Med.121,439-459.

Lo Gerfo,P.,Krupey,J.,Hansen,H.J.(1971):New Engl.
J.Med.285,138-141.
Mach,J.H.(1975):Bull.Cancer 62,445-452.
Meeker,W.R.:(1973):Arch.Surg.107,266-273
V ider,M.,Kashmiri,R.,Meeker,W.R.,Moses,B.,Maruyama,
Y.(1975):Am.J.Roentgen.Rad.Ther.Nucl.Med.124
Gold,P.,Freedman,S.O.(1975):J.Am.Med.Assoc.234,190-
192.

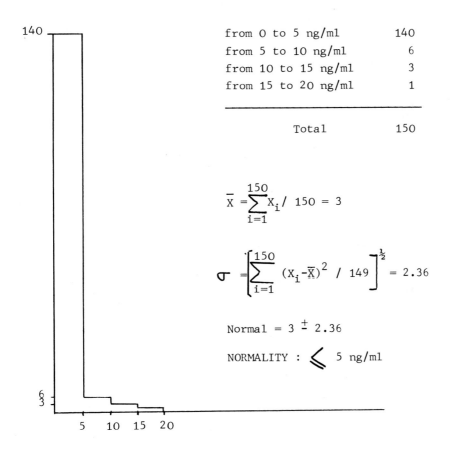

from 0 to 5 ng/ml	140
from 5 to 10 ng/ml	6
from 10 to 15 ng/ml	3
from 15 to 20 ng/ml	1
Total	150

$$\bar{X} = \sum_{i=1}^{150} X_i / 150 = 3$$

$$\sigma = \left[\sum_{i=1}^{150} (X_i - \bar{X})^2 / 149 \right]^{\frac{1}{2}} = 2.36$$

Normal $= 3 \pm 2.36$

NORMALITY : $\leqslant$ 5 ng/ml

Fig.1 Values of CEA in 150 normal persons with CIS-
kit.

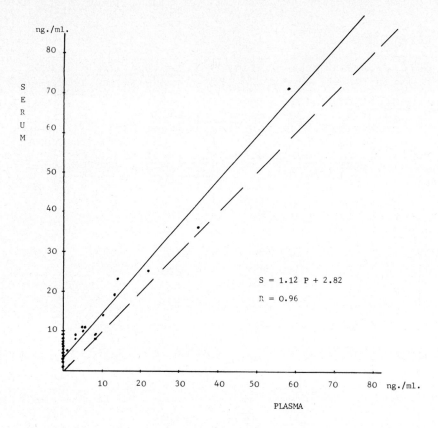

S = 1.12 P + 2.82

R = 0.96

Fig.2 Correlation Line between serum and plasma levels.

BREAST CANCER CYTOSOL CARCINOEMBRYONIC ANTIGEN (CEA) AND ESTROGEN RECEPTOR ACTIVITY (ER)

H. Rochman, E. Conniff, E. De Sombre and R. Blough

Department of Pathology, Ben May Laboratory for Cancer Research and the Biomedical Computation Facilities, University of Chicago, Chicago, U.S.A.

The results indicate that 77% of patients having the minimum estrogen receptor concentration required for a response to endocrine therapy possess high levels of CEA activity. If these elevated tumor CEA levels are reflected in the blood levels then the estrogen receptor assay of the primary tumor could help define these breast cancer patients most likely to be aided by routine plasma CEA assay.

Elevated peripheral blood CEA levels have been found in 47% (1) to 67% (2) of patients with breast cancer. Since breast cancer tissue also contains increased CEA activity (3) it can be assumed that the rise in serum CEA originates from the malignancy. The fact that serum CEA levels correlate with a response to treatment (4) would support such an assumption. It would seem therefore that serial CEA measurements may assist in the management of some patients with breast cancer. To further define this group of patients, breast cancer cytosol was examined for CEA and estrogen receptor activity.

METHODS

Estrogen receptor concentrations were determined by sedimentation analysis (5); cut off values for the positive group, > 750 fmoles/g postmenopausal and > 250 fmoles/g for premenopausal, are based on the minimum required for patient response to endocrine therapy. Cytosol CEA assay was performed by the Hansen-Z-gel technique (6). Cytosol CEA of non-malignant breast tissue was < 20 ng per ml. In all, 261 tissue samples from 252 patients with breast cancer were studied. Sixty-four samples were primary breast cancers from premenopausal patients; 14, metastases from premenopausal patients; 134 were primaries from postmenopausal patients; and 49 were metastases from postmenopausal patients.

275

RESULTS

Cytosol CEA activity for the four categories of patients are shown in Figures 1-4. The frequency of elevated CEA was similar for all categories (58-64%) and also the mean values were not significantly different. Therefore, unlike estrogen receptor binding, CEA of breast cancer tissue is not influenced by the menopausal status. Seventy-seven per cent of the 71 ER + patients had elevated cytosol CEA, whereas only 54% of ER − cases showed elevations, Fig. 5, and this was highly significant (Chi-Square test, $P < 0.01$); further, there was little difference when primaries and metastases were compared. Also, the mean CEA of ER + patients were significantly greater than the mean CEA of ER − patients for all categories (307 - 643 versus 140 - 224 ng per ml); student's t-tests using log transformed data, $P < 0.02$.

Conceivably many factors contribute to the blood levels of a biochemical species originating from tumor tissue and this probably includes tumor load, its vascularity and the concentration of the biochemical species in the tumor cell. In the present study cytosol CEA was examined and the results indicate that tumor tissue that contains significant levels of estrogen receptor binding protein is more likely also to have elevated tumor CEA, ie. ER + tumors more frequently show an elevated cytosol CEA than ER − tumors. Should the raised cytosol CEA be reflected in the blood levels then it could be expected that plasma CEA of ER + patients would more frequently be elevated; if so, this would help specify those patients for whom routine assay of CEA would be most beneficial for monitoring progress of disease, response to treatment, and also possible early detection of recurrence.

REFERENCES

(1) Laurence, D. J. R., Stevens, N., Bettelheim, R. et al. (1972): Brit. Med. J. 3, 605.

(2) Lo Gerfo, P., Krupey, J. and Hansen, H. J. (1971): New Engl. J. Med. 285, 138.

(3) Menendez-Botet, C. J., Hisselbaum, J. S., Fleisher, M. et al. (1976): Clin. Chem. 22, 1366.

(4) Steward, A. M., Nixon, D., Zamchek, N. and Aisenberg, A. (1974): Cancer 33, 1246.

(5) Jensen, E. V., Smith, S. and De Sombre, E. R. (1976): J. Steroid Biochem. 7, 911.

(6) Hansen, H. J., Snyder, J. J., Miller, E. et al. (1974): Hum. Pathol. 5, 139.

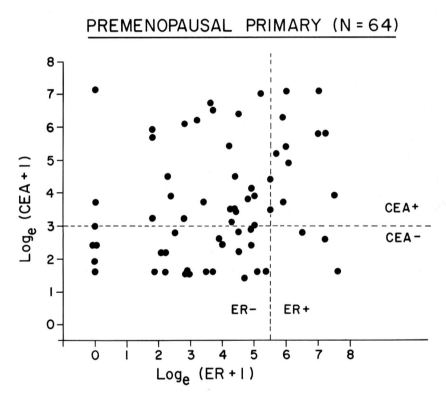

Fig. 1 CEA and ER activities of primary breast cancer tissue: premenopausal patients.

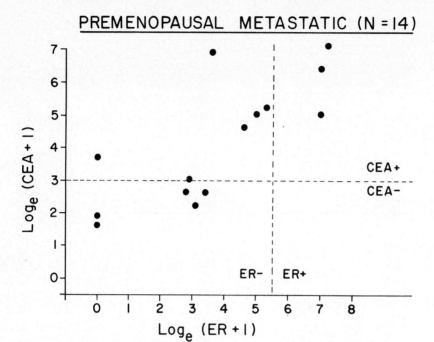

Fig. 2 CEA and ER activities of metastatic tissue from premenopausal patients with breast cancer.

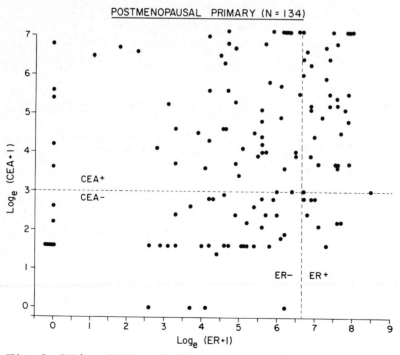

Fig. 3 CEA and ER activities of primary breast cancer tissue:
postmenopausal patients.

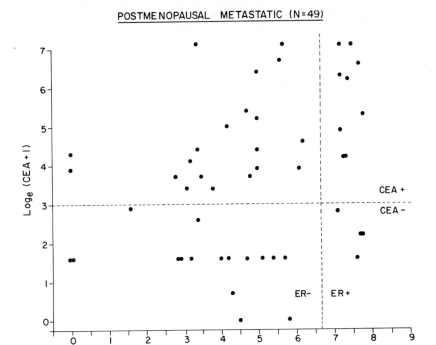

Fig. 4 CEA and ER activities of metastatic tissue from post-menopausal patients with breast cancer.

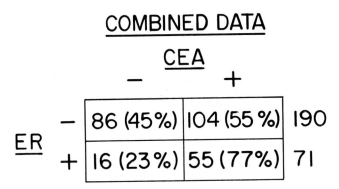

Fig. 5 Correlates ER and CEA for all samples examined.

CARCINOEMBRYONIC ANTIGEN IN BREAST CANCER CYTOSOL : RELATIONSHIP
WITH OESTRADIOL RECEPTORS AND PLASMA CEA

M.Francoual , M.Namer, J.L.Moll, G.Milano, C.Bonet, C.M.Lalanne
and B.P.Krebs

Centre Antoine Lacassagne, 36 Voie Romaine, 06054 Nice Cedex, France

The measurement of Oestradiol Receptors (ER) in breast cancer
cytosol has been routinely carried out since October 1976 at this
Center. These tumours were either primary cancer (46 patients) or
biopsies from skin metastasis (40 cases). In addition, plasma carcinoembryonic antigen (CEA) levels are estimated in these cases in order
to monitor the effect of treatment. The aim of this work was to
study the correlation between (i) CEA in cytosol and receptors,
(ii) Plasma CEA and receptors, (iii) Plasma CEA and cytosol CEA.

MATERIAL AND METHODS

The specimens are taken either during mammectomy or tumorectomy
when the cancer is primary or by biopsy of skin metastasis. In table
1 are shown, methods, units and positivity threshold of the different
assays. The statistic analysis is performed by the distribution free
test of MANN and WITHNEY.

TABLE 1 Methods

	Methods	Units	Threshold of positivity
Oestradiol receptors	McGuire et al.	fmoles/ mg proteins	More than 8
CEA in plasma	Sorin, Meriadec et al.	ng/ml	More than 5
CEA in cytosol	Sorin, Meriadec et al.	ng/ml proteins	More than 5
Total Proteins	Lowry	ng/ml	

Table 2 shows the general repartition of positivity for both
CEA and receptors.

TABLE 2   Estradiol receptors and CEA levels in cytosol

		Nb	Percentage
Estradiol receptors positive	Primary	23	50
	Metastasis	16	39
CEA level positive	Primary	26	56.5
	Metastasis	18	45

Correlation between CEA in cytosol and Estradiol receptors

As shown in fig.1, no statistically significant difference
exists in the cytosol CEA level between primary tumours and skin
metastases.
In contrast, if our population of primary and metastatic
samples is classified only according to the presence or absence
of receptors, the difference is very significant (p < 0.001) (Fig.2).
This is also true for primary tumours and metastases analysed
separately. On these two figures is represented the median for the
different groups.

Correlation between plasma CEA and ER

The incidence of positive plasma CEA level in our population
closely ressembles data in the literature: i.e. 20.5% in localized
tumours, 58% in disseminated diseases. For primary tumours as well
as for metastases there is no relationship between plasma CEA and
presence of ER.

Correlation between plasma CEA and cytosol CEA

Plasma CEA is not related with cytosol CEA in localized tumours
(p < 0.001): since one patient out of five has CEA in plasma while
three patients out of five have CEA in cytosol in primary tumours.
Concerning metastases there is no statistically significant difference
between CEA in plasma and CEA in cytosol.

CONCLUSIONS

Simultaneous measurement of ER and CEA in breast tumours
primary and skin metastasis has shown the following points.
1. Primary tumours are much more often secretor of CEA than
is reflected in the serum level (fig.3).
2. Although metastases are not more often secretant than
primary tumours. But all metastases of one patient are not secretors,
however their CEA production is accurately reflected in the plasma
(fig.3).
3. For primary tumours and metastases there exists a close
relationship between the ability to synthetize CEA and the presence

of ER. The combination of CEA with the ER is statistically significant but not sufficiently accurate for either test to suffice alone.

REFERENCES

(1) McGuire, W.L., Carbone, P.P., Sears, M.E., Eschen, G.C.(1975) :
    Estrogen Receptors in Human Breast Cancer. An Overview , Raven
    Press, New York, 1975.pp.1-7 .
(2) Meriadec, B., Martin, F., Guerin,J., Henry,R., Klipping,C.(1973):
    Bull. Cancer, 60, 403.

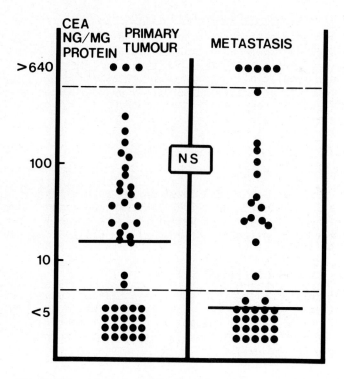

Fig.1 There is no statistically significant difference between CEA
content of primary tumour and metastasis.

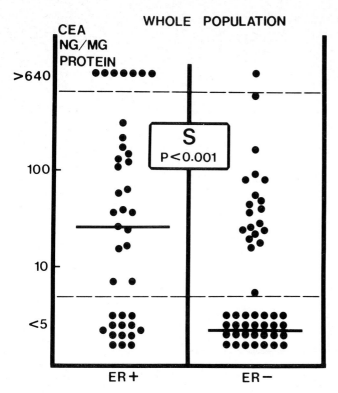

Fig.2 There is a significant association between presence of estradiol receptors and CEA content of the tumour.

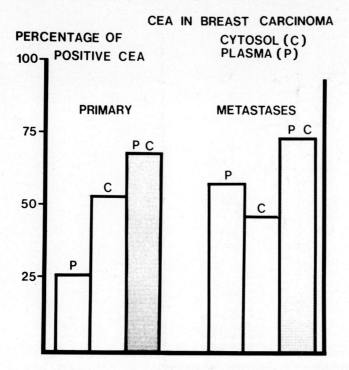

CEA IN BREAST CARCINOMA

Fig.3 In the primary , CEA is more often elevated than in plasma. In contrast, it appears that metastases are heterogenous concerning CEA content because plasma levels are more often positive than a sample of one metastasis.

COMPARISON OF PREGNANCY-ASSOCIATED MACROGLOBU LIN (PAM) AND CARCINOEMBRYONIC ANTIGEN (CEA) IN PRE-CLINICAL DETECTION OF METASTASES FROM MAMMARY CANCERS*

J. Maxwell Anderson, W. H. Stimson, G. Gettinby, R. W. Burt and S. K. Jhunjhunwala

Surgical Division and Radioimmunoassay Laboratory, Royal Infirmary, Glasgow.   Department of Biochemistry and Department of Mathematics, University of Strathclyde, Glasgow.

Accurate detection of micrometastases from mammary cancers (1, 2, 3) by pregnancy-associatedα - macroglobulin α_2-glycoprotein (PAM), a glycoprotein (4, 5) characteristically elevated in the blood of pregnant women, (6, 7) has been reported. Studies of carcinoembryonic antigen (CEA) (8, 9) suggest that it might also be an indicator in this context.   The PAM study has been extended (10) and a direct comparison of the detective properties of PAM is now made with those of CEA in mammary cancer bearers followed for up to 9 years after mastectomy.

DESIGN OF STUDY

Thirty patients bearing stage 1 or 2 mammary cancers, resectable and apparently localised to the breast or to the breast and axilla were entered to the study sequentially and without further selection. Eleven were treated by mastectomy alone, 16 by mastectomy plus radiotherapy and 3 by mastectomy plus radiotherapy and stimulatory immunotherapy by cancer autografts (11, 12).   Sera were obtained by centrifugation of clotted venous blood samples within 2 hours of withdrawal and immediately stored at -50°C in coded 1ml vials. Matching coded samples were used subsequently for determining PAM by an enzyme-linked immunoassay (3) and CEA by radio-immunoassay (4).   Baseline values for CEA and PAM were calculated for each patient, except one in the case of CEA, as the average of 3 or 4 weekly measurements immediately after patients entered the study.   Percentage changes from the baselines were obtained at intervals of 3 months or more frequently for 8-37 (median, 21) months.

RESULTS

Eleven patients aged 42-78 (median, 51) years have developed

*Supported by donations from Eli Lilly and Company and the Lister Social Club of Glasgow Royal Infirmary and by a Cancer Research Campaign grant (WHS).

macrometastases while 19 aged 46-70 (median, 55) years remain well and free from disease upon clinical, general biochemical, radiographic and scintigraphic screening. The macrometastases developed in the mastectomy scars or in the axillary/supraclavicular lymph nodes in 4 cases and in bones, alone or with other sites, in 7 cases. Of the other sites 3 were in liver, 4 in lungs and 1 in brain. A clear difference has emerged between the maximum PAM rises of the 11 patients who have developed metastases and of the 19 who remain clinically well. All in the metastatic group had elevations of serum PAM in the range 57-1 800% above baselines (Table 1) BEFORE metastases were detected by the conventional clinical and special methods, only one being less than 75%.

TABLE 1 Individual maximum percentage increases for PAM and CEA in the metastatic and clinically well patients.

Detector	Metastatic					Clinically Well					p in Mann-Whitney U test
PAM	125	90	57	144	777	40	27	1	26	8	< 0.01
	76	1 056	198	150	162	16	0	28	5	0	
	1 800					0	29	92	15	63	
						316	122	182	169		
CEA	60	39	83	1 184	50	85	371	15	26	48	N. S.
	47	107	0—	445	--	86	79	0	730	0	
	73					57	44	26	243	26	
						114	81	88	229		

In the clinically well patients PAM rises of 1-316% occurred; in 5 subjects the rises exceeded 75% and subsequently fell towards baselines. The difference between individual maximum PAM rises in the two groups was statistically significant with $p < 0.01$ in a Mann-Whitney U test. The result of a previous preliminary assessment (1) on the same patients was similar when a comparison of the wholeprofiles of PAM changes in the two groups was examined by attempting to develop a method of constructing zero-constrained regression lines.

The percentage changes of CEA from baselines have been assessed in the same way (Table 1). Rises exceeded 75% in 4 of 10 metastatic patients and in 2 of these there were two later observations below the 75% level before metastases were detected. Ten of the clinically well group had single rises exceeding 75%, 7 fell close to baselines later, 1 remained close to the 75% level and 1 main-

tained a rise of 230%. The difference between the individual maximum percentage CEA rises in the 2 groups is not significant in a
Mann-Whitney U test. When a rise in CEA of >45% is examined for
discrimination between metastatic and clinically well patients, 8 of
10 patients with metastases would be correctly detected but 12 of 19
patients remaining well would be incorrectly suspected of harbouring
active metastases. A discriminant analysis to obtain a weighted
combination of the individual maximum percentage PAM and CEA
rises which might separate the well and the metastatic patients more
clearly did not reduce the misclassifications obtained with PAM alone.
The optimal discriminant function was

$$7.07e^{-x_1/170} - 1.16e^{-x_2/170}$$

where x_1 is the maximum percentage rise in PAM and x_2 is the maximum percentage rise in CEA. The exponential transformation was
used to preserve the difference in means between the well and the
metastatic groups and to give equality of covariances. This gave 1
out of 10 misclassifications in the metastatic group and 5 out of 19 in
the well group.

TABLE 2 Performance of tests.

DISCRIMINANT	SENSITIVITY %	SPECIFICITY %
PAM >75%	91	74
CEA >75%	40	47
CEA >45%	80	37
PAM + CEA	91	74

Thus as shown in Table 2, using a discriminant of a 75% rise from
baseline the test sensitivity (percentage of correct classifications in
the metastatic group) is 91% for PAM and 40% for CEA while the test
specificity (percentage of correct classifications in the well group) is
74% for PAM and 47% for CEA. With a 45% rise as the discriminant
for CEA the test sensitivity becomes 80% and the specificity falls to
37%. The combined discriminant for PAM and CEA has a test sensitivity of 91% and a specificity of 74%.
    No significant correlations were found between the absolute
values of PAM and CEA, or between their incremental changes.

DISCUSSION

    The interpretation of variations in biochemical detectors of
microcancers is more difficult than at first appears. Variations in a
detector characteristic of established macrometastases do not
necessarily mean they will be found at a micrometastatic stage and

conversely variations noted with micrometastases may be absent at a macrometastatic stage. Also normal ranges of values for most potential detectors are imperfectly established and statements based upon the proportions of "abnormal" values obtained should be viewed with caution. These difficulties can be managed by frequent sequential measurement of the detectors, by the use of index numerals for changes from baseline values in individuals acting as their own controls and by retrospective comparison of results in patients remaining clinically well with those developing metastases. This approach was put to the test in this study, purposely restricted in size to reduce the chances of error in handling large bodies of data and to ensure close personal clinical control within a single centre. The requirement of index numeration for reliable values was met in each subject of this study by using the mean value of several measurements at the start of surveillance. The approach to the problems of the reliability of the assays at low values of the putative detectors is an integral feature of the experimental design since the detective significance of variations from such levels, particularly for CEA is unknown. The lowest level of sensitivity of the PAM assay is 100ng/ml, which is well below the microgram levels found in the blood of most females.

The difference in PAM profiles between the metastatic and the clinically well groups allow the definitive conclusion that PAM often detects growing metastases from mammary cancers. However the odds that a rise of 75% or more in serum PAM might be followed by a fall with maintenance of the clinically well status, are 6 to 17 in this series. Further clarification of the time sequence of PAM changes may help to identify those with potentially lethal metastases. Comparison of PAM measurements with those of CEA discloses a much wider range of accurate detection by PAM, which is not approached by reducing the discriminant level for CEA to a 45% rise from baselines or by the optimal combination of the PAM and the CEA data. The possibility that CEA might detect the growth of hepatic metastases has not been investigated.

Although the wide range of normal PAM values does not allow its use in diagnosis, the rises of serum PAM described here alert us to the presence of otherwise undetected micrometastases of mammary cancers as previously suggested (1, 2, 3) and PAM is clearly superior to CEA as a detector of such micrometastases with growth potential. This study demonstrates the value of incorporating into experimental designs percentage changes from well-controlled individual baselines and that of valid comparisons of patients remaining clinically well with those developing metastases.

ACKNOWLEDGEMENT

Dr. J. G. Ratcliffe contributed valuable discussions upon the study.

REFERENCES

(1) Anderson, J. M., Stimson, W. H., Kelly, F. (1976): Brit. J. Surg., 63, 819.
(2) Stimson, W. H., (1975): Lancet, i, 777.
(3) Stimson, W. H., (1975): J. Clin. Path., 28, 868.
(4) Stimson, W. H., Eubank-Scott, L., (1972): FEBS Lett., 23, 298.
(5) Von Schoultz, B., Stigbrand, T., (1973): Acta obstet. gynec. Scand., 52, 51.
(6) Stimson, W. H., (1975): J. Reprod. Fert., 43, 579.
(7) Von Schoultz, B., (1974): Amer. J. Obstet. Gynec., 119, 792.
(8) Chu, T. M., Nemoto, T., (1973): J. Natl. Cancer Inst., 51, 1119.
(9) Coombes, R. C., Powles, T. J., Gazet, J. C., Ford, H. T., Sloane, J. P., Laurence, D. J. R., Neville, A. M., (1977): Lancet, i, 132.
(10) Anderson, J. M., Stimson, W. H., Kibby, M. R., (in press): Proceedings of the 4th Eli Lilly Vinca Alkaloid Symposium.
(11) Anderson, J. M., Gettinby, G., Kelly, F., Wood, S. E., (1977): Cancer, 40, 30.
(12) Anderson, J. M., Gettinby, G., (in press): Proceedings IABS Symposium.
(13) Stimson, W. H., Sinclair, J. M., (1974): FEBS Lett., 47, 190.
(14) Laurence, D. J. R., Stevens, U., Bettelheim, R., Darcy, D., Leese, C., Tuberville, C., Alekander, P., Johns, E. W., (1972): Br. Med. J., iii, 605.

PRIMARY BREAST CANCER-ASSOCIATED ANTIGEN (S)

A.Bartorelli and R.Accinni

Istituto Ricerche Cardiovascolari "G.Sisini", II Clinica Medica dell'Univer‾
sità e II Cattedra di Radiologia dell'Università, Via F.Sforza 35, Milano.

In the last ten years the results of several clinical trials and many techniques for the detection of CEA in body fluids have been published. In all these case-lists CEA seems to be present not only in patients with adeno-carcinomas of the gastroenteric tract, and even more in their metastases,but also in several tumours in different sites, both entodermic and not entodermic (1-6). Pancreas, lung, prostate, ovary and breast seemed the organs which, above all in the presence of distant metastases, supplied the highest rate of positivity with the different CEA tests (7). As a matter of fact, it was possible to hypothesize in all these neoplastic forms, and even more so in their metastases, of CEA, i.e. that antigen extracted for the first time by Gold and Freedman from liver metastases of colon adenocarcinoma. But it was also possible to set forth the hypothesis of several antigens, associated to the various types of primitive adenocarcinoma, which, in the liver metastatic site, would differentiate themselves with an "immunological shift", due to the site and/or the metabolic medium of the site itself, towards the CEA immuno-logical determinants.

In the case-list which was studied with our technique (8), only 10 out of 80 cases of breast adenocarcinoma turned out positive. All these ten cases showed liver metastases, while no breast cancer without liver metastases ever turned out positive in our CEA test (7).

Therefore our working hypothesis was the following: the liver meta-stasis site should enhance the positivity of our test for each kind of pathology, and this was not due to a higher level of circulating CEA, but to an increased cross-reactivity of the circulating "metastatic" antigens with the CEA anti-body. Had this hypothesis been valid, in primitive breast carcinomas, never positive to our CEA test, there should have been tumour-associated antigens with a low, but anyhow present, cross-reaction with the CEA antibody. Only if this cross-reaction were present, the hepatic metastatic location would have been able to increase it, and thus cause the CEA test positivities which we observed in the cases of liver metastases from breast adenocarcinoma (9).

Therefore our aims were the following: 1) to use the labelled CEA-anti-CEA radioimmunological system as "monitor" to detect, in the extracts of breast primitive carcinoma, the presence of antigens cross-reacting with the CEA antibodies; 2) to point out the absence of these antigens in the non neoplastic breast tissues; 3) to show the immunochemical differences between

290

these antigens and CEA; 4) to purify, to label these antigens and prepare antisera for the possible working out of a radioimmunological test.

In our previous papers (9,10) we showed the presence in the 3 M KCl extracts of primitive breast carcinomas, of an antigenic pool (Crude Breast Cancer: CBC), absent in non neoplastic breast tissues (Normal Crude Breast: NCB) able to inhibit the binding capacity of the ^{125}I CEA-anti CEA system. The purification steps of this material with gel filtration, and ion exchange chromatography suggested the presence of an antigenic pool, present at three different molarities of phosphate buffer (0.025 M, 0.05 and 0.1 M) with a maximum CEA activity at 0.05 M.

The antisera raised with CBC and NBC confirm the presence in CBC of CEA-like antigenic determinants, absent in NCB. Only the anti-CBC antisera are able to bind, even at low titers, ^{125}I CEA.

The extraction with 1 N HCl O$_4$ followed by a further extraction with 3M KCl, according to the modalities adopted by us for CEA preparation, was performed on hepatic metastases of colon adenocarcinoma, on breast primitive carcinoma and on non-neoplastic normal tissues. C.CEA (crude CEA), CBC and NCB, thus obtained, could be compared among themselves. The ion exchange chromatography of these three crude extracts shows that C.CEA inhibits the binding capacity on the ^{125}I CEA-anti CEA system at all molarities of phosphate buffer with a maximum at 0.05 M. On the contrary CBC brings about an inhibition 30 less and only at three molarities (0.025 M, 0.05 M and 0.1 M). This crude extract, as well as that obtained by the only extraction with 3M KCl, elicits the maximum inhibition at 0.05 M. No inhibition at any molarity can be observed with NCB.

The antisera raised with C.CEA, CBC and NBC by means of 1 N HClO$_4$ extraction, confirm the previous data when incubated with ^{125}I CEA. Anti-NCB antisera show no binding capacity, while anti-CBC antisera bind, though at very low titers, ^{125}I CEA. Anti C.CEA antisera bind ^{125}I CEA at titers 70-100 times higher than anti-CBC antisera.

As a confirmation of this the agar double diffusion points out with images of partial identity the cross reaction among these antigenic pools and their antisera.

Further purifications of CBC on a molecular sieve did not allow us obtaining a material to be labelled which would meet the characteristics required for a possible radioimmunoassay. The presence, after labelling, of very high "blanks" (the "blank" of each labelling fraction was checked by adding normal rabbit serum, diluted in the same way, instead of each antibody) was one of the drawbacks of these preparations from perchloric acid and 3 M KCl extracts. Among all extractions attempted that with 3M KCl followed by 80% saturated (NH$_4$)$_2$ SO$_4$ was that which allowed us to obtain the best results.

The extraction and the steps of partial purification both on a molecular sieve and ion exchange were monitored with the two available radioimmunological systems, labelled CEA-anti-CEA and labelled CEA anti-CBC. Fig. 1 shows the final steps after ion exchange chromatography of CBC and NCB,

eluted at 0.05 M, both on Sephadex G 100 and G 200. The two radioimmunological systems recognize two different zones of maximum inhibition of the
binding capacity. Worth mentioning is the fact that the two systems give almost no response on the NCB eluate, where, on the other hand, no "zone"
differentiation can be observed.

The most active fractions on the labelled CEA-anti-CBC system were
therefore pooled and concentrated: this material was termed BCA (Breast
Cancer Antigen(s). After labelling with Na ^{125}I and gel filtration on G 200,
12,000 cpm of each elution fraction were incubated with the different antisera available (Fig. 2). Anti-CBC antiserum, absorbed and non absorbed
with NCB, shows a maximum binding capacity when diluted 1:7,000 on the
apex of the first peak which will be therefore called "labelled BCA". It is
worth mentioning that this antiserum bound labelled CEA only when diluted
1:320. The anti-NCB antiserum which, diluted 1:320, slightly binds labelled
CEA, after absorption with NCB shows no more any binding capacity at whatever dilution. Confirming both the cross-reaction and the differences among
CEA and BCA anti-CEA and anti C.CEA antisera which bind labelled CEA
at very high titers (1:200 ,000 and 1:20,000 respectively) are able to bind
7% of labelled BCA only when concentrated 1:800.

Finally it worth mentioning the blank values, very low and present
only in the very first elution fractions, comparable to those obtained by label
ling CEA.

With labelled BCA as tracer, and anti-CBC antisera absorbed with
NCB, we performed inhibition curves by employing as standard the different
antigenic preparations available (Fig. 3). The radioimmunological system
labelled BCA anti-CBC recognizes CBC only at microgram values; NCB and
C.CEA do not show, at these concentrations, any inhibition of the binding
capacity.

When BCA and CEA are challenged as standard against the system
labelled BCA-anti-CBC the sensitivity of the system increases remarkably.
In fact only a few nanograms of BCA are required to inhibit the binding
capacity, while CEA standard does not bring about any drop of the binding
capacity.

The antigenic pool associated with the primitive breast carcinomas
seems to show a slight cross-reaction with CEA and this property allowed
us to study it in the initial phase. The immunochemical differences between
these antigens and the experiments under way with anti-BCA antisera allow
the hope of the working out of an immunological test with satisfactory specificity for breast carcinomas.

REFERENCES

(1)   Burtin, P., Sabine, M.C. and Chavanel, G. (1972): Int. J. Cancer,
       10, 72.
(2)   Burtin, P., Martin, F., Sabine, M.C. et al. (1972): J. Natl. Cancer
       Inst., 48, 25.

(3)   Kupchick, H.Z. and Zamcheck, N. (1972): Gastroenterology, 63, 95.
(4)   Laurence, J.R., Stevens, U., Bettelheim, R., Darcy, D., Leese,C., Turberville, C., Alexander, P., Johns, E.W. and Munro Neville, A. (1972): Brit. Med. J., 3, 605.
(5)   Lo Gerfo, P. and Herter, F.P. (1972): J. Surg. Oncol., 4, 1.
(6)   Pusztaszeri, G. and Mach, J.P. (1973): Immunochemistry, 10, 197.
(7)   Mor, C., Orefice, S., Rocco, F., Ferrara, R., Biancardi, C., Accinni, R. and Bartorelli, A. (1977): Neoplasma, 24, 345.
(8)   Bartorelli, A., Accinni, R., Golferini, A., Mistretta, A.P., Tassi, G.C., De Barbieri, A., Mor, C., Leonetti, G., Orefice, S. and Rocco, F. (1973): Boll. Ist. Sieroter. Milan., 52, 333.
(9)   Accinni, R., Bartorelli, A., Ferrara, R. and Biancardi, C. (1977): Experientia, 33, 88.
(10)   Bartorelli, A. and Accinni, R. (1977): Experientia, 33, 85.
(11)   Mistretta, A.P., Bartorelli, A., Golferini, A., Tassi, G.C., De Barbieri, A. and Accinni, R. (1974): Experientia, 30, 1209.

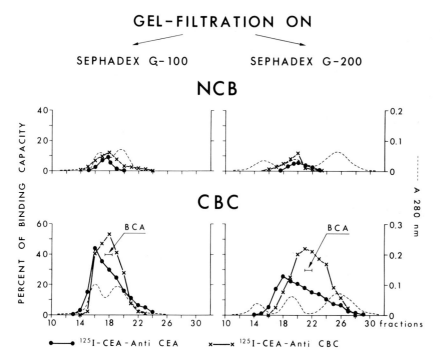

Fig. 1 Purification on Sephadex G–100 and Sephadex G–200 of Crude Breast Cancer (CBC) and Normal Crude Breast (NCB) by ion–exchange chromatography eluted at 0.05 M. Each fraction (100 μl) is monitored with ^{125}I CEA–anti–CEA (●—●) and ^{125}I CEA anti–CBC (×—×) radioimmunological system. The most active fractions on the ^{125}I CEA–anti–CBC system was termed BCA (Breast Cancer Antigen(s)).

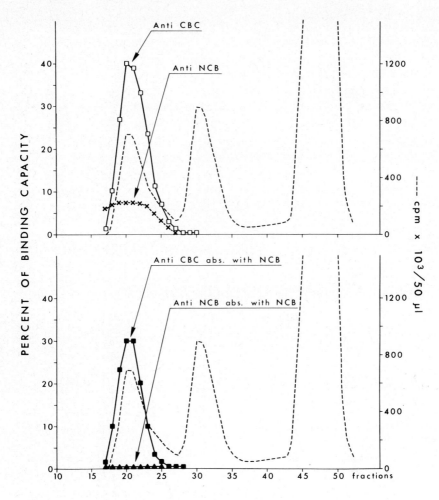

Fig. 2 Labelling of BCA. Elution profiles after gel filtration on Sephadex G-200. See the text.

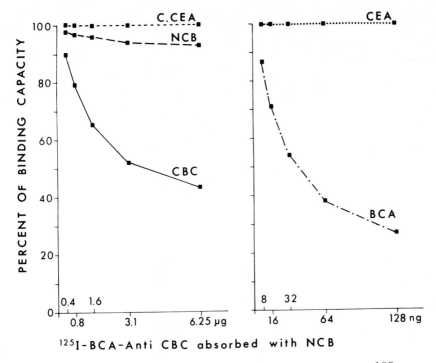

Fig. 3 Inhibition curves of the binding capacity of the RIA ^{125}I BCA–anti-CBC absorbed with NCB system. See the text.

DISCUSSION

BURTIN P. (Villejuif) : Did you measure the inhibition by plasma from breast cancer females in your system?

BARTORELLI A. (Milano) : We only measured pooled serum from females with and without breast cancer. The difference is significant but we have not,yet, individuals results.

STUDY OF THE CASEINE-LIKE MATERIAL IMMUNOREACTIVITY IN 150 PRIMARY BREAST TUMORS*

M. Assicot, T. Assicot, G. Voglino and C. Bohuon

Unité de Biologie Clinique et Expérimentale
Institut Gustave-Roussy, Villejuif.

INTRODUCTION

Casein, a milk protein, is present in quantities measurable by radioimmunoassay, in sera of normal women during pregnancy and lactation and in sera of bearers of breast cancer and other various cancers (1,2). This finding of casein as a possible breast tumor marker was questioned by further studies which were unable to demonstrate a significant increase of casein circulating levels in breast cancers (3). This discrepancy may be explained, in great part, by the high degree of heterogeneity of human casein and hence by the nature of the antibody and tracer used in the radioimmunoassay of this milk protein complex. Moreover, the immunoreactivity processes of "normal" and "neoplastic" caseins may involve reported differences in physico-chemical properties between these proteins (4).

We report here the results of caseine-like material measurements in normal, benign and malignant breast cytosols.

MATERIAL AND METHOD

Tissue preparation

Tumor samples were obtained from patients enduring mastectomy or biopsy. Within 15 min. of excision, tissues were dissected free of fat, weighed, minced and homogenized in 3 vol of ice-cold 0.01M Tris-buffer (pH 7.4) containing 12 mM dithiothreitol and 10 % of glycerol. The homegenate was immediately centrifuged at 105,000 x g for 60 min. The cytosol used for assay was sometimes stored at -80° up to 3 weeks. Protein concentration was determined according to the method of Lowry et al. (5) using crystalline bovine serum albumine as a standard.

Antiserum preparation

Rabbits were immunized with purified casein obtained from human milk by acid precipitation at pH 4.6 (6). The precipitate was freeze-dried, ether defatted and submitted to Ultrogel chromatography (A C A 54) to eliminate α - lactalbumine. Approximately 250 μg of protein were homogenized in complete Freund's adjuvant and I.D. injected in about 20 sites along the rabbit's backbone. A booster injection was given 6 weeks later. After 4 more weeks, the animals

* Supported by INSERM (Grant ATP 24-75-47)

were bled and the sera stored in small aliquots at -20°. The antiserum was adsorbed against at 10-fold excess of normal male serum and was
used in radioimmunoassay at a 1:30,000 dilution.

Preparation of radiolabelled casein

Labelling of casein was effected by a modification of the procedure of Hunster and Greenwood (7). All reagents were dissolved in
sodium phosphate buffer 0.05 M, pH 7.5 - 15 µl of buffer, 1mCi of
Na^{125}I (Amersham) in 10 µl, 25 µg of chloramine T in 15 µl were added
successively to 5µg of casein in 10 µl. The oxydation was stopped
after 30 sec with 50 µg of metabisulfite in 10 µl. Labelled protein
was purified by chromatography on Sephadex G-100 (0.6 x 18 cm) in
0.05 M phosphate buffer, pH 7.5, containing 0.2 % bovine albumin.
Specific activities were generally 50 - 80 µCi/µg. Because of the
great instability of the labelled preparation, labelling was effected
just prior to assay.

Casein assay

A double antibody solid phase method was used in the radioimmunoassay. The incubation mixture consisted of labelled casein, (approximately 10,000 cpm), 0.1 ml of tumor cytosol and a 1:30,000 dilution
of antiserum, in a final volume of 0.4 ml of 0.05 M phosphate buffer
with 0.5 % bovine serum albumine and 0.05 % of NaN$_3$. 0.1 ml of a pool
of normal male serum was added to each standard tube. The mixture was
allowed to stand overnight at room temperature. Then 0.5 ml of a sus-
pension of an anti-rabbit gamma-globulin immunoadsorbent was added.
The mixture was shaken by gentle rotation for 4 H at room temperature.
The precipitate was collected by centrifugation, washed and counted
directly in a gamma scintillation-counter.

RESULTS

Tumors were obtained from new consulters coming to the hospital
for investigation or treatment. 148 cytosols preparations were examined from women 18-80 year-old with primary breast tumors. Grading of
all the tumors and axillary lymph-node involvement was analysed by
histological examination.

The histologically benign tumors consisted of 13 fibroadenomas,
3 cystosarcoma phyllodes and 3 sclerocystic diseases. The "normal"
breast tissues were obtained from the ill breast of women with mammary carcinomas.

Fig. 1 shows the results of assays for human casein in cytosols.
Five of 6 normal breast tissues had a casein level below 2 ng/mg
protein while the measured level reached 10.6 ng in 1 case. 17 of
19 specimens of benign breast tumor had not detectable casein or had
values ≤ 2 ng/mg protein. 2 patients had a level between 2 and
3.8 ng/mg protein. Since 24 of 25 (96 %) non-malignant tissues ranged
under 4 ng/mg protein, this value has been choosen as the upper limit
of normality.

Positive levels of casein were found in 14.8 % of 148 women with primary mammary carcinoma. 19 patients had a level between 4 and 20 ng/mg protein. The casein level was raised over 100 ng/mg protein in 3 cases. The highest value (117 ng/mg protein) was found in a tumor where necrosis areas were large.

At last, casein was measured in the tumor cytosols from patients with sarcoma (5) and melanoma (3). None of these 8 specimens showed a positive level of casein.

DISCUSSION

In this study only 15 % of the 148 breast primary tumor specimens exhibited increased casein levels. No histological or clinical characteristic could be correlated to the presence of casein in these tumors. These results agree with those reported by Monaco et al. (3) who found 17 % (8 out of 47) breast cancer tumors positive for casein by radioimmunoassay. Hurlimann et al. (8), using immunofluorescence techniques found a similar frequency of casein positivity (5 of 43 cancer tumors examined). Besides, in our study on the basis of a more limited number of cases, no benign breast tumor or other malignant tissue exhibited increased casein levels. In our knowledge nor former data are available, about the presence of casein in other cancer tissues but breast tumor specimens.

Looking forward at a clinical usefulness, it can be noticed that a cancer marker has to be detected in the serum and not only in the tumor itself. In fact, a systematic approach correlating tissue and serum casein levels in the same patient has not been made. However two previous reports may give interesting indications. Zangerle et al. (2) found 15 % of casein positivity in the serum of breast cancer patients at the onset of clinical course. At the opposite, Monaco et al. (3) reported elevated casein levels in non-malignant disease states (renal failure, inflammation) and more seldom in serum samples from breast cancer patients. In all these experiments, anti-casein preparation were obtained from purified fractions corresponding to various types of milk casein. Hence, differences in the antisera reactivity and specificity might be responsible for the failure to detect casein-like material observed in some cancer patients.

In our opinion, it is not excluded that the observed immunoreactivity might be due to some inflammatory proteins and not related to the cancer.

REFERENCES

(1) Hendrick, J.C. and Franchimont, P. (1974) : Europ, J. Cancer, 10, 725.
(2) Zangerle, P.F., Hendrick, A., Thirion, A. and Franchimont, P. (1976) : in Cancer Related Antigens, edited by Franchimont. North-Holland. p 61.

(3) Monaco, M.E., Bronzert, D.A., Tormey, D.C., Waalkes, P. and
    Lippman, M.E. (1977) : Cancer Res., 37, 749
(4) Hendrick, J.C., Thirion, A. and Franchimont, P. (1976) : in
    Cancer Related Antigens, edited by Franchimont, North-Holland
    p 51
(5) Lowry, O.H., Rosebrough, N.J., Farr, A.L. and Randall, R.J.
    (1951) : J. biol. Chem., 193, 265.
(6) Malpress, F.H. and Hytten, F.E. (1974) : Biochem. J., 91, 130
(7) Hunter, W. and Greenwood, F. (1962) : Nature, 194, 495
(8) Hurlimann, J., Lichaa, M. and Ozzello, L. (1976) : Cancer Res.,
    36, 1284.

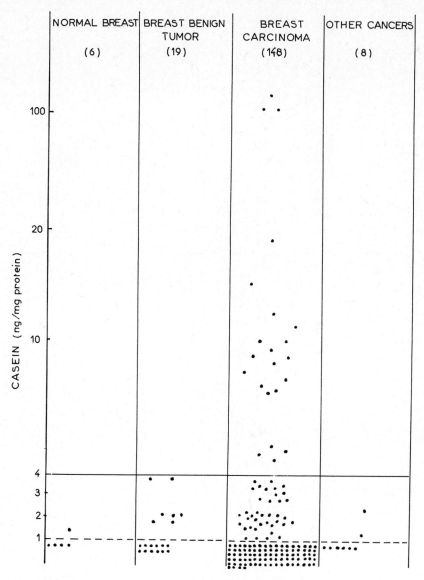

CASEIN LEVELS IN NORMAL AND ABNORMAL HUMAN
TISSUES

Fig. 1 Casein levels in normal and abnormal human tissues.

DISCUSSION

BOUNAMOUX Y. (Bâle): It is well known that fibrinogen and fragments of fibrinogen can cross react in casein radioimmunoassay. Have you taken care of this?

ASSICOT M.(Villejuif): We have not investigated that particular point; Franchimont's group has shown that fibrinogen and fragment D and E of fibrinogen had no effect on the system.

SIZARET P. (Lyon) : How many precipitating lines have you found in immunoelectrophoresis? You have shown us 25 fractions in normal electrophoresis.

ASSICOT M.(Villejuif): We have partial cross reaction with the different caseins. Immunoelectrophoretic analysis of human whole casein showed two precipiting lines with our anti-casein serum.

SIZARET P. (Lyon): My opinion is that as long as your assay is not monospecified, you cannot drawn any conclusion.

CARCINOEMBRYONIC ANTIGEN IN CANCER OF THE FEMALE GENITAL TRACT. A CLINICAL APPRAISAL.*

S. K. Khoo

University of Queensland Department of Obstetrics and Gynaecology, Brisbane, Australia.

The important impetus to our present understanding of tumour associated antigens as diagnostic markers in human cancer was the demonstration of carcinoembryonic antigen (CEA). In a series of tolerance and absorption experiments, Gold and Freedman (1) showed the interesting relationship of CEA to embryonic tissues in colonic cancer. The development of sensitive radioimmunoassay methods for the measurement of quantitative levels in blood (2) led to a proliferation of studies directed to the immunobiological and clinical aspects of CEA and an intensified search for other onco-fetal antigens.

Although the originally-held idea that CEA was specific to colonic cancer was not confirmed, the detection of CEA in tumours of other body systems has opened up a new field of cancer immunodiagnosis The clinical significance of CEA, however, has been blurred by its detection in serum of some patients with non-cancerous conditions.

Requirements as a useful circulating tumour marker appear to be met by CEA in several respects. CEA, a surface membrane glycoprotein is continually shed and released into the circulation and other biological fluids its level in serum is related to the amount and extent of tumour, and is rapidly cleared after complete removal of the tumour. This information has produced a growing interest in the application of CEA to clinical practice How useful a contribution the measurement of CEA makes to the management of cancer remains to be fully determined.

In the present review, attention is focused on CEA in tumours of the female genital tract, with emphasis given to its clinical application and problems of interpretation.

PATIENTS AND METHODS

Our results are based on a 6-year study of 459 women with cancer of the ovary, uterine cervix and body. Close followup was carried out at the Queensland Radium Institute. Diagnosis in each instance was made by histological examination of the tumour and detailed assessment provided by a Consultative Clinic which consisted of gynaecologists, radiotherapists and medical oncologists. Further data were obtained from 568 patients with other cancers, 178 with

* Support by grants from the National Health and Medical Research Council of Australia and the Queensland Cancer Fund.

intra-epithelial cancer of the cervix, 821 patients with benign conditions, and 360 control subjects - a total of 2,386 patients were studied.

In this study, the double-antibody radioimmunoassay was used (5). 0.025 ml of serum was sampled without perchloric acid extraction and immune complexes of CEA and goat anti-CEA were precipitated with rabbit anti-goat serum. This assay, although less specific than the Z-gel assay, is more applicable to a smaller serum volume and provides a greater facility for multiple assays. To date, nearly 6,000 tests have been performed. Prior extraction with perchloric acid was used in tissue studies.

RESULTS AND COMMENTS

General considerations

There is a wide distribution of CEA in serum and tissues, differences between cancerous and non-cancerous conditions appear to be quantitative rather than qualitative. In our studies (21)the highest tissue content of CEA was found in tumours, especially those of the gastrointestinal tract. Tissue CEA content in female genital tract tumours was low; the mean value of 75 ng per g wet weight was lower than that in the gastrointestinal tract of the early fetus but higher than that of the adult. Similarly, a general survey of CEA in serum, at the level of 5 ng per ml, showed a clear gradation of CEA-positivity in patients with cancer at a stage when the tumours were clinically evident (Fig. 1). On the basis of these results, the 'CEA-associated cancers' defined as those which gave a 50% or greater incidence of positive CEA results are as follows, in order of frequency: gastrointestinal, lung, breast and female genital tract. However, consideration has to be given to some CEA-positivity in health and benign diseases (Fig. 2.). In inflammatory conditions of the bowel, liver and pancreas, although the levels were usually low, the rates of positivity were significantly high, between 25 and 64%. However, in the absence of these conditions, CEA estimation is diagnostically useful because its detection in subjects with no apparent disease or those with benign gynaecological conditions was less than 5%.

The CEA of colonic tumour origin, a complex glycoprotein macromolecule of about 200,000 Daltons (6) was reported to show some heterogeneity by accepted physicochemical and immunochemical parameters (7). However, less is known of CEA in other types of tumours. Recently, CEA in squamous carcinoma of the cervix was found to be immunologically identical to colonic CEA, although the molecule appeared to be much larger (8). Our findings of CEA in ascitic fluid and tumour tissue obtained from patients with ovarian cancer also demonstrated immunological similarity with colonic tumour CEA. Its elution profile on gel chromatography suggested 200,000 Daltons in molecular size, and after ^{125}I-iodination, the peak radioactivity coincided with that of colonic tumour CEA.

Detection in intraepithelial carcinoma

The expression of CEA during the process of malignant transformation remains intriguing, particularly in the intraepithelial phase, an easily identifiable lesion in the uterine cervix. Most studies reported the detection of CEA in serum in about 30% of patients with intraepithelial carcinoma (so-called pre-invasive). Van Nagell and co-workers (9) showed the relation of CEA levels to the amount of disease and the presence of glandular extension, as well as to residual disease after conization. Our findings in 178 patients (Fig. 3) revealed a correlation between the rate of CEA-positivity and serum levels and the extent of intraepithelial changes in the uterine cervix. Whether the detection of CEA in the pre-invasive stage of cancer is a feature of the malignant potential of the disease, however, remains to be evaluated. The lack of clear-cut tumour specificity of CEA was shown in 2 further groups of women (Table 1).

TABLE 1   Serum CEA levels in women during pregnancy and with minor problems

| | Percentage Positive Results | |
	5 - 10 ng/ml	>10 ng/ml
Pregnant Women (121)		
First trimester	20	0
Second trimester	29	0
Third trimester	53	5
Women attending cytology clinic in Brisbane No cervical neoplasia found (149)		
'Erosion and cervicitis'	8*	5*

*   Majority aged over 50 years, and smokers.
     Most repeat tests negative

Pregnancy was associated with low CEA levels, the incidence increased from 20% in the first trimester to 53% in the third trimester. Women with minor cervical problems of 'erosion and cervicitis', after assessment at the Cytology Clinic, also showed a 13% incidence of CEA-positive results. The majority of these women were over 50 years and smokers; the influence of these factors has been alluded (20) to and could explain the transient detection of CEA in some of them. Nevertheless, there were a few women with CEA-positive results without identifiable cause.

Detection in invasive carcinoma

There is general agreement that CEA is frequently detectable in serum and plasma of patients with invasive cancer of the female genital tract (10,11).Of the 3 onco-fetal antigens surveyed in our studies, only CEA was of diagnostic value in cancers of the ovary, cervix and body (Table 2). CEA was detectable in 61% of patients with ovarian cancer, 60% with cervical cancer, and 77% with body cancer. Although the incidence of CEA-positivity in patients with trophoblastic neoplasms (hydatidiform mole and choriocarcinoma) was 52%, the marker of choice in this tumour type is undoubtedly β-subunit chorionic gonadotrophin (βHCG) which was detected in 100% of patients.

TABLE 2 Detection of circulating tumour markers in female genital cancer

	Percentage Positive Results			
	Ovary (213)	Uterine Cervix (185)	Uterine Body (61)	Tropho-blast (85)
Carcinoembryonic antigen	61	60	77	52
Alphafetoprotein	17*	1*	3*	-
β-Subunit chorionic gonadotrophin	11+	-	-	100

* Low levels in advanced epithelial tumours, high levels in germ cell tumours.
+ Only in germ cell tumours (teratoma)
( ) Number of patients

The use of alphafetoprotein (AFP) and β-HCG was restricted to germ cell tumours of the ovary. Highly elevated AFP levels were obtained in patients with these tumours, especially those containing yolk sac or immature glial elements, and low levels of β-HCG were sometimes found in patients with malignant teratoma. However, low levels of AFP were also detected in some patients with advanced epithelial tumours metastatic to the liver.

It is quite clear that the frequency of detection and level of CEA in serum are dependent on the extent of tumour spread. In our series, this relationship held for cancers of the ovary, cervix and body (Table 3).

TABLE 3 Serum CEA levels in relation to stage in cancer of ovary, uterine cervix and body

Stage of Disease	% Incidence of Positive Results (High Levels > 20 ng per ml)*		
	Ovary (213)	Cervix (185)	Body (61)
I	50 (2)	57 (16)	36
II	40 (10)	62 (26)	39
III	75 (25)	50 (33)	81
IV	73 (52)	75 (50)	90

For patients with localized disease (stage I and II), the incidence of positive results was much higher in cancers of the ovary and cervix than in those of the body, possibly because the tumour in cancer of the body was usually small in amount and exophytic. In the presence of dissemination, higher CEA levels were often obtained, and a level exceeding 20 ng per ml usually indicated metastatic disease involving the liver.

CEA in ascitic fluid

Antigenic proteins, continually being produced and shed from the tumour cells in an intraperitoneal tumour, would be expected to appear in the peritoneal fluid. Such is the case with CEA in ovarian cancer which often presents with ascitic fluid. In our study of the frequency of detection of CEA in serum and ascitic fluid obtained simultaneously in 38 patients, 18 patients showed CEA in both types of fluid, with a correlation between serum and ascitic fluid levels. The notable feature was the detection of CEA in only one type of fluid in 15 patients. In the 6 patients with a positive result in serum, the pelvis was usually 'frozen', with the tumour extending to the bowel and pelvic walls. This suggests an easier access of CEA to the circulation than to the peritoneal cavity. On the other hand, in the 9 patients with a positive result in ascitic fluid, the tumour was often found to infiltrate widely the peritoneal surface and omentum. On the basis of these findings, the practice of culdocentesis to obtain peritoneal fluid for the measurement of CEA should increase the diagnostic accuracy in patients with suspected ovarian cancer or those under followup.

Detection of residual and metastatic tumour

The followup of genital cancer in women is often bedevilled by an inability to assess the adequacy of treatment. Several suggestions for the use of serial CEA levels in gastrointestinal cancer have been made - postoperative rate of disappearance in prognosis (12), determination of postoperative residual or metastatic tumour, especially to the liver (3), and monitoring of disease and effects of treatment (13). However, caution in interpretation is necessary in each instance because of 'missed' progressions of disease and 'false positive' CEA results in some patients (4, 14).

In female genital cancer, we have shown the rapid return of CEA levels to negative after complete excision of tumour (15). For example, CEA disappeared completely from the serum 2 weeks following radical hysterectomy for cancer of the cervix, whereas when the same type of cancer was treated by radiotherapy, CEA levels fluctuated markedly for more than 12 weeks before becoming negative. The latter observation is interpreted as a result of less rapid changes in the tumour mass induced by radionecrosis.

We were particularly interested in serum CEA levels in patients with residual ovarian cancer, after the diagnosis and assessment of the tumour had been made at operation. Some prognostic significance was shown in patients followed for at least 12 months, the CEA level on first presentation being directly related to subsequent tumour behaviour (Table 4). Whereas 38% of CEA-negative patients showed no evidence of disease, the corresponding figure in those with high CEA levels was only 19%.

306

TABLE 4   Relation of initial CEA level to subsequent prognosis in
patients with residual ovarian tumour

| | Prognosis (Percentage of patients) | | |
	NED	ISQ	Pro-death
Undetectable CEA	38	32	30
Low CEA levels (5 - 10 ng per ml)	35	22	43
High CEA levels (> 10 ng per ml)	19	28	53

NED: No evidence of disease,   ISQ: Disease unchanged,
Pro-death: Progressive disease leading to death

Features influencing CEA detection in residual tumour

It is difficult to appreciate why and how some tumours, known
to be present as residual masses in the body were not associated with
detectable CEA. In our series of 130 patients with ovarian cancer
the influence of the following features were evaluated: clinical
stage which was either III or IV, histological type, site of tumour
in the body, organs involved by tumour, estimated tumour volume, and
age of the patient. Three interesting points were revealed in the
analysis. Firstly, despite the known presence of tumour, only 64%
of patients showed CEA in the serum. Secondly, there were no differences in the distribution of CEA-positive and CEA-negative patients
in relation to the features studied. That certain tumours do not
produce CEA is thus a likely reason for the failure to detect CEA in
serum. Thirdly, a correlation between serum CEA levels and the site
of tumour, organs involved and estimated tumour volume was found among
CEA-positive patients. Whilst no differences in distribution were
apparent between CEA-negative and low CEA-positive patients, there was
a preponderance of patients with high CEA levels when the tumour was
located in the pelvis and abdomen (44%) and when the tumour had infiltrated the peritoneum and greater omentum (46%).

Monitoring of tumour and treatment

Problems in management such as the inability to detect small
postoperative recurrences and the relative difficulty to assess the
impact of further therapy are particularly increased in ovarian cancer,
a disease where the tumour is inaccessible to examination. Even if
the tumour appears to be completely resected, at least one-third will
develop recurrent tumour. The use of a CEA NOMOGRAM (16), which measured the observed CEA level against the 95% confidence limits, allowed
a correct call of tumour recurrence in 22 of 25 patients with gastrointestinal cancer; this antedated the other investigations by 3 or
more months. The usefulness of serial CEA levels in monitoring less
rapid changes in tumour mass was shown in our 10-month study of 25
patients with ovarian cancer who received chemotherapy (17). In
general, rapidly falling CEA levels were associated with a favourable
tumour response, and rising or elevated levels with progressive tumour

growth. However, the paradoxical fall in CEA levels in some patients in the terminal phase of cancer, although not a clinical problem, raises the possibility of disturbance of CEA release and clearance.

Prompt recognition of recurrence is not often possible during longterm followup and late detection is given as a reason for poor survival. The use of tumour markers, in particular CEA, was previously found to be of assistance in some but not other studies (18, 19). In order to define the predictive value of serial monthly estimations of CEA, 213 patients with ovarian cancer were prospectively followed over 5 years. Assessment was made in 3 groups of patients: those with no residual tumour, those with a minimal tumour, and those with a large tumour. The treatment protocol after surgery consisted of radiotherapy and subsequent intermittent chemotherapy in the first 2 groups, and chemotherapy in the third.

If the 'non-CEA-producing' tumours - 35.2% in this series - were excluded, the patterns of CEA levels were useful in predicting tumour behaviour. This was shown especially in patients with no residual tumour at the beginning of the study (Table 5).

TABLE 5   Predictive value of serial CEA levels in longterm followup of ovarian cancer.

No apparent residual tumour (58 patients)

Serial serum levels	Tumour Status		
	Free	Recurrence	Progressive-Death
Rapid disappearance remaining negative (13)	13	-	-
Persistently low levels (8)	8	-	-
Re-appearance after initial disappearance (12)	7 (5)*	4	1
No detection throughout (25)	25	-	-

*   Transient

In general, a rapid disappearance of CEA in serum or low levels was associated with a good prognosis; all 21 patients showed no evidence of tumour. The re-appearance of CEA indicated recurrent or progressive tumour in 5 of 12 patients. To date, the others showed no evidence of tumour, but CEA was only transiently detectable in 5. The predictive value in patients with minimal residual tumour was more variable. However, a good prognosis was again associated with CEA patterns showing, not only a rapid disappearance, but also a delayed fall or persistently low levels. All 11 patients were either free of disease or had residual disease under control. The re-appearance of CEA was observed in another 11 patients, and 8 had developed recurrence or had progressive disease. However, no evidence of tumour was found in 3 despite close surveillance. The interpretation of the re-

appearance of CEA in the absence of tumour is uncertain at present.
Transient detection may reflect the influence of chemotherapy on
selected tumour cell populations or extraneous effects such as smoking. Perhaps, in some of these patients, tumour recurrence has remained occult, and the period of observation is not sufficiently long
to allow detection by the conventional means. Table 6 shows the CEA
patterns in the presence of a large residual tumour where the serial
CEA levels were more variable and complex, and their interpretation
more difficult.

TABLE 6   Predictive value of serial CEA levels in longterm followup
of ovarian cancer

Large residual tumour (110 patients)

Serial serum levels	Tumour status			
	NED	Res-R	Res-ISQ	Prog.-D
Rapid disappearance remaining negative (8)	2	1	3	2
Delayed fall (2)	-	-	2	-
Persistently low levels	4	1	13	2
Re-appearance after initial disappearance (27)	1	1 (1)*	4 (2)*	21
Persistently high or rapidly rising levels (26)	-	-	2	24
No detection throughout (27)	6	4	5	12

* - Transient;   NED - No evidence of disease;   Res-R - Residual response;   Res-ISQ - Residual unchanged;   Prog-D - Progressive/Death.

In general, patterns showing a rapid disappearance of CEA, delayed fall, and persistently low levels, were frequently associated
with a more favourable prognosis. In the majority of these patients
(18 of 30) the residual tumour had remained unchanged, and another
8 patients showed tumour response, some of which were complete. However, there were 4 patients who continued to deteriorate or had died.
The pattern showing a reappearance of CEA was generally associated
with deterioration -13 patients had progressive disease and 8 had
died. An exception to the expected prediction of the CEA levels was
observed in 6 patients - the residual tumour was unchanged in 4 and
had responded to treatment in another 2; but the detection of CEA
was transient in some. Patterns of persistently high or rapidly rising CEA levels were predictive of progressive tumour activity with
greater precision, in 24 of 26 patients.

It is therefore timely, on the basis of current information, to
consider the use of CEA levels in continuing management. Whether
asymptomatic patients with genital tract cancer who show rising CEA
levels without other evidence of recurrence can derive benefit from
further treatment such as 'second-look' surgery or chemotherapy is

being determined. Early reports in gastrointestinal cancer are encouraging (16). In the individual patient, attention given to the
sequential changes in CEA levels has allowed an earlier institution
of treatment in some cases. This is illustrated in Fig. 4.

The patient had a stage II squamous cell carcinoma of the cervix,
treated initially by radiotherapy. A marked rise in CEA level led
immediately to the detection of a vaginal recurrence which was treated by Wertheim hysterectomy. A subsequent rise, signalling the appearance of a recurrence in the obturator region, was promptly followed by chemoimmunotherapy. The patient had remained well; the much
lower CEA levels detected periodically thereafter, probably reflected
the gradual response of the tumour.

CONCLUSION

Of the difficulties in the management of female genital tract
cancer, some are special to these tumours and others are common to
all tumours. In general terms, CEA is the most useful tumour marker
available. Its estimation in blood can provide some assistance when
the diagnosis of the primary tumour is in doubt, but the problem of
nonspecificity, especially within the range of 5 - 10 ng per ml, has
to be considered. Its value in the monitoring of disease has been
enhanced by the knowledge that a proportion of tumours do not produce
CEA, the time taken for CEA to disappear from the circulation is influenced by the therapeutic modality, and serum levels are related to
the site and volume of CEA-producing tumours. However, the transient
detection of CEA in the absence of a clinical tumour and 'false negative' results remain to be clarified. The CEA assay provides a useful guide to longterm followup of intrapelvic tumours such as of the
genital tract because these tumours are not easily accessible to examination. However, interpretation in the full knowledge of the
clinical situation is important.

ACKNOWLEDGEMENT

The collaboration with Professor E. Mackay and the staff of the
Queensland Radium Institute is greatly appreciated. The CEA and anti-
CEA reagents for the radioimmunoassay were kindly donated by Doctors
P. Gold and P. Burtin.

REFERENCES

(1)   Gold, P., and Freedman, S. O. (1965): J. exp. Med., 121: 439.
(2)   Thomson, D. M. P., Krupey, J., Freedman, S. O., and Gold, P.
       (1969): Proceedings, National Academy Science, U.S.A., 64: 161.
(3)   Zamcheck, N. (1975): Cancer, 36: 2460.
(4)   Martin, E. W., Kibbey, W. E., DiVecchia, L., Anderson, G.,
       Catalano, P., and Minton, J. P. (1976): Cancer, 37: 62.
(5)   MacSween, J. M., Warner, N. L., Bankhurst, A. D., and Mackay,
       I. R. (1972): Brit. J. Cancer, 26: 356.
(6)   Krupey, J., Wilson, T., Freedman, S. O., and Gold, P. (1972):
       Immunochemistry, 9: 617.
(7)   Banjo, C., Shuster, J., and Gold, P. (1974): Cancer Res., 34:
       2114.

(8) Goldenberg, D. M., Pletsch, Q. A., and Van Nagell, J. R. (1976): Gynec. Oncol., 4: 204.
(9) Van Nagell, J. R., Meeker, W. R., Parker, J. C., Kashmiri, R., and McCollum, V. (1976): Amer. J. Obstet. Gynec., 126: 1.
(10) Reynoso, G., Chu, T. M., Guinan, P., and Murphy, G. P. (1972): Cancer, 30: 1.
(11) Van Nagell, J. R., Meeker, W. R., Parker, J. C., and Harralson, J. D. (1975): Cancer, 35: 1372.
(12) Lo Gerfo, D., Krupey, J., Herter, F. (1972): Amer. J. Surg., 123: 127.
(13) Holyoke, E. D., Chu, T. M., and Murphy, G. P. (1975): Cancer, 35: 830.
(14) Meeker, W. R. Jr., Kashmiri, R., Hamler, L., Clapp, W., and Griffen, W. O. Jr. (1973): Arch. Surg., 197: 266.
(15) Khoo, S. K., and Mackay, E. V. (1973): Aust. N.Z. J. Obstet. Gynaec., 13: 1.
(16) Martin, E. W. Jr., James, K. K., Hurtubise, P. E., Catalano, P., and Minton, J. P. (1977): Cancer, 39: 440.
(17) Khoo, S. K., and Mackay, E. V. (1976): Brit. J. Obstet. Gynaec., 83: 753.
(18) Khoo, S. K., and Mackay, E. V. (1974): Cancer, 34: 542.
(19) Samaan, N. A., Smith, J. P., Rutledge, F. N., and Schultz, P. N. (1976): Amer. J. Obstet. Gynec., 126: 186.
(20) Stevens, D. P., Mackay, I. R., and Busselton Population Studies Group (1973): Lancet, 2: 1238.
(21) Khoo, S. K., Warner, N. L., Lie, J. T., and Mackay, I. R. (1973): Int. J. Cancer, 11: 681.

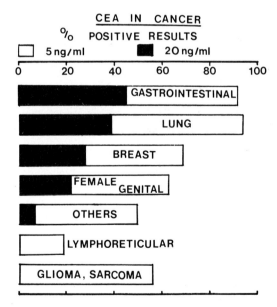

Fig. 1. Survey of CEA-positivity in serum of patients with various cancers at a stage when the tumour is clinically evident, showing the 'CEA-associated' cancers.

311

CEA IN HEALTH AND BENIGN DISEASES

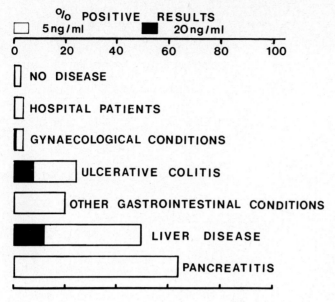

Fig. 2. Survey of CEA-positivity in serum of patients with non-cancerous conditions and subjects with no apparent disease.

SERUM CEA AND NEOPLASIA OF THE CERVIX

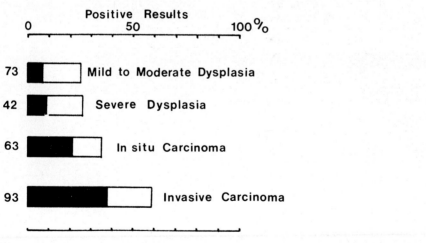

Fig. 3. CEA-positivity in serum of patients with intraepithelial and invasive cancer of the uterine cervix.

312

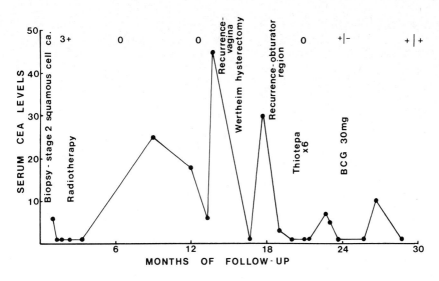

Fig. 4. Case study of a patient with Stage II sqaumous cell carcinoma of the cervix, showing rise in CEA levels in relation to detection of recurrence and treatment.

DISCUSSION

SEPPALA M.(Helsinki): You had a slide showing that, after surgical removal, the CEA level dropped from 50,0 ng/ml to less than 5 ng/ml within a week. If you calculate the half-life of CEA from this figure, you get less than 2 days, actually not much more than 1 day. Do you have any experience on the half-life of CEA?

KHOO S.K.(Brisbane): As far as the half-life is concerned, I think if you have a day to day estimation,that is the only way you can assess the half-life. Now with regards to the half-life , if you estimate weekly, after surgical excision, half-life could be around one to two weeks. If you mesure day to day the levels do not come down straight and are fluctuating up and down and that is why I call day to day variation.

SEPPALA M. (Helsinki): How can the CEA level show day-to-day variation if the half-life is one or two weeks?

KHOO S.K. (Brisbane): We do not know what happens in between. It will be about half a week.

SEPPALA M. (Helsinki): But blood transfusion could explain why the level dropped after operation.

KHOO S.K. (Brisbane): It could.

TALERMAN A. (Rotterdam): May I ask two questions :
1) The first concerns the association of glial elements with raised alpha-fetoprotein in your germ cell tumour. We do not have the same results.
2) The other point is : how do you explain the high incidence of raised serum CEA in patients with gynecological malignancies, as compared to other authors.

KHOO S.K. (Brisbane): To your first question, there is a big study done by the Japanese (TOSHIDA) in which he examined about 70 germ cell tumours. He has also remarked that there were two in which there were some immature glial elements with no evidence of yolk sac elements. We had, in our experience only two patients with so called immature glial elements which gave raised elevated AFP.
But in the majority, we agree, this included mainly endodermal sinus tumour.
For the second question : I think both the cut-off point you accept as positive, and the method you use, could be responsible for the increased incidence.

SEPPALA M. (Helsinki): I would like to address my question to all speakers. Has anybody performed a second-look surgery on the basis of re-elevated CEA level in gynecologic cancers?

KHOO S.K. (Brisbane): I think our experience is very limited at the present time and is only anecdotal. We had recently 3 patients with cervical cancer and the first abnormal thing was the raised CEA and at that stage, we were mainly assessing the patients more carefully, repeating the test and this went on for about 3 months. This first patient, after 3 months of observations, showed abnormal cells in the vaginal smear and then was submitted to laparotomy.
At laparotomy, the uterus and adnexa were removed and according to the pathologists there was a focus of dysplastic cells in the area of the cervix. The patient was initially treated by radiotherapy.
The second patient had a sudden elevation in CEA. She appeared perfectly well; we did the same thing and we observed a carcinoma of the splenic flexure of the colon.
The third patient had an elevation and then the levels fell back to normal and did not rise again. After curettage, abnormal cells were found in the uterus. So if the levels are substained over a period of time, I think they are more likely to be due to malignant recurrence than to other factors known to cause temporary elevations of CEA.

TALERMAN A. (Rotterdam): This already shows us how important is the fact that we must determine all these antigens serially and that single determinations are insufficient in the follow-up of these patients. They may be useful sometimes, when the levels are high, for diagnosis, but in the follow-up, I think serial determinations over a considerable time are always necessary.

DIAGNOSTIC AND PROGNOSTIC USE OF CARCINOEMBRYONIC ANTIGEN IN MALIGNANT TUMORS OF THE FEMALE GENITAL TRACT

P.HAEGELE, J.C.PETIT, D.RODIER, J.C.JANSER, M.EBER.

Centre Régional de Lutte contre le cancer Paul Strauss Strasbourg.

SUMMARY

Serum carcinoembryonic antigen (CEA) levels were determined for 204 patients with primary invasive squamous cell carcinoma of the cervix and 23 patients with recurrent squamous cell carcinoma of the cervix, for 67 patients with primary endometrial adenocarcinoma and 19 patients with recurrent endometrial adenocarcinoma and for 73 patients with recurrences or residual diseases after incomplete surgery of serous cystadenocarcinoma of the ovary. A double antibody radioimmunoassay (CIS - Saclay - France) was employed. The proportion of elevated (above 15 ng/ml) CEA levels increased from earlier stages (TI : 13 % and TII : 25 %) to later stages (TIII : 44 % and TIV : 56%) of cervical carcinoma. This low incidence of elevated serum levels of CEA at early stages was also found with endometrial cancer (TI : 15 % and TII : 27 %). The correlation between the incidence of elevated serum CEA levels and advancing stages is low in the groups of ovarian cancer (19 %) and endometrial cancer (16 %). Serial CEA assays performed on the patients with primary cervical carcinoma showed a correlation between the incidence of recurrences or the mortality rate and an elevated level before and/or after the initial treatment.

In this study, 356 patients with cervical,endometrial and ovarian carcinoma were investigated in order to evaluate the diagnostic and pronostic use of serum CEA levels, before and after surgical resection or radiotherapy of primary cancer and, in case of cervix, during the course following this treatment.

I. PATIENTS AND METHODS

A. Patient Selection and Classification

Patients admitted to hospital with primary gynecologic malignancy, histologically confirmed, were evaluated by clinical examination, by roentgenogram and by cystoscopy. Patients were staged according to the TNM classification (UICC,1972) for cervix and endometrium and to the FIGO staging system for ovary.

Patients with recurrences were considered to have had adequate primary treatment.

315

B. Serial CEA Measurements

Blood specimens for CEA were obtained prior to the onset of therapy (surgery and/or irradiation, chemotherapy) and subsequent specimens were drawn at the end of the radio-therapy or 7 days after surgery, and at intervals of 3 to 6 months in many cases.

C. Method of CEA Determinations

Serum CEA estimation were carried out by the double antibody solid phase radioimmunoassay, without perchloric extraction (Method CIS - Saclay - France). A CEA level of 10 ng/ml or greater was considered as "positive" but 15 ng/ml may be more realistic and we preferred this cut-off point for "elevated" values. The values from 5 ng/ml to 14 ng/ml were considered as borderline values.

II. RESULTS

A. CEA Levels and Disease Stage

1. Cervix (Table I)

The serum CEA values of patients with prima-ry invasive squamous cell carcinoma of the cervix in later stages of disease were higher than those in earlier stages: mean level of 7 ng/ml (0-43 ng/ml) in stage I and 40 ng/ml in stage IV (0-260 ng/ml). The percentage of values above 15 ng/ml increased from stage I (13 %) to stage IV (56 %). However in advanced stages of primary cancer and in recur-rences the proportion of low values remained important : 56 % of stage III patients, 44 % of stage IV patients and 57 % of patients with recurrences had CEA levels below 15 ng/ml.

TABLE I : Carcinoembryonic Antigen Values in 227 Patients with cervical squamous Carcinoma in Relation to the Clini-cal Stage.

Tumor Stage*	Number	Serum CEA (ng/ml)			
		0 - 4	5 - 9	10 - 14	> 15
Stage I	70	39(56%)	15(21%)	7(10%)	9(13%)
Stage II	79	30(38%)	18(23%)	11(14%)	20(25%)
Stage III	39	13(33%)	3(8%)	6(15%)	17(44%)
Stage IV	16	4(25%)	3(19%)	/	9(56%)
Recurrences	23	7(31%)	6(26%)	/	10(43%)

* TNM Classification (UICC, 1972)

In the group of patients with recurrences 2 out of 9 localized recurrences had levels about 15 ng/ml (22%) whereas

8 out of 14 regional recurrences had levels above 15 ng/ml (57 %); the mean values of CEA were respectively 6,5 ng/ml and 28 ng/ml.

2. Endometrium (Table II)

In earlier stages 15 % of stade I patients and 29 % of stage II-III patients had elevated CEA levels.

TABLE II : Carcinoembryonic ntigen Values on 86 patients with Endometrial Adenocarcinoma in Relation to the Clinical Stage.

Tumor Stage*	Number	Serum CEA (ng/ml)			
		0 - 4	5 - 9	10 - 14	⟩15
Stage I	53	25(47%)	16(30%)	4(8%)	8(15%)
Stage II	14	5(35%)	4(29%)	4(29%)	4(29%)
Recurrences	19	8(42%)	7(37%)	1(5%)	3(16%)

✳ TNM Classification (UICC, 1972)

The mean values were respectively 6,5 ng/ml (0-29) and 8 ng/ml (0-25). In the group of 19 patients with recurrences the CEA levels remained below 20 ng/nlexcept one case (136 ng/ml) and there were no differences in CEA levels between 7 localized recurrent diseases and 12 regional diseases or distant metastases; in both cases the proportion of levels below 15 ng/ml was high (84 %) and the mean value was 13 ng/ml (0-136 ng/ml).

3. Ovary (Table III).

In a group of 52 TIII-TIV patients and patients with recurrences the percentage of patients with elevated CEA levels was very low (21%) compared with a group of 21 patients with residual tumor after surgery but without clinical evident disease (14%). The mean values were respectively 15 ng/ml (0-154) and 7 ng/ml(0-25).

TABLE III : Carcinoembryonic Antigen Values in 73 Patients with Ovarian Serous Cystadenocarcinoma in Relation to the Clinical Stage.

Clinical stage		Serum CEA (ng/ml)			
		0 - 4	5 - 9	10 - 14	⟩15
No evident disease	21	9(43%)	5(24%)	4(19%)	3(14%)
TIII*- TIV* Recurrences	52	23(44%)	13(25%)	5(10%)	11(21%)

✳FIGO Staging system

317

B. CEA Levels following Primary Tumor Treatment

Following CEA values were taken once or more between the end of radiotherapy or the 7th day after resection and the 24th month after this treatment.

1. Cervix

In general, this carcinoma was treated by radiotherapy (intracavitary radium and/or external irradiation) and/or by extended hysterectomy (Wertheim or Colpohysterosalpingectomy).

Only 1 patient with stage I had elevated CEA level after treatment; this patient developed recurrence two years later. After 6 months 3 patients with initially CEA level above 10 ng/ml had recurrences whereas none of the patients with initially level below 10 ng/ml had recurrence. Besides in one patient, 15 months after treatment, the CEA increased from 0 to 37 ng and recurrence was evident 3 months later.

In stage II, 9 out of 20 patients (45%) with initial elevated values had persistent serial elevated values after treatment and developed recurrence before 2 years follow-up whereas 3 out of 10 (30%) patients with levels between 10-14 ng/ml and 3 out of 35 (9%) with levels below 10 ng/ml developed recurrence : in 4 of these 6 cases there were rising serial values.

For the stages III-IV little change in CEA level was noted after treatment. However 11 out of 23 patients (48%) with initially elevated CEA values died before 3 months, 13 out of 21 (62%) before 6 months and 14 out of 19 (74%) before 1 year, whereas in the group of patients with low values before the treatment 4 out of 19 (21%) died before 3 months, 5 out of 18 (28%) before 6 months and 10 out of 14 (71%) died before 1 year.

2. Endometrium

This carcinoma was treated by abdominal hysterectomy with pre or postoperative radiotherapy. Most of these patients had CEA values below 15 ng/ml after treatment and there was very often a lack of rise in CEA values when a recurrence appeared.

3. Ovary

Similarly, there was a great lack of correlation between increased tumor spread , evident residual disease or recurrence and increased CEA values. Low CEA levels remained stable despite progressive disease.

III. DISCUSSION

Earlier reports have schown a correlation between the amount of tumor or the extent of dissemination in multiple

318

gynecologic malignancies (1,2,3,5,7,11) and the incidence
of positive serum levels of CEA. The pronostic significance
of serum levels after treatment has been reported for female genital cancer (4,5,6,7,11) and in general a correlation
between decreasing CEA levels and decreasing tumor bulk
during treatment was found in patients in whom the cancer
was associated initially with high levels; if the treatment
appeared to be effective, there seemed to be a drop in the
serum CEA amount and inversely; a reappearance of elevated
values was concomittant to recurrence of clinical disease.
       The present data in cervical carcinoma were in gene-
ral agreement with these findings. With regard to the patients with endometrial carcinoma and ovarian cancer, the
present results were in disagreement with those of other authors
(2,5,7) who found a very high correlation between the stage
of malignancies and the frequency of elevated CEA levels.
However the failure reported here to demonstrate a good
correlation between tumor extent and positive CEA values
in case of endometrial and ovarian carcinoma is also reported by other authors (8,9). For the ovarian carcinoma it
was found (10) that CEA levels were only elevated in patients with mucinous ovarian tumors; this may perhaps explain our results with serous ovarian carcinoma.
       Besides, several patients, as in the present study,had
low CEA levels at the onset of the treatment or at time of
the recurrence; this would appear to be a limiting factor
in the use of the assay in the following of cancer.However
there is some support for the assumption that the CEA assay
would be of considerable help in patients with gynecologic
malignancies.

REFERENCES

(1)DISAIA P.J.,HAVERBACK B.T.,DYCE B.et al (1974)
     Surg.Gynecol.Obstet.138, 542
(2)DISAIA P.J.,HAVERBACK B.T.,DYCE B.et al (1975)
     Amer.J.Obstet.Gynec. 121, 159
(3)KHOO S.K.,MACKAY E.V. (1973)
     Aust.N.Z.J.Obstet.Gyn. 13, 107
(4)KHOO S.K.,MACKAY E.V. (1973)
     Aust.N.Z.J.Obstet.Gynaecol. 13, 1
(5)KHOO S.K.,MACKAY E.V. (1974)
     Cancer 34, 512-548
(6)DISAIA P.J.,MORROW C.P.,HAVERBACK B.J.et al.(1976)
     Obst.Gynec. 47, 95
(7)VAN NAGELL J.R.,MEEKER W.R.,PARKER J.C.et al.(1975)
     Cancer 35, 1372
(8)SEPPALA M.,PHIKO H.,RUOSLAHTI E. (1975)
     Cancer 35, 1377
(9)LOGERFO P., KRUPEY J., HANSEN H.(1971)
     N.Eng.J.Med. 285, 138
(10)VAN NAGELL J,PLETSCH Q.A.,GOLDENBERG D.M.(1975)
     Cancer Research 35, 1433
(11)BARRELET V., MACH J.P. (1975)
     Amer.J. Obstet. Gynec. 121, 164-168

DISCUSSION

LARRA F. (Angers): If pre-treatment CEA level is within normal range, we are unable to show an increase in CEA predictable of metastatic spread. Our opinion is that in these cases, CEA is not useful.

HAEGELE P. (Strasbourg): I agree with you. In our patients without elevated CEA before treatment, only one increase predictable for metastases was observed. In contrast, when the initial level is high, we found that CEA is a very useful marker.

MACH J.P. (Lausanne): Your comment is probably true for gynecological cancer, but we have observed in several cases of colonic carcinoma that metastases are associated with increased CEA levels, even if pre-operative CEA levels lay in the normal range.

CARCINO-EMBRYONIC ANTIGEN IN PATIENTS WITH GYNECOLOGICAL MALIGNANCIES
TREATED WITH IRRADIATION.

BOLLA M., HORIOT J.C., BORDES M., GUERRIN J., LE DORZE C.

Centre Georges-François Leclerc (Director : Pr. F. CABANNE)
DIJON, France.

INTRODUCTION

The carcino-embryonic antigen (CEA) is found in 50 % of
patients with malignancies outside of the digestive tract such as
gynecological malignancies : DISAIA (3) (4), KHOO and MACKAY (9),
BARRELET and MACH (1), DONALDSON (5)...

At the Georges-François Leclerc Tumor Institute of DIJON,
France, we have determined the serum antigen levels in patients
afflicted of gynecological malignancies because of its prognostic
significance when positive. The radio-immunologic assay of the
serum is made according to the technique of Saclay. Values above
10 ng/cc are considered positive. The determination is performed
before the course of external beam, at the end of the course of
external beam, at the time of the last curietherapy and each time
the patient is seen in follow-up.

Hereby we describe our series of 92 patients distributed
as follows :
- 60 cervical carcinomas : 52 within this group previously
untreated and who received a course of external 25 MV photon beam
therapy and uterine and vaginal curietherapy with Cesium 137,
after-loading technique.
- 29 corpus carcinomas, of which there were 13 post-surgical
patients. However, the other 16 receiwed external beam therapy,
uterine and vaginal curietherapy and extra-facial hysterectomy.
- 3 vaginal carcinomas : patients treated with radiotherapy.

RESULTS
1) Cervical carcinomas :
Within the group of previously untreated patients, the CEA
was positive in 35 % of the cases (18/52) with a mean value of
35 ng/cc and maximum and minimum values of 190 ng/cc and 10,5 ng/cc
respectively.

* Distribution of values according to the stage (FIGO)
       I B : 2/14   II B : 5/12   III B : 9/16
      ' II A : 1/6   III A : 1/2   IV   : 0/2
Although these findings suggest a higher incidence of positive
values in the more advanced stages, however we cannot be as certain
of this correlation as other authors : DISAIA (4), HAEGELE (7).

✱ Correlation of positive results and histology
- epidermoid carcinoma well differentiated............... 4/14
- epidermoid carcinoma poorly differentiated............13/30
- anaplastic... 1/2
- adenocarcinoma.. 1/3
- mesonephric carcinoma................................. 0/3

✱ Correlation of positive values and lymphangiography
- lymphangiography positive............................ 10/23
- lymphangiography negative............................ 6/27

There is a higher incidence of positive values in lymphangiography positive cases.

✱ Evolution during treatment

14 out of 18 positive tests returned to normal values at the end of treatment and have remained negative.

This has correlated well with the clinical status of the patients as they have remained free of disease though the maximum follow-up period is 12 months (table 1).

2 initially positive values became negative during the treatment but returned to positive values immediately after treatment (stage II B) while the clinical exam did not show signs of recurrent or metastatic disease : in one of these cases, the test could not be repeated as the patient expired shortly after a cerebro-vascular accident.

2 have remained positive : one stage III A apparently free of disease has subsequently shown normal values ; other patient had stage III B and received palliative therapy only.

The evolution of the negative values is interesting ; they have all remained negative even in the presence of recurrence disease in one patient stage III B.

2) Uterine carcinomas :

Of the 16 determinations pre-treatment, 3 were positive :
- one stage IV patient was treated palliatively and did not have subsequent determinations.
- two stages II patients had subsequent negative determinations and the surgical specimens showed no residual tumor.

The determination on the 13 patients after initial surgery showed :
- 3 yielded positive results
- 2 became negative by the end of treatment

3) Vaginal carcinomas :

Two of three cases were positive. Both positive cases had T2 tumors. At the end of treatment, the values were within normal limits, but one of the two cases became positive concomitantly with the development of local recurrence and metastasis.

CONCLUSION

The value of the CEA determination in patients with gynecological malignancies seems to be, when initially positive, in the correlation of its return to normal levels, coupled with a complete regression of the tumor.

The patients with irradiated cervical cancer represent a good example of the conversion to normal CEA values as soon as the treatment is completed and even before the second curietherapy is carried out.

As previously mentionned (10) a study of the CEA values as a function of time is worth doing (table 2).

The persistance of a positive value in the absence of residual disease has been noted (9) and it may correspond to a release of CEA by the disintegrating cells or to the presence of occult metastatic disease.

The frequent, repeated determinations will justify in a given case, the institution of adjuvant treatment in these patients with high risk of reccurrent or metastatic disease.

A significant number of cases, 65 % approximately in our study had normal values, which points out to the need for a search for other tumor markers.

REFERENCES

(1) BARRELET V., MACH J.P. : Variation of the carcino-embryonic antigen level in the plasma of patients with gynecologic cancers during therapy. Am. J. Obstet, Gynecol, 1975, 121, 164-168.

(2) BOLLA M., BORDES M., HORIOT J.C., JAMPOLIS S., LE DORZE C. : l'antigène carcino-embryonnaire dans les cancers du col utérin. Evolution du dosage en cours d'irradiation et dans les suites immédiates. Nouv. Presse med., 1977, 6, 2608.

(3) DISAIA P.J., MORROW C.P., HAVERBACK B.J., DYCE B.J. : Carcino-embryonic antigen in cervical and vulvar cancer patients. Serum levels and disease progress. Obstetrics and Gynecology, 1976, 47, 95-98.

(4) DISAIA P.J., MORROW C.P., HAVERBACK B.J., DYCE B.J. : Carcino-embryonic antigen in cancer of the female reproductive system. Serial plasma values correlated with disease state. Cancer, 1977, 39, 2365-2370.

(5) DONALDSON E., VAN NAGELL J.R., WOOD E.G., PLETSCH Q., GOLDENBERG D.M. : Carcino-embryonic antigen in patients treated with radiation therapy for invasive squamous cell carcinoma of the uterine cervix. Am. J. Roentgenol., 1976, 127, 829-831.

(6) GOLD Ph., FREEDMAN S.O. : Specific carcino-embryonic antigen of the human digestive system. J. Exp. Med. 1965, 122, 467-481.

(7) HAEGELE P., PETIT J.C., EBER M. : CEA et cancer du col de l'utérus. Bulletin du Cancer, 1976, 63, 4, 515, 518.

(8) HENRY R., MERIADEC B., PICO J.L., SALARD J.L. : Intérêt du dosage de l'antigène carcino-embryonnaire dans le bilan et la surveillance des cancers du sein. Nouv. Presse Méd., 1965, 5, 1233-1238.

(9) KHOO S.K., MACKAY E.V. Aust. N.Z.J. Obstet. Gynaecol. 13, 1, 1973.

(10) LARRA F., HERVE C., DAVER A., TIGORI J. : L'intérêt des anti-gènes carcino-embryonnaires dans les cancers du col et du corps utérin. Bulletin du Cancer, 1976, 63, 4, 505-514.

STAGE	NUMBER OF PATIENTS	INITIAL POSITIVE DOSAGE	POSITIVE DOSAGE at THE END OF TREATMENT	POSITIVE DOSAGE in FOLLOW-UP
I B	14	2	0	0
II A	6	1	0	0
II B	12	5	2	2
III A	2	1	1	0
III B	16	9	1	1
IV A	2	0	-	-
Total	52	18	4	2

TABLE 1

DISCUSSION

LARRA F. (Angers): Was your radiotherapy only teletherapy or associated with curietherapy and, a second question : how long do you have to wait before normalisation of CEA level in cases of successful radiotherapy?

BOLLA M. (Dijon): After teletherapy, we start the first course of curietherapy, but CEA is measured only after the second course. We found that if CEA decreases to normal level, this occurs very rapidly.

TUMOUR MARKERS IN GERM CELL TUMOURS OF GONADAL AND EXTRA-GONADAL ORIGIN *

B. Nørgaard-Pedersen

Department of Clinical Chemistry, Sønderborg Hospital,
DK-6400 Sønderborg, Denmark

INTRODUCTION

A large number of biochemical tumour markers has been described, and many of these are now used in clinical routine. However, for most of these tumour index substances the initial optimistic findings have not been confirmed in later more comprehensive studies. Ideally, a biochemical marker for monitoring malignant disease should fulfil several criteria including: 1. Adequate tumour specificity. 2. Circulating tumour marker levels should be proportional to viable tumour mass. 3. Assay methods for the marker should have adequate specificity, sensitivity and simplicity i.e. it should be easy to measure in blood or urine (2, 18). In germ cell tumours of gonadal and extragonadal origin alpha-fetoprotein (AFP) and human chorionic gonadotropin (hCG) have been shown to fulfil most of the above mentioned criteria.

The purpose of this paper is to discuss the mechanism for the neosynthesis of these tumour index substances in germ cell tumours and to give a short review on the practical clinical use of these markers.

Cellular Basis for the Neosynthesis of AFP and hCG in Germ Cell Tumours

The association of AFP with 'teratocarcinomas' of the ovary and testis was simultaneously and independently demonstrated by Abelev et al. 1967 and Masopust et al. 1967 and 1968. The basis for the reappearance of the AFP remained unexplained for a long time, but in the studies by Ballas 1972 and 1974, Wilkinson et al. 1973, Tsuchida et al. 1973 and Teilum et al. 1974 AFP was found in patients

* Supported by the Danish Cancer Society Foundation and The Medical Research Foundation for the Hospitals in Ringkøbing, Ribe and Sønderjylland's Counties.

with tumours diagnosed as specific endodermal sinus tumours (pure yolk sac tumours)(Fig. 1). Increased serum AFP levels have also been found in patients with gonadal and extragonadal germ cell tumours having vitelline components of various patterns (Fig. 2) (9, 21, 27, 29, 34, 36).

According to Teilum's classification (Fig. 3) the embryologically different forms from the multipotent stem cell of embryonal carcinoma are divided into the following three types: 1. Endodermal sinus tumour (yolk sac tumour). 2. Choriocarcinoma and 3. Teratoma (3o, 31, 32). Any combination of these three types and the embryologically undifferentiated embryonal carcinoma may occur. The cellular basis for the AFP production in germ cell tumours seems therefore to be dependent on a specific differentiation into yolk sac endoderm of the tumour cells. This AFP synthesis is thus analogous to the physiological AFP synthesis by fetal yolk sac.

By immunofluorescence microscopy several studies have demonstrated that AFP is synthesized by the yolk sac endoderm in the tumour (9, 21, 33, 36) (Fig. 4). In these studies a positive staining has been found of the cells of the viseral endoderm lining the endodermal sinuses and of the various sized intra- and extra-cytoplasmic PAS-positive hyaline globules in the tumour.

It is also well documented that gonadal and extragonadal germ cell tumours may produce hCG and contain frank trophoblastic elements on microscopy, but in the majority of cases such elements cannot be demonstrated. Recently, however, immunohistochemical techniques have demonstrated hCG in giant cell types of non-trophoblastic tumours (Fig. 5). These giant cells may be of trophoblastic origin (1o, 19, 24). Other trophoblast-specific proteins such as pregnancy specific β_1-glycoprotein (PSβG) can be identified by immunocytochemical techniques on formalin-fixed tissue (11), and it shall be interesting to see, if this protein also can be found in the giant cells.

AFP and hCG in the diagnosis, therapy and Follow Up of Patients with Germ Cell Tumours

Quantitation of AFP and hCG in blood from patients with gonadal and extragonadal germ cell tumours are important functional parameters in the classification and diagnosis of these tumours. The finding of increased levels of serum AFP in preoperative samples indicates that the histopathologist should look for EST elements in the tumour tissue. Also elevated hCG levels indicate that a search for trophoblastic elements should be carried out. And by immunohistological methods a positive staining for AFP or hCG may be found in EST tumour elements or in atypical giant cells respectively. Elevated serum AFP levels have

326

been found in some patients with no detectable EST elements, but in view of the variety of histological patterns found in germ cell tumours, it is possible that the presence of the EST elements has been missed. The use of PSβG as a marker in trophoblastic malignancy might have one inherent advantage over hCG in that PSβG like material has not been found in the non-pregnant adults, at least at the detection limit of the current assays, whereas the cross reaction between luteinizing hormone (LH) and hCG limits the sensitivity of assay directed against hCG. This cross reaction is due to immunological similarity of the α-subunits of the two hormones, and is to some extend overcome by the use of β-subunit antisera specific for hCG. A collaborative study under the auspices of the International Agency for Research on Cancer is being carried out at present to compare the levels of PSβG and hCG in the sera of patients with trophoblastic tumours. In several studies AFP has been used as a therapeutic marker (6, 7, 8, 12,14, 15, 23, 26). After radical surgery of an AFP producing gonadal or extragonadal germ cell tumour AFP disappears from the blood with a half-life of about 5 days (28) (Fig. 6). A slower disappearance rate gives suspicion of residual disease. If a patient with an AFP producing germ cell tumour is in complete remission, a recurrence is most often preceeded by a rise in serum AFP levels several months before the tumour becomes clinically apparant (26). So in most patients with AFP producing germ cell tumours the AFP serum levels generally reflects the activity of the disease (Fig. 7) however, in a few cases clinical evidence of metastatic disease may occur before rise in serum AFP levels.

In patients known or suspected to have trophoblastic tumours hCG in blood and urine has proved to be of considerable value in the diagnosis, management and subsequent follow-up (2, 18). The hCG level has also been shown to reflect the tumour burden, and both in vitro and in vivo the production rate of hCG by tumour cells has been found to be approximately 10^{-12} g/cell/day (2). Therefore, both AFP and hCG are equally important as biochemical markers for germ cell tumours (6, 21, 24, 28). The discordant behaviour of the two proteins in the same patients during progressive disease also indicates that both markers should be followed during therapy (6, 26, 28). Tumours, which are originally AFP and/or hCG producing, may recur without an associated elevation in serum levels of AFP and/or hCG, and tumours, which initially show no evidence of AFP and/or hCG synthesis, may be associated with high serum levels of one or both substances during recurrence. Germ cell tumours with raised serum levels of AFP and/or hCG seems to carry a poorer prognosis than tumours not producing AFP and/or hCG (5, 26). The reasons for this are unclear, but could be due to the presence of a specific population of cells in such tumours. It should furthermore be emphasized that these tumour markers are present in serum in a considerably higher proportion of patients with advanced disease than in patients with localized or regional disease (26).

Future Research

The clinical use of tumour markers in germ cell tumours of gonadal and extragonadal origin needs further evaluation, but in certain tumours their use is rather established now. In EST in children (infantile testis, ovary or sacrococcygeal region) AFP seems to fulfil most of the ideal criteria of a tumour marker for det management of the disease (Fig. 6).

In adult testis tumours several studies have shown the value of AFP and hCG monitoring in the diagnosis, prognosis and therapy (2o, 25, 26) (Fig. 7). However, in view of the relatively large number of patients in this group there is a need for a collaborative study in these patients, for instance under the auspices of The European Organisation for Research and Treatment on Cancer (EORTC). At least, a Danish national study has been fruitful in several aspects (26).

Also in ovarian and extragonadal germ cell tumours monitoring of AFP and hCG has proved to be clinical useful (13, 22, 28)(Fig. 8), but these tumours are relatively rare. However, the histopathologist should be aware of these tumours and order an estimation of AFP and hCG even several days after operation, since the half-life of the two markers are about 5 days and 16 hours respectively (22,15).

There is also a need for further evaluation of the immunohistological methods for detection of tumour index substances on tissue sections, so that tumour morphology can be further extended by immunochemical analysis of the neoplasm itself. We have recently found it very informative to carry out mono- and bidimensional radioimmunoelectrophoresis for AFP on 5 micron thick cryostat-cut tumour tissue specimens i.e. about o,5 µg or o,5 µl of tumour tissue. We have seen an amazingly high concentration even in patients with only marginally elevated preoperative serum AFP values (Fig. 9). It has also been possible to analyse the AFP geography within a particular tumour tissue section, and to compare these findings with the immunohistological findings.

In conclusion future research should concentrate upon comparison of the different techniques available for detection of tumour index substances. Tumour tissue culturing studies and experimental yolk sac tumours in animals have not been mentioned, but are also most important in future studies. The classification of germ cell tumours should be based upon both morphological and functional or biochemical characteristics. Finally, monitoring of AFP and hCG is important in earlier detection of recurrences or metastases, and in assessement of the rate of progression of established metastases. Furthermore, both markers may act as indicators of response to treatment and as prognostic indices.

REFERENCES

(1) Abelev, G.J., Assecritova, J.V., Kraevsky, N.A., Perova, S.D. and Perevodchikova, N.J. (1967): Int. J. Cancer, 2, 551.
(2) Bagshawe, K.D. (1974): Brit. med. Bull., 3o, 8o.
(3) Ballas, M. (1972): Amer. J. clin. Path., 57, 511.
(4) Ballas, M. (1974): Ann. Clin. Lab. Science, 4, 267.
(5) Bourgeaux, C., Martel, N., Sizaret, P. and Gourrin, J. (1976): Cancer, 38, 1658.
(6) Braunstein, G.D., McIntire, K.R. and Waldmann, T.A. (1973): Cancer, 31, 1o65.
(7) Cochran, J.S., Walsh, P.C., Porter, J.C., Nicholson, T.C., Madden, J.D. and Peters, P.C. (1975): J. Urol., 114, 549.
(8) Grigor, K.M., Detre, S.I., Kohn, J. and Neville, A.M.G. (1977): Brit. J. Cancer, 35, 52.
(9) Itoh, T., Shirai, T., Naka, A. and Matsumoto, S. (1974): GANN, 64, 215.
(1o) Heyderman, E. and Neville, A.M. (1976): Lancet, ii, 1o3.
(11) Horne, C.H.W., Towler, C.M. and Milne, G.D. (1977): J. clin. Path., 3o, 19.
(12) Kohn, J., Orr, A.M., McElwain, T.J., Bentall, M. and Peckham, M.J. (1976): Lancet, i, 433.
(13) Kurman, R.J. and Norris, H.J. (1976): Obstet. Gyn. 48, 579.
(14) Lange, P.H., McIntire, K.R., Waldmann, T.A., Hakala, T.R. and Fraley, E.E. (1976): New Engl. J. Med., 295, 222.
(15) Lange, P.H. and Fraley, E.E. (1977): New Engl. J. Med. 296, 694.
(16) Masopust, J., Kithier, K., Fuchs, V., Kotál, L. and Rádl, J. (1967): Excerpta Medica Monograph. Series pp. 3o-35.
(17) Masopust, J., Kithier, K., Rádl, J., Koutecký, J. and Kotál, F. (1968): Int. J. Cancer, 3, 364.
(18) Neville, A.M. and Cooper, E.H. (1976): Ann. clin. Biochem.,13, 283.
(19) Neville, A.M., Grigor, K. and Heyderman, E. (1976): J. clin. Path., 29, 1o26.
(2o) Newlands, E.S., Dent, J., Kardana, A., Searle, F. and Bagshawe, K.D. (1976): Lancet, ii, 744.

(21) Nørgaard-Pedersen, B., Albrechtsen, R. and Teilum, G. (1975): Acta path. microbiol. scand. Sect. A 83, 573.

(22) Nørgaard-Pedersen, B. (1976): Human Alpha-Fetoprotein. A review of recent methodological and clinical studies. Universitetsforlaget, Oslo. Scand. J. Immunol. Vol. 5, suppl.4.

(23) Nørgaard-Pedersen, B., Hertz, H., Sell, A and Tygstrup, I. (1976): Infantile Endodermal Sinus Tumours (Yolk Sac Tumours) and Alpha-Fetoprotein. In Onco-Developmental Gene Expression, 379. Eds.: W.H. Fishman and S. Sell, Academic Press, Inc.

(24) Nørgaard-Pedersen, B., Lindholm, J., Albrechtsen, R., Arends, J., Diemer, N.H., and Riishede, J. (in press 1977): Cancer.

(25) Perlin, E., Engeler, J.E., Edson, M., Houp, E., McIntire, K.R. and Waldmann, T.A. (1976): Cancer, 37, 215.

(26) Schultz, H., Sell, A., Nørgaard-Pedersen, B. and Arends, J. To be published.

(27) Scully, R.E. and McNeely, B.U. (1974): New Engl. J. Med., 291, 837.

(28) Sell, A., Søgaard, H. and Nørgaard-Pedersen, B.(1976): Int. J. Cancer, 18, 574.

(29) Talerman, A. and Haije, W.G. (1974): Cancer, 34, 1722.

(3o) Teilum, G. (1959): Cancer, 12, 1o92.

(31) Teilum, G. (1965): Acta path. microbiol. scand., 64, 4o7.

(32) Teilum, G. (1971 and 1976): Special Tumours of Ovary and Testis. Comparative Pathology and Histological Identification. Munksgaard, Copenhagen, J.B. Lippincott Comp., Philadelphia.

(33) Teilum, G., Albrechtsen, R. and Nørgaard-Pedersen, B. (1974): Acta path. microbiol. scand. Sect. A, 82, 586.

(34) Teilum, G., Albrechtsen, R. and Nørgaard-Pedersen, B. (1975): Acta path. microbiol. scand. Sect. A, 83, 8o.

(35) Tsuchida, Y., Saito, S., Ishida, M., Ohmi, K., Urano, Y., Endo, Y. and Oda, T. (1973): Cancer, 32, 917.

(36) Tsuchida, U., Endo, Y., Urano, Y. and Ishida, M. (1975): Ann. N. Y. Acad. Sci., 259, 221.

(37) Wilkinson, E.J., Friedrich, E.G. and Hosty, T.A. (1973): Am. J. Obstet. Gynecol., 116, 711.

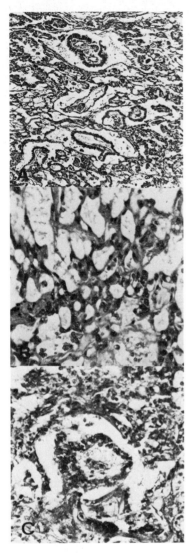

Fig. 1 Endodermal sinus tumours of the infant testis sho-
wing:
   A. Typical endodermal sinus structures (21-month-old
      boy). Serum AFP was 221o µg/l before operation.
      H.E., x 58
   B. Vacuolated network with honeycomb appearance. Same
      patient as A. H.E., x 140.
   C. Endodermal sinus structure (1o-month-old boy). Se-
      rum AFP was 2ooo µg/l before operation. H.E.,
      x 140   (Nørgaard-Pedersen et al. 1975)(21)

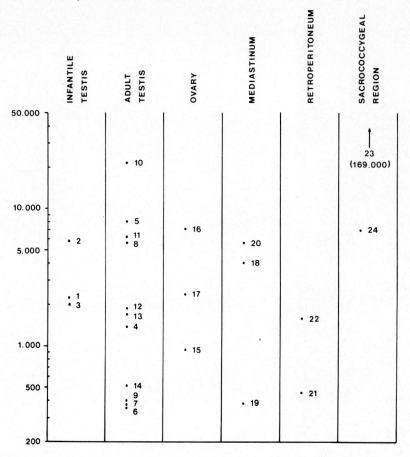

Fig. 2 Serum AFP concentration in germ cell tumours with different localization all having endodermal sinus structures in various patterns.

(Nørgaard-Pedersen et al. 1975) (21)

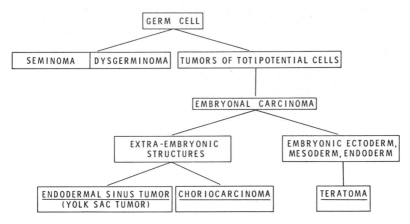

Fig. 3 Histogenesis and interrelationship of ovarian and testicular tumours of germ cell origin. In this classification the term 'embryonal carcinoma' is restricted to tumours composed of undifferentiated totipotential embryonal cells, representing the undifferentiated form of the extra-embryonic as well as embryonic tumour types.
(Teilum 1965) (31)

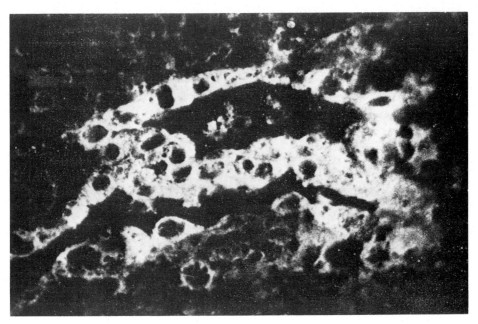

Fig. 4 Indirect immunofluorescence AFP staining of the tumour from a 23-year-old man with a right side testicular tumour. (Embryonal carcinoma of the testis with a few endodermal sinus structures). Serum AFP was 4oo µg/l before operation. A positive staining is seen of the cells lining the endodermal sinuses and of the hyaline globules.(x 390).
(Nørgaard-Pedersen et al. 1975)(21)

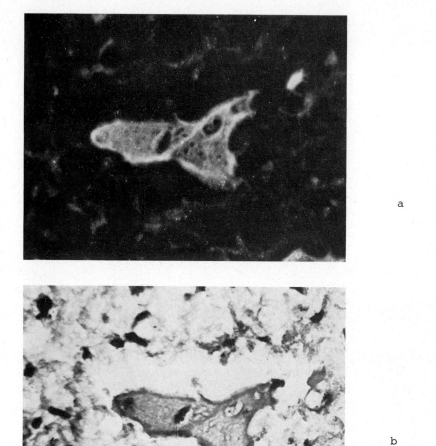

a

b

Fig. 5 a) Giant cell with positive staining for hCG by indirect immunofluorescence microscopy x 700.
b) The same area after HE x 700.
(Nørgaard-Pedersen et al. 1977)(24)

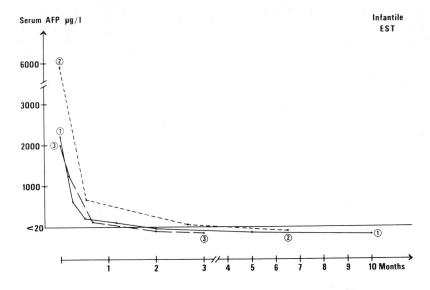

Fig. 6 Pre- and postoperative serum AFP levels in 3 cases of EST of the infantile testis.

(Nørgaard-Pedersen et al 1976)(23)

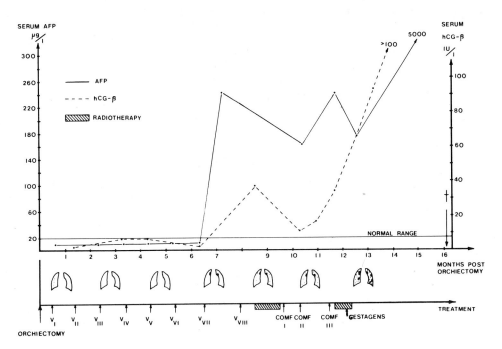

Fig. 7 Adult testis tumour (embryonal carcinoma). The figure shows an example of appearance of tumour marker synchronously with the appearance of multiple distant metastases.   (Schultz et al. 1977) (26)

335

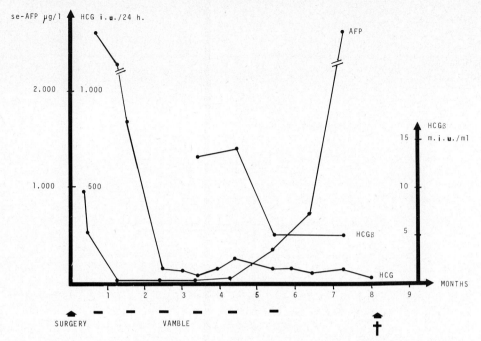

Fig. 8 Ovarian tumour of combined type (EST combined with choriocarcinoma and dysgerminoma (21-year-old woman). Serum AFP and urinary and serum hCG were followed during postoperative chemotherapy. Note the discordant effect of therapy on AFP and hCG. Postmortem histological examination showed only the EST tumour component.

(Sell et al. 1976) (28)

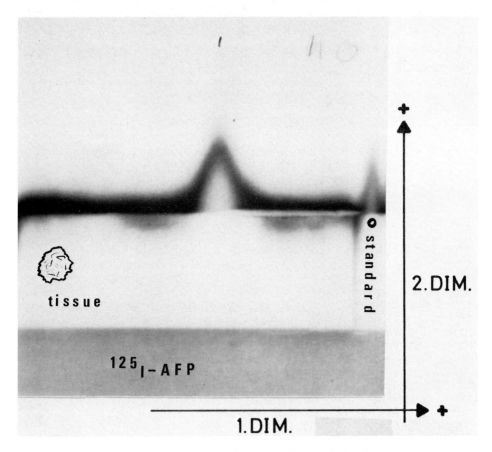

Fig. 9 Radiocrossed immunoelectrophoresis of a cryostat-cut tumour tissue specimen on a microscopic slide. A right side testicular tumour about 4 g (Embryonal carcinoma) (14-year-old boy). Serum AFP was 24 µg/l before operation, and was less than 5 µg/l 14 days after operation.
(Nørgaard-Pedersen et al. unpublished)

DISCUSSION

TALERMAN A. (Rotterdam) : Do the different histological types of endodermal sinus tumour show a specific pattern in your last technique (electrophoretic migration using microscopic slices).

NØORGARD-PEDERSEN B. (Sønderborg) : No, we have not yet had time to do so. But I agree that it is very important to use this technique to further evaluate different immunohistochemical methods.

GROPP C. (Marburg) : There have been some reports that after recurrence of the tumour, the tumour will no longer produce AFP or β HCG. Have you made the same observation?

NØORGARD-PEDERSEN B. (Sønderborg) : Yes, I have made the same observation, but you may also see the opposite.

337

ALPHAFOETOPROTEIN (AFP) IN PATIENTS WITH GERM CELL
TUMOURS AND HISTOLOGICAL PATTERNS IN GERM CELL TUMOURS
ASSOCIATED WITH RAISED SERUM AFP

A. Talerman, W.G. Haije and L. Baggerman

Depts. of Pathology and Chemical Pathology, Institute
of Radiotherapy, P.O. Box 5201, Rotterdam

Although the presence of raised serum alphafoetoprotein (AFP) in some patients with germ cell neoplasms
was noted 10 years ago (1), it is only during the last
few years that the value of AFP as a tumour marker in
this group of neoplasms has been fully recognised.
During the last few years the histological aspects of
the germ cell tumours associated with raised serum AFP
have been studied and the relationship between the
presence of Endodermal Sinus Tumour (EST) or Yolk Sac
Tumour (YST) elements within the tumour and presence of
raised serum AFP has been noted (2,3,4,5).
Five years ago we have decided to study serum AFP
in patients with germ cell tumours and to examine
whether there is a correlation between the histological
appearances of the tumour and AFP synthesis determined
by the presence of raised serum AFP.
In view of the homology between germ cell tumours
of the gonads and extragonadal sites we have decided to
include all patients with germ cell neoplasms irrespective of the location of the neoplasm.

PATIENTS AND METHODS

In the first 18 months of the study AFP was
determined by counter-immunodiffusion using a slight
modification of the method of Alpert et al (6), which
detects levels of serum AFP in excess of 140 ng/ml.
During the following $3\frac{1}{2}$ years in addition to counter-
immunodiffusion we have been using radio-immunoassay
capable of detecting AFP with an accuracy of a few
ng/ml. In addition to this for high values we have been
using Partigen plates of Behringwerke AG Marburg Lahn
and modifications of Laurell's rocket technique (7).
Serum AFP of 20 ng/ml was considered as the upper
limit of normal. In the past five years serum AFP has
been determined in 259 patients with malignant gonadal
and extragonadal germ cell neoplasms. Whenever possible
serial determinations were performed.
The histological appearances of all the tumours in
patients whose serum AFP was determined were reviewed

338

either before, or in conjunction with the AFP determinations.

The testicular tumours were classified according to the modified classification proposed by the British Testicular Tumour Panel (8) and according to the classification proposed by Dixon and Moore (9) in both cases modified by the inclusion of EST (YST) as a specific entity. The criteria used for diagnosis of EST were those described by Teilum (10).

RESULTS

Table 1 shows an overview of the material under study.

TABLE 1   Patients with malignant germ cell tumours who had serum AFP determinations

	No. of cases
Testicular tumours	220
Ovarian tumours	26
Mediastinal tumours	7
Retroperitoneal tumours	5
Pineal tumours	1
Total	259

Table 2 shows serum AFP in patients with testicular tumours whose serum AFP was determined either pre-operatively or in the immediate postoperative period.

TABLE 2   Serum AFP in patients with testicular germ cell tumours

	No. of cases	Serum AFP
Seminoma	26	Normal
Embryonal carcinoma + Teratoma	7	Normal
Embryonal carcinoma	2	Normal
Embryonal carcinoma	2	Slightly raised
EST + other types of germ cell tumour	14	Raised
Choriocarcinoma + Teratoma	3	Normal

In patients with testicular germ cell tumours with definite evidence of metastatic disease and whose serum AFP was determined a considerable time after orchiectomy only patients whose metastases contained EST were found to have raised serum AFP.

All patients with testicular germ cell tumours and no evidence of active disease had normal levels of serum AFP at all times irrespective of the histological appearances of the tumour.

Table 3 shows serum AFP in patients with malignant ovarian germ cell tumours. It shows that only patients with EST had elevated serum AFP. The patient with malignant or immature teratoma had a large tumour, which was studied inadequately. It was first diagnosed as mature teratoma. When the tumour recurred 3 months later the patient was referred for treatment to our Institute and review of the histology revealed both mature and immature elements. The specimen was by that time discarded and more material was not available for study. The patient did not respond to radiotherapy and died with metastases and recurrences 5 months after excision of the ovarian tumour. Autopsy was not permitted.

TABLE 3   Serum AFP in patients with malignant ovarian germ cell tumours

	No. of cases	Serum AFP
Mixed germ cell tumours containing EST	12	Raised
Pure EST	4	Raised
Dysgerminoma	6	Normal
Teratoma (mature and immature)	1	Raised

Serum AFP was also determined in 50 patients with testicular, paratesticular and ovarian tumours which were not of germ cell origin and was normal in all cases.

Table 4 shows serum AFP in patients with extra-gonadal germ cell tumours. The patients with tumours composed of EST, have raised serum AFP. The patient with the primitive germ cell tumour, a young man of 21 years, had a highly malignant poorly differentiated mediastinal tumour. The biopsy was inadequate both in quantity and quality. The tumour could only be identified as a poorly differentiated embryonal germ cell tumour. There was no response to therapy and the patient died within 6 months of diagnosis. Autopsy was not permitted.

Figure 1 shows serial serum AFP determinations in a 17-year-old girl with a large mixed germ cell tumour containing EST. The serum AFP was determined on the 11th postoperative day and was 2200 ng/ml. It returned to normal 7 weeks after the operation and remained normal for 4 months when at first a slight and then more rapid gradual rise was noted, although the patient was treated with triple chemotherapy.

TABLE 4   Serum AFP in patients with malignant extra-gonadal germ cell tumours

	No. of cases	Serum AFP
Mediastinum		
EST	3	Raised
Primitive germ cell tumour	1	Raised
Seminoma	3	Normal
Retroperitoneum		
EST + Embryonal carcinoma	1	Raised
Seminoma	4	Normal
Pineal		
Seminoma (germinoma)	1	Normal

Clinically there was no evidence of disease for further 5 months, but high levels of serum AFP were present when a small mass was noted in the abdomen. One month later a laparotomy was performed and tumour deposits composed entirely of EST were excised from the abdominal cavity. Although a slight fall in serum AFP was noted after the second operation soon a sustained rise occurred indicating that the disease was far from being eradicated. This rise continued until the patient's death 20 months after the original operation. This figure illustrates the value of serial serum AFP determinations in the early detection of recurrent disease, in the assessment of lack of response to therapy and in demonstrating that the disease was not eradicated by the excision of metastases during the second operation.

DISCUSSION

The results of the present study indicate that in patients with germ cell neoplasms, it is those with tumours which are composed of, or contain EST, who have consistently elevated levels of serum AFP. The serum AFP levels in these patients are usually high or very high and can be measured in 100's or 1000's ng/ml.

Apart from two patients with embryonal carcinoma, who have had slightly raised levels (< 60 ng/ml), and from two patients with raised serum AFP whose tumours could not be studied adequately all patients with tumours which did not contain EST had normal serum AFP. It is considered that the two patients with embryonal carcinoma may have had small foci of EST within the tumour, which in spite of a thorough study of the material available escaped detection and that these foci may have been responsible for the slight elevation of serum AFP.

The results of the present study further confirm the value of AFP as a good and reliable tumour marker in patients with germ cell tumours composed of, or containing EST, and the importance of serial determinations of serum AFP in these patients for assessing whether after the initial treatment the disease has been eradicated, for early detection of metastases and recurrences, and for assessment of the efficacy of therapy.

REFERENCES

(1) Abelev, G.I., Assecritova, I.V., Kraevsky, N.A., Perova, S.D. and Perevodchikova, N.I. (1967): Int.J.Cancer, 2, 551.
(2) Ballas, M. (1972): Amer.J.Clin.Path., 57, 511.
(3) Tsushida, Y., Saito, S., Ishida, M., Ohni, K., Urano, Y., Endo, Y. and Oda, T. (1973): Cancer, 32, 917.
(4) Talerman, A. and Haije, W.G. (1974): Cancer, 34, 1722.
(5) Nørgaard-Pedersen, B., Albrechtsen, R. and Teilum, G. (1975): Acta Path.Microbiol.Scand. Sect.A, 83, 573.
(6) Alpert, E., Herschberg, R., Schur, P.H. and Isselbacher, K.J. (1971): Gastroenterology, 61, 137.
(7) Laurell, C.B. (1965): Analyt.Biochem., 10, 358.
(8) Pugh, R.C.B. (1972): The Panel Classification. In Pugh R.C.B. Pathology of the testis. Blackwell Scientific Publications, Oxford, pp.144-146.
(9) Dixon, F.J. and Moore, R.A. (1952): Tumors of the male sex organs. Atlas of Tumor Pathology. Section 8. Fascicles 31b and 32. Armed Forces Institute of Pathology, Washington D.C. pp.50-53.
(10) Teilum, G. (1965): Acta Path.Microbiol.Scand. 64, 407.

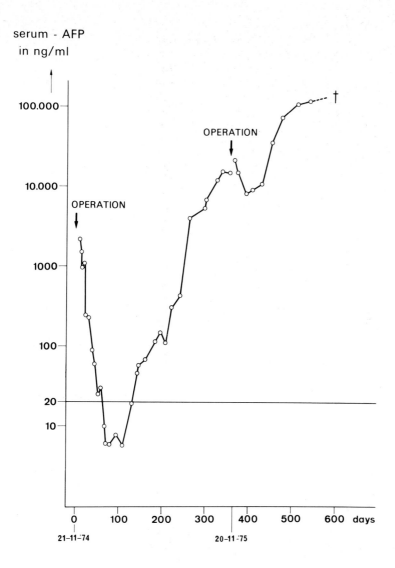

Fig. 1   Serial serum AFP determinations (logarithmic scale) from the time of diagnosis till death in a 17-year-old girl with a mixed germ cell tumour of the ovary containing EST.

343

DISCUSSION

SEPPALA M. (Helsinki): Did you measure HCG levels in your patients?

TALERMAN A. (Rotterdam): Yes, we did in some patients who had evidence of choriocarcinomatus elements in the tumours and we found in a number of cases a discordance between AFP and HCG in the serum. But we have found that in patients who had histological evidence of choriocarcinomatus elements within the tumours there was invariably raised beta sub-unit of HCG.

SEPPALA M. (Helsinki): Is it necessary to see morphological evidence for chorionic like tissues before you assayed for HCG, or can you find HCG in the absence of any morphological indications?

TALERMAN A. (Rotterdam): Yes, you can. But high levels were only found in cases where we found choriocarcinomatus elements. I fully agree that we do find cases with small elevations of beta sub-unit in patients with no histological evidence of choriocarcinoma, although we found some of these large multinucleate cells, which we believe are of syncytiothrophoblastic origin.
Another point which I would like to mention is : we have studied CEA in a number of these cases, and we have found that the levels of CEA were normal in all these cases.

LALANNE C.M. (Nice): If you find HCG , do you think it is a chorio-epitelioma even if you do not find trosphoblastic cells under the microscope.

TALERMAN A. (Rotterdam): No, I don't,because we know that inappro-priate secretion of hormone does occur in a number of tumours; we have seen tumours of the eosophagus, of the uterus associated with production of HCG in considerable amounts, so I do not think that we always can demonstrate histologically the presence of cho-riocarinomatus elements . But I must say that in the seminomas, we do find that there is a number of cases where you see large syncy-tiothrophoblastic giant cells and in these cases, you tend to have slightly elevated level of HCG. On the other hand, we do not find any evidence that patients with these seminomas have a worse progno-sis than the general population of patients with seminoma.

HCGβ SUBUNIT RADIOIMMUNOASSAY IN CERVICAL, ENDOMETRIAL, AND OVARIAN CANCER*

M. Seppälä and E.-M. Rutanen

Department of Obstetrics and Gynecology, University Central Hospital, 00290 Helsinki 29, Finland

Elevated serum levels of human chorionic gonadotropin (hCG) have been reported to occur in various types of nontrophoblastic tumors (1,2). In these studies hCG was measured by radioimmunoassay employing antiserum against the β-subunit of hCG (3). In order to evaluate the clinical significance of hCG measurements in the management of nontrophoblastic gynecologic cancer we used the hCGβ subunit radioimmunoassay in 380 patients with benign or malignant tumors of the genital tract.

MATERIALS AND METHODS

Patients

Our series included 380 patients with gynecologic disease. There were 276 cancer patients and 104 patients with various non-cancerous states including endometriosis (15 cases), adenomyosis (6 cases), myomas (33 cases), ovarian simple cyst (9 cases), serous cyst (7 cases), mucinous cyst (20 cases), and dermoid cyst (14 cases). Malignant tumors were cancer of the vulva (8 cases), the vagina (6 cases), the cervix (111 cases), the endometrium (125 cases), and the ovary (26 cases). The tumors were grouped according to the International Federation of Gynecology and Obstetrics classification. Serum samples from 116 healthy adults including 15 postmenopausal women were also studied.

In all cases the first serum sample was taken before treatment. Additional specimens were obtained in 66 cases after radical surgery and in 18 cases after chemo- and/or radiotherapy. The patients were followed-up for 6 to 22 months after treatment.

HCG subunit radioimmunoassay

We used the NICHD (Bethesda, Md., U.S.A.) radioimmunoassay kit for hCGβ subunit using the SB6 antiserum (3). The 2nd International Standard Preparation for hCG served as the standard (Fig. 1). The standards were made up with 10 % normal human serum, and the serum samples tested at 1:10 dilution. The sensitivity of the assay varied

*This study was carried out under contract with the Association of the Finnish Life Insurance Companies and also supported by the Finnish Cancer Society.

between 5 and 10 mIU/ml. A positive reading gave an inhibition greater than 2 standard deviations of mean zero binding.

Human luteinizing hormone (hLH) radioimmunoassay

All specimens were also run by hLH radioimmunoassay (NIAMDD, Bethesda, Md.) so as to find out if there is any relationship between hLH and hCG concentrations. The human pituitary FSH/LH standard LER 907 was used as reference preparation.

RESULTS

Normal individuals

None of the healthy individuals including 15 postmenopausal women had any detectable hCG in serum.

Nonmalignant tumors

A positive recording was obtained in 15 of 104 patients (14 %). In all cases the hCG elevation was slight, the values fluctuating between 7 and 21 mIU/ml. In this group hCG-positive patients were significantly older than hCG-negative patients.

Gynecologic cancer

Positive hCG reactions were found in 48 of 276 cancer patients (17 %). Elevated levels varied between 8 and 66 mIU/ml. No significant difference was found in the occurrence of hCG-positivity in patients with cervical, endometrial and ovarian cancer, and hCG was demonstrated in early as well as in advanced stages of malignant disease. We found no correlation between hCG level and the spread of the tumor, and no significant difference was noted in the age distribution between hCG-positive and hCG-negative patients.

Radical surgery, chemo- and/or radiotherapy

After radical surgery including hysterectomy and ovariectomy hCG disappeared from circulation in 11 of 17 cancer patients (35 %). All these patients were tumor free during the follow-up period. Six patients remained hCG-positive: one of them had a clinical tumor (Fig. 2).

Conversion from hCG-negative to positive took place in 7 of 48 patients (15 %) after radical surgery, and 41 patients remained hCG-negative. While 7 patients had signs of clinical recurrence, only one of them was hCG-positive at the time clinical tumor was identified (Fig. 3).

Four hCG-positive cancer patients remained hCG-positive after chemo- and/or radiotherapy. All had residual tumor 2 to 8 months later. Four out of 10 initially hCG-negative patients became hCG-positive after chemo- and/or radiotherapy. Residual tumor was present in 5 of 10 hCG-negative and 2 of 4 hCG-positive cases.

346

Comparison between hCG and hLH levels

The human pituitary FSH/LH standard LER 907 inhibited in our hCGβ radioimmunoassay when the levels exceeded 500 ng/ml. In the total series of 380 patients there were altogether 3 patients who were hCG-positive and whose hLH levels were in excess of 500 ng LER 907/ml. One of them had cancer and 2 had benign tumors. In these cases positive hCG-readings may have been attributed to hLH cross-reaction. However, hCG was demonstrated in 61 other patients whose serum hLH concentration was below the crossreacting level, and there were 8 other patients whose serum hLH concentration was in excess of 500 ng LER 907/ml, but still no hCG was found.

DISCUSSION

We found hCG immunoreactivity in serum of 64 patients with gynecologic tumors. This reactivity was not related to hLH in general, but in 3 cases hLH crossreaction was likely. There was no significant difference in the hCG-positivity rate between malignant (17 %) and nonmalignant (14 %) diseases, but none of 116 healthy adults including postmenopausal women showed any demonstrable hCG in serum. Our results suggest that hCG can hardly serve as a tumor marker for nontrophoblastic gynecologic cancer under the test conditions generally employed. This was further supported by the fact that there were 7 patients in whom hCG appeared for the first time after radical surgery. However, in certain cancer patients hCG disappeared from serum after surgery and in those cases monitoring by hCG may be feasible. We now look forward to seeing whether hCG reappears in these patients before recurrent tumor is clinically manifest.

REFERENCES

(1)   Braunstein, G.D., Vaitukaitis, J.L., Carbone, P.P. and Ross, G.T. (1973) : Ann. Intern. Med., 78, 39.
(2)   Tormey, D.C., Waalkes, T.P. and Simon, R.M. (1977) : Cancer, 39, 2391.
(3)   Vaitukaitis, J.L., Braunstein, G.D. and Ross, G.T. (1972) : Am. J. Obstet. Gynecol., 113, 751.

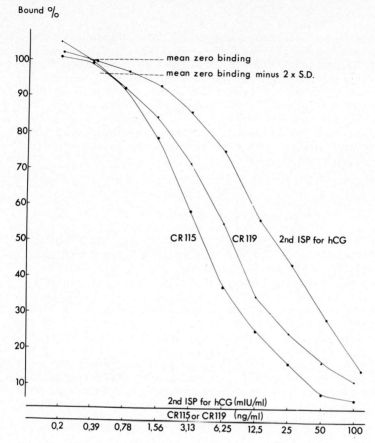

Fig. 1 Radioimmunoassay of hCG using antiserum against the β-subunit of hCG (SB6) and labeled hCG (CR 119). Abbreviations are : CR 115 : β-subunit of hCG ; CR 119 : purified hCG.

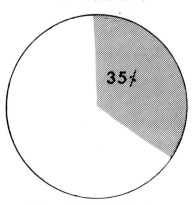

HCG-positive gynecological cancer N= 17

OPERATION

35ʸ

AFTER TREATMENT

HCG-negative
11 cases,
no clinical tumor

HCG-positive
clinical tumor
in 1/6 cases

FIG. 2

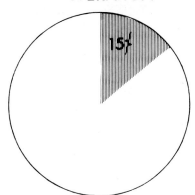

HCG-negative gynecological cancer N=48

OPERATION

15ʸ

AFTER TREATMENT

HCG-negative
clinical tumor
in 6/41 cases

HCG-positive
clinical tumor
in 1/7 cases

FIG. 3

Fig. 2 The effect of radical surgery on serum hCG in initially hCG-positive cancer patients. Shaded area indicates the proportion of hCG-positivity after operation.

Fig. 3 The effect of radical surgery on serum hCG in initially hCG-negative cancer patients. Shaded area indicates the proportion of hCG-positivity after operation.

DISCUSSION

KHOO S.K. (Brisbane): Have you tried to correlate the positive results with the age of patients.

SEPPALA M. (Helsinki): Yes, in those patients who had benign tumours HCG positive patients were significantly older than HCG negative patients. This age difference was not seen in cancer patients.

KHOO S.K. (Brisbane): What is the usual range of results you get for positivity.

SEPPALA M. (Helsinki): From 7 to 66 milliunits per ml.

KHOO S.K. (Brisbane): What is your level of cut-off?

SEPPALA M. (Helsinki): The cut-off level varies between 3 and 10 mIU/ml; it depends on the assay and how old your labelled antigen is.

KHOO S.K. (Brisbane): For instance, the majority is not highly elevated.

SEPPALA M. (Helsinki): No.

KHOO S.K. (Brisbane): The third question : We have also had some interest in Beta sub-unit of HCG and we use ng and I think this made comparison very difficult.
Is there any international standard that could give us some possibility to compare results.

SEPPALA M. (Helsinki): The levels were calculated according to the Second International Standard of HCG from MRC, Holly Hill, London. We correlated these results with the NIH standard CR-119, which is a pure HCG preparation in ng terms, and 1 ng of it is equivalent to 3 mIU of the International Standard.

KHOO S.K. (Brisbane): What do you think about clinical usefulness?

SEPPALA M. (Helsinki): We must wait and see if the originally HCG positive patients who turned to negative will re-express HCG and, if so, how it correlates with tumour recurrence.

LALANNE C.M. (Nice): We have seen on one of your slides that you perform also some CEA assays. How does this correlated with HCG results?

SEPPALA M. (Helsinki): We think CEA is better.

TUMOUR MARKERS AND ENDOMETRIAL CANCER : IN VITRO STUDIES

J. Hustin, J.C. Hendrick, A. Thirion, A. Reuter,
R. Lambotte and P. Franchimont

Departments of Gynecology and Radioimmunology, University
of Liège, Belgium

Endometrial cancer is thought to be many cases hormone dependent (1). This has prompted the use of progestational agents as adjunct therapy for advanced cases or in conjunction with preoperative radiotherapy (2).
Besides, we have already mentioned that in this type of neoplasm, one or several tumour markers could be detected in the plasma of about 70 % of patients (3).
Whether hormonal treatment can induce an alteration in the pattern of production of cancerous antigens, is, at the present time, still undefined. We have thus deemed interesting to investigate in this respect the in vitro behaviour of endometrial cancers previously submitted to high dosage progestogen treatment.

MATERIAL AND METHODS

We have performed simultaneous assays of carcino-embryonic antigen (CEA), alpha-fetoprotein (AFP), human chorionic gonadotrophin in its undissociated form
(u. HCG) or as its β subunit (β.HCG) and kappa casein
(K. CAS.). The methodology used has already been published in detail elsewhere (4). The assays were performed on plasma samples and culture media. Results were expressed as ng/ml serum or ng/ml medium.
Explants of endometrial cancers were grown in organ culture according to previously described techniques (5). Every other day, the medium was collected and subsequently assayed. Simultaneously, the explants were fixed and processed for histological evaluation of viability.
The series of endometrial cancers comprised 27 patients. Fourteen had received no treatment at the time of obtention of tissue and serum ; the other thirteen, on the contrary had received one gm medroxyprogesterone acetate* I.M. per week for two weeks at least.

* Medroxyprogesterone acetate : Depo-Provera (R) -
  Upjohn C° Puurs, Belgium

RESULTS

1. Serum values

In both series (i.e. Untreated and treated cancers)
the percentage of positive cases for one antigen at least,
appeared similar : CEA in values higher than 10 ng/ml was
found in three untreated cases and two treated cases.
Undissociated HCG was present in values higher than
1 ng/ml in 30 % of all cases with an even distribution between series. There was only one untreated case with a serum value of 1.69 ng/ml of   HCG. At last, no AFP could
be detected in any case while K.cas. was detected in 6
cases (3 treated and 3 untreated) in values higher than
25 ng/ml.

2. In vitro studies

Provided adequate survival was obtained, the liberation of tumour markers in the culture medium could be assayed at various intervals for one week. The behaviour
of the explants was similar whether previously hormone
treated or not. After 6 hours, CEA could often be detected in the medium in large quantities. This antigen was
apparently liberated in much smaller amounts during the
next three days. Then an important increase in the production was observed. At the end of one week CEA levels
in the medium often equated those found after the first
six hours (Fig. 1). This evolution could be observed in 13
cases (9 treated and 4 untreated). K.cas and u.HCG were
sometimes liberated in large amounts during the first
day. Their in vitro production fell then rapidly and was
unnoticeable after one week (Fig. 2). At last the only
case with a significant plasma value of β.HCG displayed a
production pattern similar to that of CEA : after an initial decrease, the amount of the β subunit increased again
to attain 6 ng/ml after 5 days in vitro.

COMMENTS

Within the scope of this limited experiment, it appears that high dosage progestogen treatment does not
modify the production of tumour markers by endometrial
carcinoma.
Moreover, progestogen treated cancer behave in vitro exactly like untreated cancers. In this respect, it is note-
worthy that a significant in vitro release of CEA could be
demonstrated in 13 cases, that is more often than the positivity of serum assays could predict. Now we have already
observed that tissue values of CEA were higher than 100
ng/mg protein in one half of our cases, suggesting thus an
impairment of blood release in many patients (3). The organ culture technique may have thus rendered more directly
apparent the genomic derepression eventually involved in

the synthesis of CEA. But we must not forget that for K-Casein and u.HCG, the situation was always different and that their in vitro production was small and restricted to the first day. This might point to the possibility of altered conditions of good viability. This hypothesis is now currently investigated by simultaneous experiments with different culture media and for prolonged periods of time.

REFERENCES

(1) Sall, S.and Calanog, A. (1972) : Am. J. Obstet. Gynecol., 114/2, 153.

(2) Anderson, D.G. (1972) : Am. J. Obstet. Gynecol.,113/2 195.

(3) Hustin, J., Thirion, A., Reuter, A., Hendrick, J.C. and Franchimont, P. (1977) : Proceedings, Second Symposium on Endometrial Cancer, M.G. Brush and J.B. King Eds (in press).

(4) Franchimont, P. (1976) : Cancer related antigens, North Holland Publishing C° Amsterdam.

(5) Hustin, J. (1975) : Brit. J. Obstet. Gynaec., 82, 493.

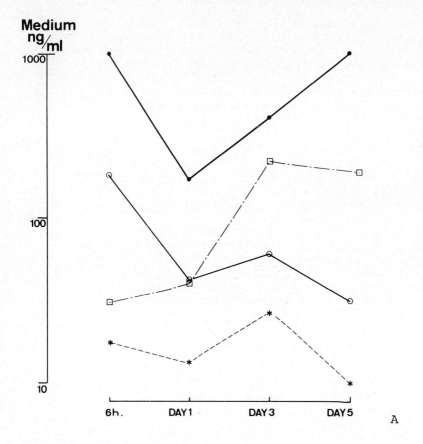

Fig. 1A. CEA liberation in the culture medium: untreated
cancers (n = 4).

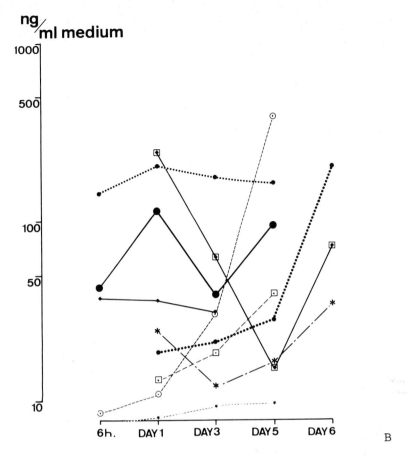

Fig. 1B. CEA liberation in the culture medium: progesto-
gen-treated cancers (n = 9). The similarity of behaviour
between both series is evident.

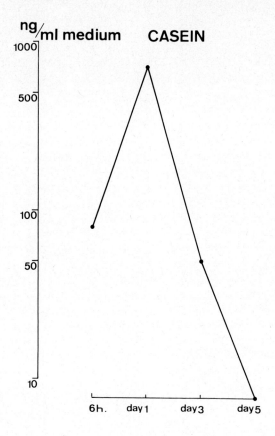

Fig. 2   K-cas release in vitro. After the first day of
culture the amount of K-cas decreases rapidly
and reaches zero at the end of the experiment.

IMMUNOHISTOLOGICAL AND RADIOIMMUNOLOGICAL STUDY OF THE β SUBUNIT OF THE CHORIONIC GONADOTROPHIC HORMONE: CLINICAL INFLUENCE

D. Bellet, J.M. Arrang, G. Contesso and C. Bohuon

Institut Gustave Roussy - 16 bis av., P.V. Couturier - 94800 Villejuif, France

INTRODUCTION

Patients bearing a trophoblastic tumor, either placental or testicular, are now monitored by a radioimmunoassay (RIA) of the β-subunit of the human chorionic gonadotropin (β-HCG) (1). The specificity and the constant occurence of this molecule, free or bound to the α-subunit, lead to consider β-HCG as an excellent marker for this type of tumor. Immunohistochemical (2) and radioimmunological studies (3) show the presence of β-subunits on tumoral cells in the serum of patients bearing nontrophoblastic malignant tumors, thus giving indications for new chemical uses of this compound.

In order to point out the interest of βHCG in various localizations, mammary tumors have been studied both by radioimmunology and immunohistochemistry. Other various non trophoblastic types of tumor were examined only from an immunohistochemical point of view : testicular tumors were paid a special attention as one knows that a number of seminomas and dysembryomas excrete HCG in serum (4).

METERIALS AND METHODS

RIA : The RIA were performed on sera stored at -20°C using a double-antibody method. The cross-reaction between LH and the specific anti-β-HCG antiserum (AC 78 from Bio Endo, Montréal) ranges below 5 %. The method sensitivity is 0.5 mUI/ml and the positivity ground level raises to 7 mUI/ml. The second international standard is used as a reference.

IMMUNOHISTOCHEMISTRY

The immunohistochemical technique uses peroxydase as a labelling compound. The specific antiserum was prepared by injection of highly purified β-HCG to rabbits (β-HCG, batch CG 113 fro Dr BIALLY, Bethesda Md). Three sections per tumor were investigated : the first one, treated with a normal rabbit serum was used as a negative

:: This work was supported by Clinical Research Grant N° FC 77 A2 from the Institute Gustave-Roussy.

reference ; the second slide, after treatment by an absorbed immunserum controled by radioimmunology for immunoreactivity loss, was
the absolute control ; finally, the third section was exposed to
the specific anti-β-HCG antiserum (5).

PATIENTS

RIA were performed on sera from 140 patients with benign
mammary tumors (119 of them were pre-menopaused patients) and from
85 bearers of a malignant mammary tumor (19 pre-menopaused patients).

Sections concerning 37 mammary adenocarcinomas, 2 masto-
sis, 1 fibroadenoma, 5 uterin and 2 pancreatic adenocarcinomas, 5
dysembryomas, 1 lymphode metastasis from one of these dysembryomas,
and 9 pure seminomas with acute clinical problems.

RESULTS

The RIA results in sera from patients with a mammary
malignant tumor (table 1) display a generally slight increase in
β-HCG rates for 22 % of the post-menopaused and 26 % of the pre-
menopaused patients. For the benign mammary tumor bearers, these
figures become 4.7 and 1.6 % respectively.

Table I

	mammary tumor	number of cases	number of cases with increased rates of β-HCG	%
Pre-menopaused patients	benign	119	2	1.6
	malignant	19	5	26
Post-menopaused patients	benign	21	1	4.7
	malignant	66	15	22

The immunohistochemical results are summarized in table II.
Thirty seven cases of malignant mammary tumors were studied : 2 of
them displayed isolated tumoral cells sharply labelled on their cytoplasm. Four out of the 9 seminomas were immunoperoxidase positive on
rare cells, mostly of syncytial aspect, sometimes with a seminal morphology. A labelling on tumoral islets was observed in 2 of 5 dysembryomas and, in a third case, if no labelling was detected on the
tumor itself, labelled cells were found in a lymphnot metastasis.

No positive reaction was observed on benign mammary tumors,
prostatic adenocarcinomas or uterus tumors.

Table II   Immunoperoxydase localyzation of β-HCG on non trophoblastic
tumors

Tumor	Number of cases	+	-
Mastosis	2	0	2
Fibroadenoma	1	0	1
Breast adenocarcinoma	37	2	35
Cervix adenocarcinoma	5	0	5
Pancreas adenocarinoma	2	0	2
Testis seminoma	9	4	5
Testis dysembryoma	5	2	3
	61	8	53

DISCUSSION

Two problems arise from radioimmunological methods used
in this type of study : the first one deals with the upper limit of
normality, depending on the antibody used in the experiment. After
checking a normal sample of 31 menopaused women where serum β-HCG
never reached 6 mUI/ml, the upper limit of normality was set at
7 mUI/ml.

The second problem concerns the specificity of such an
assay. Although a very specific antibody has been used, it might be
able to recognize a free molecule, chemically close to β-subunit.
That is why it is interesting to compare RIA results to immunochemical data. The latter technique overcome the specificity problem with
a strict methodology and the constant use of an absorbed immunserum
as a control. On the other hand, the small number of sections observed for each case and the fact that only a few cells or isolated
tumoral islets synthesize or store β-HCG may acount for the low figure
of labelling positivity.

Considering these remarks on the results' value, the
clinical interest of β -HCG, if one excepts trophoblastic tumor monitoring, moves towards two directions. Like other molecules (CEA for
instance) β -HCG can take place among the tumor "markers", especially
for mammary tumors. However, the reported results make it obvious
that β-HCG is not, as previously understated by ACEVEDO and al. (6),
an universal marker for cancerous cells.

It seems more realistic to operate immunohistochemical
techniques for non-trophoblastic testicular tumors. In these tumors,
the presence of β -HCG producing cells is interesting for the prognosis,
as an unfavourable clinical evolution is related to the presence of
these cells, and for the therapy as it is most likely that chemotherapy should then replace radiotherapy.

Thus, the clinical use of β-HCG tends to widen out with new investigational methods. Other studies, namely immunological ones, will define precisely the role and the importance of the HCG β-subunit.

ACKNOWLEDGEMENTS

We thank Doctor Burtin for helpful assistance and G. Re-coules, G. Bertin, M.C. Sabine and G. Chavanel for pre-cious technical aid.

REFERENCES

(1) JONES W.B., LEWIS J.L., LEHR M. (1975) : Monitor of chemotherapy in gestational trophoblastic neoplasm by RIA of the β subunit of HCG. Ann. J. of Obst. and gyn. , Vol. 125 n° 5, 669-673.
(2) NAUGTON M.A., MERRILL D.A, Mc MANUS L., FINLN L.M., BERMAN E., WHITE M.J. and HERNANDEZ A.M. (1975) : Localization of the β chain of human chorionic gonadotropin on human tumor cells and placental cells, Cancer Research, 35, 1887-1890.
(3) BRAUNSTEIN G.D., VARTUKNAITIS J.L., CARBONE P.P. and ROSS G.T. (1973) : Ectopic productions of human chorionic gonadotropin by neo-plasms, Ann. Intern. Med. 78, 39-45.
(4) NEWLANDS E.S., DENT J., KARDANOR A., SEARLE F., BAGSHAWE K.D. (1976):Serum α Fetoprotein and HCG in patients with testicular tumors. Lancet 1976 iib 44.
(5) HEYDERMAN E., NEVILLE A.M. (1976): Immunoperoxydase of pregnancy protein. Lancet 1976 ii 744.
(6) ACEVEDO H.F., SLIFKIN H., POUCHET G.R., and RAKSHAN M.(1976) : Human chorionic gonadotropin in Cancer cells. Third international symposium on detection and prevention of cancer. New York 1976.

DISCUSSION

KREBS B.P. (Nice) : One may not propose the radioimmunoassay of the β subunits of HCG as test in other cancers than those known to produce specifically this molecule. In fact, plasma of young women, during midcycle ovulatory LH peak, and post-menopausal or castrated women, inhibit in radioimmunoassay of β HCG in such a manner that the threshold proposed by Franchimont and generally used is too low. Therefore, hormonotherapy with central acting drugs decreases pituitary gonadotrophins and also cross reaction in β IICG radioimmunoassay. This comment is true for all antisera with more than 1% cross reaction.

TALERMAN A. (Rotterdam): I think that we cannot change the histological criteria and classification, or change the nomenclature just because we see a few cells stained by immunoperoxidase for HCG.

BELLET D. (Villejuif): This question is actually discussed by the pathologists. From the clinical point of view, this fact is important to be known because the prognosis is worse and chemotherapy may be proposed.

TALERMAN A. (Rotterdam): In a very large study of testicular tumours by the British Testicular Tumour Panel, there was no evidence that in seminoma with syncytiotrophoblastic giant cells the prognosis was worse.

NØORGARD-PEDERSEN B. (Sønderborg): I agree with Dr.Talerman.

ARDIET C.(Lyon): Dr. Bellet, have you an idea concerning reciprocal value of HCG and β HCG radioimmunoassay in choriocarcinoma.

BELLET D. (Villejuif): Both are interesting, especially if HCG falls below 100 mUI/ml; it is useful in monitoring the end of chemotherapy.

CARCINOEMBRYONIC ANTIGEN IN UROTHELIAL CANCER

K.D. Bagshawe and F. Searle

Department of Medical Oncology, Charing Cross Hospital (Fulham),
Fulham Palace Road, London W6 8 RF, England.

The results which have accrued in the study of carcinoembryonic
antigen in urothelial disease, although perhaps disappointing in the
potential application to clinical management, have nevertheless
important implications for the understanding of the metabolism,
antigenic structure and cellular origin of carcinoembryonic antigen.
A review of the literature on urinary carcinoembryonic antigen
suggests that the serial assay of samples obtained under carefully
controlled conditions without concomitant infection may be useful
in following patients with T2-T4 disease undergoing radiotherapy. The
information available on the chemical structure of the carcinoembryonic antigen-like substances in urine and its implication for the
antigenicity of the molecule will be discussed.

The first reports by Hall et al (1)on the measurement of carcinoembryonic antigen (CEA) or CEA-like substances in dialysed urine
suggested a CEA positivity in 20/30 histologically proved active
transitional cell carcinomasin males. The normal female population
presented a generally higher mean urinary CEA concentration than the
normal male population after random sampling. The elevation was
traced by these workers (2) and by Wahren et al (3) to the contamination of the urine by vaginal or cervical secretions or both.   The
presence of certain bacteria such as enterococci, E. coli, proteus
and ∝-streptococci did not interfere with the CEA assay, but high
urinary levels were encountered when symptomatic urinary infections
with inflammation of transitional epithelium were present. The CEA or
CEA-like substances present in urinesfrom infected bladders gave a
line of identity on Ouchterlony immunodiffusion with standard CEA material.(1)   When urine was collected from ileal conduits, large
quantities of CEA-like substances were detectable. However, if urine
were collected simultaneously from the ureters and ileal stoma, the
CEA content of ureteric urine could be normal while that of the stoma
urine was raised.(2) It was therefore concluded that ileal conduit
urine vitiates the CEA result.   It was also noted that urine which
had been collected in an artificial bladder contained CEA-like
activity.(3)

To circumvent the difficulties encountered in sampling urine,
levels of CEA in serum or plasma were estimated in patients with
bladder cancers.   Plasma CEA, according to Coombes et al (4) appeared
to show no consistent correlation with stage of disease; patients

with no detectable cancer at time of sampling and patients with disseminated disease both had over 50% of their samples within the normal range. Fraser et al (5) reported serum CEA >3.5 ng/ml in only 7/90 patients with active vesical carcinoma; 5 of these had Jewitt's stage O lesions, 2 had more extensive tumours.

Returning to urinary CEA levels, there were generally concurring reports on the correlation between the extent of tumour at presentation and the likelihood of urinary CEA positivity, but differing reports on histological grading and levels of CEA encountered. Thus Hall et al (1) noted that urinary CEA levels were independent of the size, extent and differentiation of the tumour; some small T_1 tumours can be associated with as high levels of CEA as large invasive T4 tumours. Although later results (2) indicated that higher CEA levels tended to occur in association with more invasive tumours, the degree of differentiation did not effect the distribution of levels encountered. Guinan et al (6) considered that tumour mass and /or surface area are directly related to urinary CEA levels, but their results, though numerous, are drawn from a relatively small number of patients. Meanwhile Fraser (5) found that while only 32/59 patients with superficially invasive transitional cell carcinoma (Jewitt's stage O,A or B1) were positive, 29/41 were positive with invasive carcinoma. (Jewitt's stage B2, C,D) indicating progression. These workers also correlated a greater number of positive CEA results (23/29) with less differentiated grade 3-4 tumours than with well differentiated grade 1-2 tumours (22/48).

Whatever the final conclusions regarding the extent of tumour and CEA level, the consensus of opinion seems to be that biopsy at cystoscopy remains the most accurate method of diagnosis.

Attention was now turned to serial urinary CEA measurements as an adjunct to therapy. Wahren et al (3) studied a series of patients at clinical stage T3, and T4 with a high histologic grade of malignancy: these are a sub-set of patients who mostly receive radiation treatment. 34 previously untreated patients and 33 patients with recurrent disease comprised the group; a control group consisted of 15 samples of urine from patients undergoing irradiation for carcinoma of the prostate, the target area including an area of normal bladder. All samples were perchloric-acid-extracted before assay.

The initial urinary CEA level decreased in 24/25 patients of Stage T2-T4 who belonged to a group free of detectable tumour at cystoscopy 4 months after treatment. In contrast the 15 samples of urine from patients undergoing irradiation for carcinoma of the prostate remained normal throughout.

As indicated, in advanced disease resection by an ileal conduit is often constructed or uretersigmoidostomy performed. Unfortunately, this vitiates the further use of CEA for monitoring as the CEA will be elevated owing to gastrointestinal secretions. Go et al (7) have measured CEA-like intestinal secretions using an intestinal perfusion technique, demonstrating that secretory rates for CEA were 10-fold higher in the colon than in the ileum.

363

From monitoring healthy individuals who had been exposed to urinary carcinogens (8) it was concluded that CEA measurements were probably less valuable than urinary cytology for monitoring a population at risk.

Although the clinical use of CEA in bladder cancer is restricted to a sub-set of patients for whom serial monitoring may be useful, namely those at clinical stage T2 to T4 before ileal conduit, a number of observations have accrued from the pursuit of these studies which are relevant to the structure of the CEA molecule.

The fact exists that in urothelial cancer, prior to metastatic invasion, there are often high levels of CEA-like activity in the urine, but no detectable CEA in the serum. By contrast, in many non-urothelial malignant diseases, there may be high circulating levels of CEA but no detectable urinary activity. Since proteins with molecular weight below 68,000 tend to be excreted in the urine, it seems at first sight surprising that, in conditions where serum CEA may be circulating at levels of 2,000 µg/litre, there is no leakage of any partially degraded, partially active fragments into the urine. The studies of Schuster et al (9) on the metabolic breakdown of iodine-labelled CEA injected into dogs have established a rapid uptake of circulatory CEA by the liver, probably by the hepatocytes. A slight amount of immunological activity could be assayed if urine samples were collected within 10 minutes of injection, the activity being polydisperse in a molecular weight range of 20,000 - 50,000. It is known from chemical studies (10) that the molecule can be largely desialylated without great loss of immunological activity, however the disulphide bonds must remain intact. It is possible to postulate the existence of a determinant composed of functional groups, perhaps comprised of both protein and carbohydrate residues, not necessarily adjacent in the molecule and therefore conformationally dependent, which no longer exists when the molecule is degraded below a molecular weight of 60,000.

In principle, in considering the CEA-like activity expressed/during urethelial disease, we have a model system to study the concepts that there are antigenic determinants on the CEA molecule which are organ specific and tumour specific. The most extensive biochemical study available of the urinary CEA-like materials was undertaken by Nery et al (11) who found CEA-like activity in two molecular weight regions in glycoprotein materials isolated from the urine of patients with bladder cancer. The higher molecular weight material (2×10^7) was designated UCEA-3, the lower molecular weight material (2×10^5) UCEA-1.

U-CEA-3 was not convertible into UCEA-1 by dispersion procedures with glycine-hydrochloric acid, an observation borne out by Wu et al (12). UCEA-3 contained immunoglobulin as well as some form of CEA-determinant carrying molecule.

UCEA-1 was chemically very similar to perchloric acid-extracted colonic cancer derived CEA, being no more heterogenous than different preparations of CEA by the criteria of electrophoresis in borate-buffered urea, centrifugation on caesium-chloride density gradient, isolectric focussing and DEAE cellulose chromatography. However, although considerable purification of UCEA-1 was achieved by repeated gelfiltration on Sephadex G-200 followed by electrophoresis on cellogel, radioimmunoassay showed that the final product contained 3% w/w of the antigenic activity of an equal weight of standard carcinoembryonic antigens: it would be interesting to know whether this carried the same form of determinant as the low-activity material in colon-derived carcinoembryonic antigen preparations which is not bound to concanavalin-A-sepharose.

If there exists a colonic organ-specific determinant, as suggested by Mori et al (13) there is presumably no reason for this to be present in material derived from bladder epithelium. It would be interesting to know if there are data available on the reaction of UCEA-1 with antisera believed to be directed at this determinant.

The question whether the CEA molecule has a tumour-specific determinant is more difficult. One could argue that with colonic cancer tissue extracts and urothelial cancer tissue extracts it should be possible to produce antisera giving a line of identity which is not shared by precipitation reactions with extracts from ulcerative colitis-derived material or from urines from bladders with inflamed epithelium. If the material were available from surgical resection, it would be intriguing to compare antisera from animals rendered tolerant to ulcerative colitis tissue extracts and then immunised with conventional CEA, with antisera from animals rendered tolerant to dialysed concentrates of urine from infected bladders, then injected with urine concentrated from patients with urothelial cancers, with of course appropriate absorption. It certainly seems that the dominant determinant of CEA will not manifest the difference. Indeed, it appears likely from the recent work of Todd et al (14) on CEA-like material from colonic lavage of healthy individuals that cancer specificity, if it exists, will reside in very subtle alterations in the antigenic determinant. The main observable difference between the perchloric-acid-extracted CEA-like material from colonic lavage and standard CEA appeared to be a lower amount of total galactose and a higher amount of terminal acetylglucosamine. Although minor differences could be observed in the radioimmunoassay inhibition curves, these were no greater than those observed for different preparations of CEA from tumour tissue or serum samples. Suppose that the antigenic determinants mainly responsible for CEA activity involves at least one functional group from a carbohydrate residue on a side chain: numerical differences in specific immunological activity may reside in the proportion of completely identical side-chains in a given molecule. Edgington et al (15) demonstrated systematic differences in binding of CEA and CEA-S to a panel of antisera which could reflect conformational differences or density of antigenic determinants.

It could be even more difficult to resolve the problem if side-chains which are not completely identical can simulate the antigenic determinant sufficiently well to be partially bound by a given

365

population of antibodies which will have an average binding constant. Unfortunately such differences do exist between pairs of antisera and labelled antigens used for radioimmunoassay which show themselves in the numerical values obtained for some 20% of non-extracted sera (after correction for immunological potency between standards) and in our experience are not necessarily associated with increasing clinical specificity for either set of reagents.

In conclusion, the study of urinary CEA-like molecules and indeed CEA-like materials from other non-colonic sources is potentially likely to assist the search for more specificity in the CEA assay and the concomitant need to strive towards the best inter-laboratory standardisation possible for routine requests.

REFERENCES

(1) Hall, R.R., Laurence, D.J.R., Darcy, D., Stevens, V., James,R., and Neville, A.M. (1972): British Medical Journal, 3, 609.

(2) Hall, R.R., Laurence, D.J.R., Neville, A.M. and Wallace, D.M., (1973): British Journal of Urology, 88.

(3) Wahren, B., Edsmyr, F. and Zimmerman, R. (1975): Cancer, 36,1490.

(4) Coombes, G.B., Hall, R.R., Laurence, D.J.R. and Neville,A.M. (1975): British Journal of Cancer, 31, 135.

(5) Fraser, R.A., Ravry, M.J., Segura, J.W. and Go, V.L.W. (1975): Journal of Urology, 114, 226.

(6) Guinan, P., John, T., Sadonghi, N., Ablin, R.J. and Bush, I. (1975): Journal of Urology, 111, 350.

(7) Go, V.L.W., Ammon, H.V., Holtermuller, K.H., Kray, E. and Phillips, S.F. (1975): Cancer, 36, 2346.

(8) Turner, A.G., Palmer, H., Powell, M.E. and Neville, A.M. (1976): Lancet, i, 308.

(9) Schuster, J., Silverman, M. and Gold, P. (1973): Cancer Research, 33, 65.

(10) Coligan, J.E., Henkart, P.A., Todd, C.W. and Terry, W.D. (1973): Immunochemistry, 10, 591.

(11) Nery, R., Barsoum, A.L., Bullman, H. and Neville, A.M. (1974): Biochemical Journal, 139, 431.

(12) Wu, J.T., Madsen, A. and Bray, P.F. (1974): Journal of the National Cancer Institute, 53(6), 1589.

(13) Mori, T., Shimano, T., Lee, P., Fujimoto, N. and Kosaki, G., (1977): Proceedings of 5th IRGP Meeting. In Press.

(14) Egan, M.L., Pritchard, D.G., Todd, C.W. and Go, V.L.W.
(1977): Cancer Research, 37, 2638.

(15) Edgington, T.S., Plow, E.F., Charkin, C.I., Deheer, A.T. and
Nakamura, R.M. (1976): Bulletin du Cancer, 63(4), 673.

DISCUSSION

COOPER E.H. (Leeds): I would like to say that CEA is disappointing
as regard to bladder carcinoma. We are examining a natural product,
Beta 2 Microglobulin. In active T1, the levels are a little bit
higher than normal, but people are old. But the fascinating thing
is this : if you consider T4 lesion and if you are lucky enough to
have T4 surviving up a year or 18 months, they seem to begin to fall
into three classes : (i) those with Beta 2 microglobulin essentially
normal, (ii) those whose Beta 2 is on a high range, (iii) those with
levels in an intermediate range.
This suggests that they may be a chemical stratification of the
tumour. There is no stoicheiometric relationship between tumour
mass and the marker. This is more likely to be an indication of
certain behaviour of the tumour.

CATTAN A. (Reims): Did you have any data on the prognosis value of
Beta 2 Microglobulin in bladder carcinoma?

COOPER E.H. (Leeds): This is far too premature for the moment.

BJORKLUND B.(Stockholm): We have heard to-day that in urinary infections, there are elevation of both CEA and TPA. I do not understand
why this is so. I know that the common infections do not produce
TPA in vitro. We have seen in foetuses that TPA is concentrated
tremendously in fetal urine but the bladder wall does not contain
more TPA than serum. So, obviously something happens during the
infection which causes the bladder to produce CEA and TPA. It could
be a proliferation or a change of type of proliferation. This needs
to be explored because we know nothing about it.

ZIMMERMAN R. (Stockholm): We found high CEA levels in the urine of
patients with long standing urinary infections. Nevertheless, we
have tried to induce CEA activity in a bladder cell line T24 with
different bacteria strains but we did not succeed.
Using immunofluorescence test on smears from bladder washings, we
found that in highly differentiated tumours it exists a higher incidence of cells containing CEA.

THE CLINICAL VALUE OF CARCINOEMBRYONIC ANTIGEN (CEA) IN HAEMATURIA AND UROTHELIAL CARCINOMA

R. W. GLASHAN and E. HIGGINS *

Department of Urology, Huddersfield Royal Infirmary, Huddersfield, Yorkshire, England.

Since carcinoembryonic antigen (CEA) was first described (1), numerous studies have shown that plasma CEA can be raised in a wide variety of neoplastic and non-neoplastic conditions (2). This communication describes a prospective clinical evaluation of CEA in haematuria and urothelial carcinoma, between 1973 – 76, initiated at the request of the Medical Research Council and the Department of Health and Social Security, London.

PATIENTS AND METHODS

Two hundred and sixteen patients, presenting with haematuria to the Urological Departments at the Huddersfield Royal Infirmary and the Royal Marsden Hospital, over a period of 18 months, had plasma and urine CEA levels estimated in addition to the routine urological investigations. Urinary infection was diagnosed if there were greater than 25 WBC per HPF and greater than 100,000 organisms/ml on urine culture. These studies were extended for 3 years to include patients with proven urothelial malignancy until a total of 325 patients had been evaluated in the following groups:

(a) 216 patients with undiagnosed haematuria (93 were found to have tumours),

(b) 138 patients with T_1 tumours,

(c) 64 patients with advanced urothelial carcinoma (T_2, T_3 and T_4 categories).

The bladder tumours were categorised according to the U.I.C.C. classification in 1974 but the CEA levels throughout the trial were not revealed to the clinicians until all the studies had been completed. On the basis of previous experience (3) (4), a plasma CEA $<$ 40 ng/ml was considered normal in both males and females but, in the urine, values $<$ 35 ng/ml in males and $<$ 110 ng/ml in females were taken as being normal.

* Supported by a grant from the Medical Research Council, London.

CEA AND HAEMATURIA

A total of 216 patients, 159 male and 57 female, who complained of haematuria, were investigated to see if there was any relationship between the diagnosis and levels of plasma and urinary CEA. A definite diagnosis was made in 213 cases who were divided into 3 groups as in Table 1.

TABLE 1   Diagnosis of cases presenting with haematuria.

Urinary tract infection with no evidence of urothelial carcinoma	38	(18%)
Urothelial carcinoma	93	(44%)
Other urological conditions with no evidence of infection	82	(38%)
	213	

CEA levels were studied to assess whether they could differentiate between benign and malignant urothelial conditions but plasma CEA was found to have no diagnostic value as it was raised in only 4 out of 93 patients with carcinoma, although all 4 patients did have invasive growths. In the presence of urinary infection, the plasma CEA was always normal.

TABLE 2   CEA levels related to diagnosis.

Diagnosis	No. of Patients	Plasma CEA		Urinary CEA		
		Normal	Raised	Normal	Raised	
Infected	38	38	0	13	25	(66%)
Carcinoma	93	89	4	*36	*21	(37%)
Other	82	80	2	77	5	(6%)
	213	207	6	126	51	

* Tumour and no infection present.

Urinary CEA levels were raised in 66% of patients with urinary infection (25 out of 38) and in 37% of patients with proven urothelial tumours and sterile urine. A knowledge of the urinary CEA level would seem to contribute little to the diagnosis of patients presenting with haematuria.

CEA AND T_1 TUMOURS

In this group, 138 patients with T_1 tumours had serial plasma and urinary CEA levels studied over a 3 year period. Altogether 784 plasma samples were analysed but only 13 (1.7%) were found to be raised and, therefore, plasma CEA was of no help in the T_1 group. Urinary CEA levels could be related to cystoscopy findings on 538 occasions as shown in Table 3.

TABLE 3   Urinary CEA in relation to cystoscopies in T_1 tumours.

| | Cystoscopies | | | | |
	FEMALES	MALES	TOTAL	CEA RAISED	
TUMOUR	68	188	256	6	2.4%
NO TUMOUR	70	212	282	29	10%
			538		

Tumours were seen at 256 cystoscopies with a raised CEA on 43 occasions, but, when active urinary infection was excluded, CEA was only raised 6 times (2.4%). In the remaining 282 cystoscopies the CEA was raised 56 times but only on 29 occasions (10%) when there was no infection present. In conclusion, urinary CEA was raised more often in bladders which were apparently clear of tumour, though the number of raised CEA levels was small, and, clinically of no value.

CEA IN ADVANCED UROTHELIAL CARCINOMA

In this group, there were 64 patients with advanced transitional cell carcinoma, (categories T_2 T_3 and T_4), at the time of the initial cystoscopy and assessment prior to treatment being instituted. Plasma and urine CEA levels were estimated before and after treatment on a serial basis until death or the conclusion of the investigation in 1976. Table 4 shows the distribution of the patients by sex and tumour category.

TABLE 4   Categories of advanced urothelial carcinoma.

	T_2	T_3	T_4	
Female	5	7	2	14
Male	14	29	7	50
	19	36	9	64

Four out of 64 patients (6%) had a plasma level 40 ng/ml initially. Two of these were T_4 growths, the other 2 being T_3 tumours (both male), who died within 3 months, suggesting they were probably understaged. In a further patient, the plasma CEA rose as the bladder carcinoma progressed and all 5 patients with a raised plasma CEA eventually died from the bladder carcinoma.

Urinary infection is known to alter urinary CEA levels (3) (5) (6) and, therefore, patients with a proven infection prior to treatment were excluded from this study. The distribution of the tumour categories in patients with a sterile urine is shown in Table 5.

TABLE 5 Categories of advanced urothelial carcinoma with sterile urine.

	T_2	T_3	T_4	
Female	4	4	1	9
Male	12	24	4	40
	16	28	5	49

Four of the 16 T_2 tumours (25%) had raised CEA levels, 3 falling to normal following treatment (1 transurethral resection and 2 radiotherapy) whilst the fourth patient's urine showed a progressively rising CEA until death occurred 2 years later.

TABLE 6 Urinary CEA in advanced bladder tumours.

	Patients	CEA RAISED
T_2	16	4 (25%)
T_3	28	14 (50%)
T_4	5	2 (40%)
	49	20

In the T_3 group, 14 out of 28 (50%) patients had initially a raised CEA level but 6 of these returned to normal following satisfactory treatment of the tumours (5 with radiotherapy and 1 with chemotherapy) In 6 other patients, CEA in the urine rose until the patients died of their bladder malignancies and the remaining 2 patients developed persistantly high but variable levels associated with intractable infections following radiotherapy. Finally, in 5 T_4 tumours, the urinary CEA was only raised in 2 patients despite the fact that all 5 progressed to an early death.

In conclusion, in 64 cases of advanced bladder cancer, only 4 patients showed a level of plasma CEA > 40 ng/ml and so plasma CEA is of little diagnostic value. Twenty out of 49 patients with a sterile urine showed a raised urinary CEA level (> 35 ng/ml in men and > 110 ng/ml in women) before treatment, 9 of these (45%) returning to normal when the tumours were satisfactorily treated as judged by repeated cystoscopic examinations. In a further 9 patients (45%), the urinary CEA rose despite treatment and, in each case, the local disease had progressed.

CONCLUSIONS

Plasma and urine CEA levels were studied over a period of three years in 325 patients with urological disease. The following conclusions have emerged

1. CEA is of no diagnostic value in haematuria, but urinary infection can raise urine CEA levels.

2. CEA is of no value in the diagnosis or follow-up of T_1 category tumours.

3. Studies of plasma CEA in 64 cases with advanced bladder carcinoma were of no value in reaching a diagnosis or in the assessment of metastatic disease.

4. Urinary CEA can be raised by urothelial carcinoma but is not a reliable diagnostic or prognostic index.

ACKNOWLEDGMENT

We would like to express our gratitude to the Institute of Cancer Research, London for the CEA estimations.

REFERENCES

(1) Gold, P. and Freedman, S.O. (1965): _Journal of Experimental Medicine, 121_, 439 – 462

(2) Neville, A.M. and Cooper, E.H. (1976): _Annals of Clinical Biochemistry, 13_, 283 – 305

(3) Hall, R.R. Laurence, D.J.R., Neville, A.M. and Wallace, D.M. (1973): _British Journal of Urology, 45_, 88 – 92

(4) Turner, A.G., Carter, S., Higgins, E., Glashan, R.W. and Neville, A.M. (1977): _British Journal of Urology, 49_, 61 – 66

(5) Coombes, G.B., Hall, R.R., Laurence, D.J.R. and Neville, A.M. (1975): _British Journal of Cancer, 31_, 135 – 142

(6) Guinan, P., Dubin, A., Bush, I., Alsheik, H. and Ablin, R.J. (1975): _Oncology, 32_, 158 – 168

DISCUSSION

BLAKE K.E. (Pittsburg): Have you had any experience with the Makari test in bladder tumours.

GLASHAN R.W. (Huddersfield): No, I have not.

MAC DONALD E.A. (Nice): May I ask whether you tried looking at CEA in tumour biopsies.

GLASHAN R.W. (Huddersfield): No.

MAC DONALD E.A. (Nice): Did you analyse the survival of those few patients who did have raised CEA levels in either the serum or in urine. Was it your feeling that this small group of tumours had disseminated disease earlier or had a poorer prognosis.

GLASHAN R.W. (Huddersfield): I think the answer to your two questions must be negative. The results may be interesting for the laboratory but not the clinical field.

TALERMAN A. (Rotterdam): Did you find differences concerning the histology of the tumours.

GLASHAN R.W. (Huddersfield): No, there was no correlation.

TISSUE POLYPEPTIDE ANTIGEN (TPA) AND CYTOLOGY IN CANCER OF THE
URINARY BLADDER

S. Isacson and Å. Andrén-Sandberg

Department of Surgery, Central Hospital, Halmstad, Sweden

Tissue polypeptide antigen (TPA) was originally described by
Björklund and Björklund in 1957 (1). TPA is an antigenic polypeptide
occurring in the membranes of human cancer cells and can be demonstrated in serum and urine by a modified hemagglutination inhibition
micro-technique (2). Since 1973 we have been closely watching the
TPA in serum and urine and the clinical course in patients with
different types of cancer (3, 4). A comparison of the TPA in urine
with cytologic findings in the urinary tract in cases of histologically verified bladder carcinoma is briefly outlined below.

MATERIAL AND METHODS

The control group consisted of 88 patients without malignant
disease or existing infection, including infection of the urinary
tract. The group with urinary tract infection verified by culture
of urine consisted of 39 patients. The samples examined for TPA and
those used for culture were always taken from one and the same specimen. None of the patients had any other known infection or malignant disease. All the 9 patients with urinary tract calculi were
controls.

The clinical material consisted of 27 patients (3 women, 24
men) with histologically verified bladder carcinoma. They ranged in
age from 31 to 90 years with a median age of 73 years. The patients
are divided into subgroups according to recommendations of l´Union
Internationale Contre le Cancer (UICC). On clinical staging 14 cases were classified as T 1, 5 as T 2, 6 as T 3, and 2 as T 4. The
histopathological grading showed that 8 patients had tumours with
mild anaplasia, i.e. grade 1. Six tumours showed marked anaplasia,
grade 3, and the rest were grade 2. Urine specimens were collected
on three different preoperative days and examined for cells, TPA,
and cultured for bacteria. TPA was determined with a modified hemagglutination inhibition micro-technique (2).

RESULTS AND COMMENTS

To assess the upper limit of what should be regarded as the
normal range of TPA in the urine, we examined samples from 88 patients without malignant disease or existing infection, including
the urinary tract (Fig. 1). 69 patients showed a TPA value of less

374

than 0.095 U/ml, 12 persons 0.095 and 7 persons 0.19 U/ml. The highest value was thus 0.19 U/ml. We regard this as indicating that a TPA value of less than 0.19 is normal, a value of 0.19 being a borderline value that deserves further investigation. Values of 0.38 or higher we regard as abnormally high. It is known from studies of other tumour markers, such as CEA, that infection can give false positive values. We therefore tested 39 patients with urinary tract infection verified by culture of the urine. 19 of the 39 patients had values above 0.19 U/ml. This means that about 50 per cent had pathological values. This implies that if the urine is infected, a high value of TPA in urine is of no help in the diagnosis of carcinoma of the bladder.

In 9 patients with urinary tract calculi the TPA values were invariably low and the highest value was 0.095. The results indicate that urinary calculi do not cause an inflammation reaction severe enough to influence the concentration of TPA in the urine.

Urine samples from 27 patients with histologically verified bladder carcinoma were examined for TPA and cells in the urine. Figure 2 shows the most abnormal TPA value of the 3 specimens from each patient. 23 of the patients had pathologically high values, i.e. 0.19 U/ml and 4 patients a borderline value. If we relate the TPA values to clinical and histopathological staging, we find the borderline values to be in the groups with the lowest degrees of staging (Fig. 3). If the material be regarded as a whole, it can be concluded that the earlier clinical stages are dominating, and that tumours with marked anaplasia constitute only about 20 per cent. When we compare TPA and the cytological findings in the patients with bladder carcinoma, we find that 16 patients had a cytologic diagnosis of cancer, compared with 23 with pathologically high values in the urine (Fig. 4). None of the patients had a really normal TPA, but in 3 cytologic studies showed nothing remarkable. When both tests were taken together, the results were pathological in 85 per cent of the patients, and in the remaining 15 per cent disease was suspected and indicated further control.

CONCLUSION

In conclusion, the results indicate that the diagnostic accuracy of bladder carcinoma can be increased by determination of TPA in the urine. Such determination combined with cytologic examination of urine provides a fairly simple and safe test combination for following up patients with bladder carcinoma, but it should not exclude or replace cystoscopy. It also seems that the two tests together can be used for screening for bladder carcinoma in persons occupied in certain industries, in which the risk of this type of cancer is great.

REFERENCES

(1) Björklund, B. and Björklund, V. (1957): Int. Arch. Allergy Appl. Immunol. 10:153-184.
(2) Björklund, B. and Paulsson, J.E. (1962): J. Immunol. 89:759-766
(3) Isacson, S., Lindblad, C., Nistor, L. and Risholm, L. (1974): XI International Cancer Congress. Florence, 1974. Abstract.
(4) Andrén-Sandberg, Å. and Isacson, S. (1976): Third International Symposium on Detection and Prevention of Cancer. New York, 1976. In press.

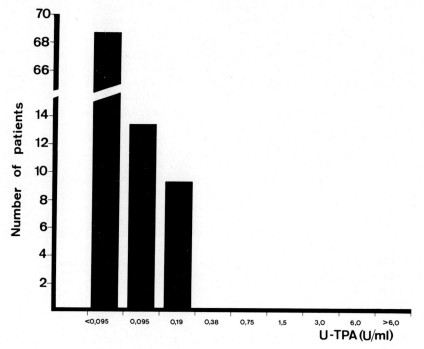

Fig. 1   U-TPA in the controls.

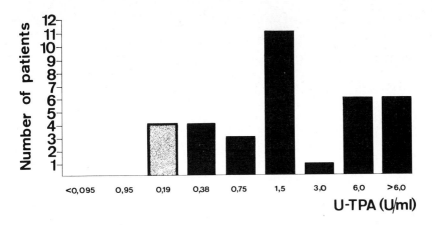

Fig. 2   U-TPA in 27 patients with histologically verified bladder carcinoma.

U-TPA-values	T (Clinical stage)				G (Pathological stage)		
	1	2	3	4	1	2	3
Normal (≤ 0,18 U/ml) Border line (0,19–0,37 U/ml) Pathologic (≥ 0,38 U/ml)	4 10	5	6	2	1 7	3 10	6

Fig. 3   U-TPA in relation to clinical and pathological stage.

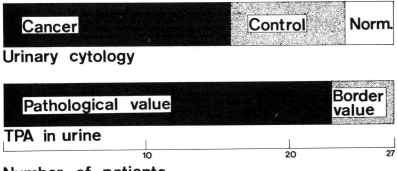

Fig. 4   Urinary cytology and U-TPA in patients with histologically verified bladder carcinoma.

CHARACTERIZATION OF CEA-LIKE MATERIAL IN BLADDER CARCINOMA

Rolf Zimmerman and Sten Hammarström

Department of Virology, National Bacteriological Laboratory, and
Department of Immunology, University of Stockholm, Stockholm, Sweden

Patients with urothelial carcinoma show increased levels of CEA-activity in serum and urine (1,5,6,7,8).

The purpose of this investigation was to purify CEA-like material from urinary bladder carcinoma and to compare its immunological and physico-chemical properties with colon cancer CEA.

MATERIAL AND METHODS

Purification: Local recurrent transitional cell carcinoma of urinary bladder from two individuals were obtained at autopsy and pooled. Tumor tissue (460 g wet weight) was homogenized in water and precipitated with perchloric acid (1 M, final concentration). The PCA soluble material was then fractionated on a Sepharose 4B column (90x 5 cm) in 0.05 M NaH_2PO_4, pH 5.0 containing 0.15 M NaCl. CEA-activity was monitored by radioimmunoassay using the Hoffmann-La Roche Z-gel kit (Figure 1). Three CEA-active pools (I, II and III) were collected. Each pool was then passed over a Concanavalin A-Sepharose affinity chromatography column and eluted with methyl-α-D-mannoside (10 and 50 mg/ml). All bound material was eluted at the lower sugar concentration. The eluted fractions were finally fractionated on an anti CEA immunoadsorbent column prepared by conjugating the IgG-fraction of a spleen absorbed sheep anti CEA serum to cyanogen bromide activated Sepharose 4B (2). Bound material was eluted with 6 M guanidine HCl, dialysed and lyophilized. Material eluted from the immunoadsorbent column (fractions IB b, IIB b and IIIB b) was labelled with $Na^{125}I$ using the chloramine T-method (2).

Reference CEA, anti-CEA and anti-NCA sera: Reference CEA was purified from liver metastases of colo-rectal cancer as earlier described (3). Rabbit and sheep anti-CEA sera were absorbed with A+B erythrocytes and PCA-extract of human spleen and were found not to precipitate with purified NCA or BGP I (2) or with PCA extract of normal lung, spleen or colon. Immunosorbent purified monkey anti-CEA antibodies were prepared from a pool of four unabsorbed monkey anti-CEA serum (4). No crossreaction with NCA or BGP I was seen at 10^3 times higher concentration than was needed for 50% inhibition with CEA using an enzyme linked immunoadsorbent assay (4). Anti-NCA serum was from rabbit injected with semipurified spleen NCA and absorbed with PCA extract of one colon tumor with very low CEA and NCA content (3). The specificity of the antiserum for NCA has been documented (3).

Analytical methods: The ability of anti-CEA and anti-NCA serum to precipitate ^{125}I-labelled purified CEA-like material from bladder carcinoma fractionated on a Sephacryl S-200 column (90x1 cm) was determined. Antibody bound material was separated from nonbound material either by the addition of sheep anti rabbit IgG covalently bound to cellulose particles or by the addition of carrier IgG and saturated $(NH_4)_2SO_4$ (monkey anti-CEA antibodies).

Size heterogeneity and molecular weights were determined by gradient polyacrylamide gel electrophoresis in sodium dodecylsulphate after complete reduction using a discontinuous buffer system (2). The analyses were performed with ^{125}I-labelled material using autoradiography. Molecular weights were determined from the mobility of standard proteins (slope calculated by linear regression).

Table I.

Purification of CEA from primary bladder cancer

		Dry weight mg	Specific activity µg CEA/mg	Total activity µg CEA
PCA-soluble		521	0.23	117.2
Sepharose 4B	I	60	1.54	92.4
	II	119	0.32	38.7
	III	73	0.65	47.5
Con A-Sepharose	IA	40	0.78	31.2
	IB	7.2	6.00	43.2
	IIA	79	0.12	9.5
	IIB	24	0.70	16.9
	IIIA	59	0.05	2.8
	IIIB	6.2	2.40	14.9
Anti-CEA-immuno-adsorbent	IB a	5.1	<0.03	<0.15
	b	–	–	7.5
	IIB a	17	<0.03	<0.5
	b	1.1	1.46	1.60
	IIIB a	4.8	<0.03	<0.15
	b	–	–	5.5

RESULTS

The recovery, specific activity (ug CEA-equivalent/mg material) and total CEA-equivalent activity obtained during purification of bladder cancer "CEA" are summarized in Table I. Figure 1 shows the elution profile on Sepharose 4B gelfiltration of the PCA-soluble fraction of bladder tumor. Several points are of interest: i) the CEA-content in bladder tumors is very low. Only about 0.2% of the dry weight of the PCA soluble fraction appears to constitute CEA. CEA-measurement of 4 other individual bladder tumors gave values of 100-

250 ug CEA-equivalent/kg tumor wet weight. The values should be compared with 25-100 mg CEA/kg tumor wet weight for liver metastases of colo-rectal cancer. ii) two peaks of CEA-activity was obtained when the PCA-extract of bladder tumor was fractionated on Sepharose 4B. iii) the specific activity increased during purification. Thus, the PCA-soluble fraction contained 0.23 ug CEA-equivalents/mg, Sepharose 4B fraction I 1.54 ug CEA-equivalents/mg, Con A-Sepharose eluted fraction (IB) 6.0 ug CEA-equivalents/mg and anti-CEA immunoadsorbent eluted fraction (IB b) > 75 ug CEA-equivalents/mg. The dry weight of the latter fraction was too small to be determined accurately but was less than 100 ug. Increase in specific activity during purification was also observed for the other two Sepharose 4B fractions. iiii) no CEA-active material (<0.03 ug CEA-equivalents/mg) passed the anti-CEA immunoadsorbent column.

Figures 2 and 3 show the elution profiles on Sephacryl S-200 of immunoadsorbent purified bladder cancer "CEA" fractions (IB b and IIIB b, Table I). The materials were labelled with ^{125}I in order to enable detection. As can be seen from the radioactivity profiles both fractions are heterogeneous with respect to molecular size indicating several populations of macromolecules. The S-200 fractions were analysed for material reacting with anti-CEA and anti-NCA sera using either anti rabbit IgG antibodies or $(NH_4)_2SO_4$ to precipitate antibody bound material (Figures 2 and 3). The following results were obtained: i) both fractions contained macromolecules precipitating with specific anti CEA sera (monkey anti-CEA and spleen absorbed rabbit anti-CEA serum) which eluted at the same position as reference CEA. However, only about 16 and 14% respectively of the total radioactivity of fractions IB b and IIIB b were precipitated by the specific CEA antisera. ii) specific anti-NCA serum precipitated about 15% of the radioactivity in fraction IB b and about 35% in fraction IIIB b. Anti-NCA reactive material showed considerable size heterogeneity. iii) unabsorbed anti-CEA serum precipitated a higher percentage of the material in each fraction then either of the specific antisera alone. In fact the percentage of radioactivity precipitated by unabsorbed anti-CEA serum corresponded closely to the sum of the radioactivity precipitated by specific anti-CEA and anti-NCA serum.

SDS-PAGE analyses of ^{125}I-labelled fractions IB b and IIIB b revealed the presence of several components in each fraction. Fraction IB b contained bands with the following apparent molecular weights: 175,000; 115-150,000 broad zone; 74,000 and 53,000. Fraction IIIB b contained the following bands: 175,000; 115-140,000 broad zone; 74,000; 53,000; 44,000 and 25-27,000. Colon cancer CEA and the CEA-related normal adult components, NCA and biliary glycoprotein I (BGP I), gave apparent molecular weights of 175,000+8,000; 115-125,000 and 83,000+4,000 respectively when analysed by this method (2).

DISCUSSION

This study shows that small amounts of CEA-like material can be purified from local bladder carcinomas using a purification procedure similar to that adopted for colon cancer CEA. The final product after immunoadsorbent purification appeared to be a mixture of several molecular species. Two species were tentatively identified: 1) material identical with colon cancer CEA with respect to molecular size (gel filtration and SDS-PAGE), PCA solubility and ability to bind to Concanavalin A and most importantly the ability to bind to specific monkey anti-CEA serum. This antiserum was shown not to react with CEA-related normal components even when assayed with a highly sensitive enzyme linked immunoadsorbent assay (4). 2) material with the same chromatographic and immunological properties as NCA.

It may seem surprising that NCA was isolated on the anti-CEA immunoadsorbent since the antiserum used was heavily absorbed with spleen tissue in order to remove NCA-crossreactive antibodies. The antiserum was furthermore shown to be CEA specific by immunodiffusion. The finding probably illustrates the difficulty in removing the last traces of crossreactive antibodies by absorbtion. It should be noted that only a few ug of NCA was isolated.

In addition to the two components tentatively identified the purified fractions contained four additional components with lower molecular weights. From the precipitation experiments (Figures 2 and 3) it seems likely that they are non-CEA related substances.

Further analyses are needed in order to establish whether the molecular species tentatively identified as CEA is in fact identical with colon cancer CEA. Considering the low amounts of CEA-active material isolated from bladder carcinoma it seems furthermore important to establish the tumor origin of the isolated material. Studies on bladder carcinoma cell lines may resolve this question.

ACKNOWLEDGEMENT

This work was supported by a grant from the Swedish Cancer Society (no. 706-B76-04XA).

REFERENCES

(1) Coombes, G., Hall, R., Laurence, D. and Neville, M. (1975): Brit. J. Cancer 31, 35.
(2) Hammarström, S., Svenberg, T., Hedin, A. and Sundblad, G. (1977): Scand. J. Immunol. Suppl. 6, in press.
(3) Hammarström, S., Engvall, E. and Sundblad, G. (1976): p. 24 in Boström N, Larsson T & Ljungstedt N (eds). Health Control in Detection of cancer. Scandia Int. Symposia, Almqvist & Wiksell, Stockholm.
(4) Hammarström, S., Engvall, E. and Feld, S. (1977): in Griffiths K (ed). Tumor Markers, Determination and Clinical Role, in press.
(5) Nery, R., Barsoum, A., Bullman, H. and Neville, M. (1974): Biochem. J. 139, 431.
(6) Reynoso, G., Chu, T.M., Guinan, P. and Murphy, G. (1972): Cancer 30, 1.
(7) Wahren, B., Edsmyr, F. and Zimmerman, R. (1975): Cancer 36, 1490.
(8) Wu, J., Madsen, A. and Bray, P. (1974): J. Natl. Cancer Inst. 53, 1589.

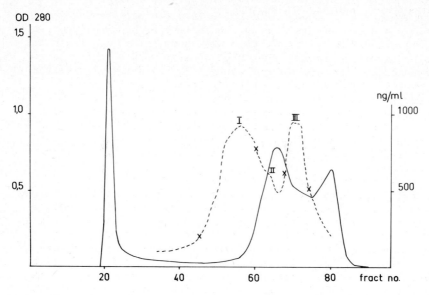

Fig. 1 Gelfiltration of the PCA-soluble fraction of bladder tumor homogenate on a Sepharose 4B column. Solid line: optical density at 280 nm. Broken line: CEA concentration in ng/ml.

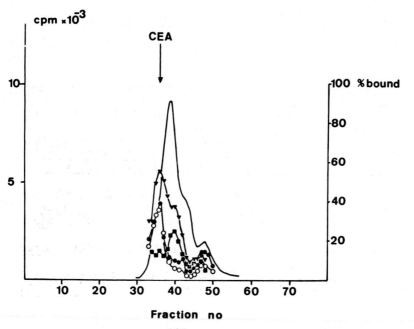

Fig. 2 Gelfiltration of ^{125}I-labelled fraction IB b (Table I) on a Sepharcyl S-200 column. Solid line: CPM/200 ul. (▼ - ▼) % radioactivity precipitated by unabsorbed rabbit anti-CEA serum. (◑--●) % radioactivity precipitated by spleen and erythrocyte absorbed rabbit anti-CEA serum. (O--O) % radioactivity precipitated by monkey anti-CEA serum. (■--■) % radioactivity precipitated by specific rabbit anti-NCA serum.

382

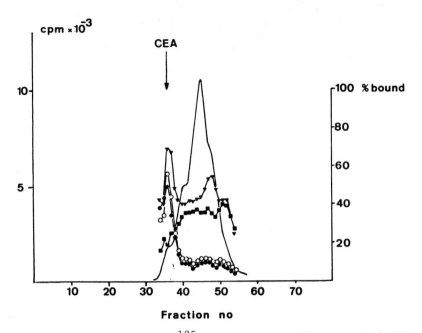

Fig. 3 Gelfiltration of ^{125}I-labelled fraction IIIB b (Table I) on a
Sephacryl S-200 column. Symbols as in Fig. 2.

CARCINOEMBRYONIC ANTIGEN DETERMINATIONS IN HEAD AND NECK CANCER

M.Schneider, F.Demard, P.Chauvel, J.Gueguen, J.Vallicioni, B.P.Krebs, A.Ramaioli

Centre Antoine Lacassagne, 36 Voie Romaine, 06054 Nice Cedex, France

LITERATURE DATA

Head and Neck cancer management is not a major field for the application of CEA measurement. Thus only one major paper from SILVERMAN et al (1) is analysed in our review.

439 patients were compared, 276 normal controls,smokers and non-smokers. Table 1 shows the incidence of positive CEA levels in the five groups.

Table 1 : Distribution of CEA levels in controls and patients with head and neck squamous carcinoma.

Groups studied	CEA level (ng/ml)			Percentage CEA elevations	
	< 5	$\geqslant 5 < 7$	$\geqslant 7$	$\% \geqslant 5$	$\% \geqslant 7$
Non Smokers	116	4	2	5	2
Smokers	134	13	7	13	5
Tumour-bearing	113	33	30	36	17
Tumour-free 2 years	95	15	6	18	5
Tumour-free 2 years	126	17	4	14	5

Silverman et al.,1976

One can notice that 36% of tumour-bearing patients are positive if 5 ng/ml is chosen as cut-off level (only 17% if 7 ng/ml). On the other hand, the author insists on the fact that the actual levels are much more elevated in cancer patients - 15 to 80 ng/ml - than in smokers (15 ng maximum) and non-smokers (10 ng maximum) control groups. In tumour-free patients, the incidence of positivity is lower, 18% if the free interval is less than 2 years, 14% if over 2 years.

Table 2 : Comparison of CEA levels and clinical tumour stage in patients with head and neck squamous carcinoma.

Tumour stage	CEA level (ng/ml)			Percentage CEA elevations	
	<5	$\geqslant5<7$	$\geqslant7$	%$\geqslant$5	%$\geqslant$7
I	17	4	5	35	19
II	32	6	2	20	5
III	39	14	7	35	12
IV	20	7	13	50	33
Distant metastases	5	2	3	50	30

Silverman et al.1976

This table shows a correlation between staging of disease and CEA levels or incidence of positive values. Silverman's team's conclusions could be summarized as follow :

i) there is no relationship between pre-operative CEA values and clinical evolution;
ii) one month after surgery, positive values return below 5ng/ml;
iii) 10 out of the 14 relapsed cases had normal CEA values;
iv) pre-treatment CEA levels fall in all cases submitted to radiotherapy;
v) there is no relationship between the CEA levels after remission and clinical status.
AMIEL et al.(2) do not find any positive values in tumours of facial bones. In contrast, in the series of 57 cases of E.N.T. tumours, they have observed 21% of positive values (more than 10 ng/ml). Nevertheless no relation was found according to tumour size or site.

POPULATION SUBMITTED TO ANALYSIS

CEA was measured (3) in plasma of 85 ENT patients.
Table 3 : Repartition of prtients in relation with tumour site and size.

Localisation	Nb	T1		T2		T3		Outside TNM
		No	N1/2/3	No	N1/2/3	No	N1/2/3	
Oral cavity	18	4	1	4	4	1	1	3
Oropharynx	20	2		1	2	1	7	7
Hypopharynx	10			1	2		4	3
Larynx	23	4		2	4	1	2	10
Miscellaneous	14	1	2	1	2	1	3	4
Total	85	11	3	9	14	4	17	27

RESULTS

Table 4 : CEA values related to tumour localisation

Localisation	CEA $<$ 5 ng/ml	CEA $>$ 5 ng/ml
Oral cavity	12	6
Oropharynx	8	12
Hypopharynx	5	5
Larynx	12	11
Miscellaneous	8	6
Total	45	40

No difference between tumour sites can be noticed, no more than with tumour spread as shown in Table 5.

Table 5 : CEA values related to tumour spread

Tumour spread		Nb	CEA $<$ 5 ng/ml	CEA $>$ 5 ng/ml
T1	No	11	4	7
	N1/2/3	3	2	1
T2	No	9	7	2
	N1/2/3	14	7	7
T3	No	4	2	2
	N1/2/3	17	9	8
Outside TNM		27	14	13

Table 6 shows that there is no association between either clinical status or death from tumour evolution :

Clinical status			CEA $<$ 5ng/ml	CEA $>$ 5ng/ml
Patients alive		Controlled	21	13
	Non controlled	Loco-regional recurrence	6	6
		Metastase	1	3
		Loco-regional recurrence + metastase	3	2
		Total	10	11
Patients dead			14	16

In our series, CEA does not act as tumour marker for assessment of therapeutic efficiency (fig.1). In fact, many discrepencies can be noticed in follow-up of patients. For example, CEA levels decrease as tumour increases and disseminates. On the other hand, in patients without clinical evidence of disease, high values were found.

CONCLUSION

In head and neck cancer, the value of CEA as tumour marker is not clearly demonstrated. No relation exists between the high levels of CEA and caracteristics of the tumour. Concerning monitoring, CEA was unable to predict local recurrence,metastatic spread or apparition of new cancer. CEA was also unable to confirm the efficiency of surgical treatment. Lastly, CEA was unable to appreciate efficiency of systemic treatment. So, in the particular field of ENT cancer, despite a great incidence of raised levels in plasma, CEA cannot be proposed as a tumour marker for diagnosis, prognosis, follow-up, prediction of local or disseminated recurrences of diseases.

REFERENCES

(1) Silverman,N.A., Alexander, J.C., Chretien,P.B. (1976) : Cancer, 37, 2204-2211.

(2) Amiel, J.L., Henry,R., Van den Broucke,C.,Pico,J.L., Meriadec,B, Froz,J.P. (1976) : Bull. Cancer , 63, 519-524.

(3) Meriadec,B., Martin,F., Guerin ,J., Henry,R.,Klipping,C.(1973): Bull.Cancer,60, 403.

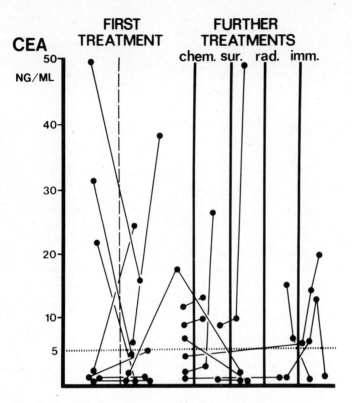

Fig.1 : CEA levels according to treatments.

DISCUSSION

COUETTE J.E. (Caen): Did you find a relationship between CEA production and histology.

SCHNEIDER M. (Nice): I cannot answer because our series was too short.

LALANNE C.M. (Nice): Could you slight elevated CEA levels be explained by smoking of alcoholism?

SCHNEIDER M.(Nice): Certainly, but we have also non-malignant lung diseases in our population.

COUETTE J.E. (Caen): In my opinion, you must not too much rely on non-specific increase of CEA due to bronchitis, cirrhosis or other non-malignant diseases. You need further examination for specific increase of CEA.

VALUE OF CARCINOEMBRYONIC ASSAY IN EARLY DETECTION OF MEDULLARY
CARCINOMA OF THE THYROID.

C. Calmettes, M.S. Moukhtar, J. Taboulet and G. Milhaud.

Unité 113 INSERM, Hôpital Saint-Antoine, Paris.

Since the demonstration that medullary carcinoma of the thyroid
(MCT) is a differenciated tumour secreting calcitonin (CT) (1)(2)(3)
(4), radioimmunoassays of this hormone have been extensively used for
the diagnosis of the disease (5)(6). Raised levels of CT in subclini-
cal forms are now considered pathognomonic of the tumour. The recent
findings of high levels of carcinoembryonic antigen (CEA) in the
plasma and tissues of patients suffering from MCT (7) and the positive correlation existing between levels of the antigen (CEA) and the
hormone (CT)(8)(9) raises the question of the value of CEA estimation
in the diagnosis and follow up of patients suffering from MCT. We
have therefore investigated CEA and CT levels in a comparatively
large series of MCT patients suffering from either hereditary or
sporadic forms of the disease.

MATERIAL AND METHODS

CT and CEA levels were measured in plasma samples obtained from
60 patients with histologically proven MCT, 6 patients with suspicion
of the sporadic form of the disease and 24 patients suffering from
the familial form. In 9 of these cases, MCT was associated with phaeo-
chromocytoma (Sipple's syndrome) and in one case with marfanoid features. In 8 cases, plasma samples were obtained before and after the
first operation. The levels of both antigen and hormone were also
measured during calcium perfusion (4 cases) and pentagastrin injection (4 cases). Perchloric extracts of tissue obtained at operation
were estimated for CEA in 4 cases.

Plasma levels of both antigen and hormone were also assayed in
20 cases of other thyroid tumours.

CT was estimated by a specific radioimmunoassay developped in
our laboratory (10) and which has been used for five years in the
diagnosis and follow up of patients suffering from medullary carcinoma of the thyroid, CEA was estimated by a commercial kit (CEA-IRE-
Sorin).

RESULTS

Normal values of CT and CEA ranged from 0 to 0.5 ng/ml for CT
and 0 to 20 ng/ml for CEA with the radioimmunoassays used.

389

Plasma levels of CEA in MCT and in other thyroid tumours are reported in figure 1. High levels of CEA are present in 75 % of cases of MCT. Values varied from 20 to 7 000 ng/ml. In trabecular cancer of the thyroid, the four cases studied showed high levels of CEA (range : 22.57 to 129 ng/ml) and in one case this abnormal level is associated with a normal level of CT. A single case of anaplastic carcinoma showed a high level of CEA (236 ng/ml). Other types of thyroid tumours are associated with normal or slightly elevated levels of CEA. In patients with clinical remission, CEA levels are within the normal range or slightly higher and in these patients CT was normal.

The close association of CEA and CT levels is apparent in figure 2, in spite of the presence of patients with high levels of CT and normal levels of CEA (left corner of figure 2). The index of correlation is 0.6548, P<0.001.

CEA and CT levels in members of a family screened for the probable occurence of hereditary MCT are reported in figure 3. In this particular family, an excellent correlation is observed between CEA and CT levels. A single exception is a patient (G.F.) where CT levels are high and CEA is normal. Three members of this family were subsequantly operated (H.C., H.M. and G.A.) and histological examination confirmed the presence of MCT.

Levels of CEA and CT measured before and after operation are reported in figure 4. Both antigen and hormone are lowered after tumour excision. Nevertheless in one case CT level does not return to normal indicating a probable incomplete removal of neoplastic tissue, while CEA returns to normal. The reverse is observed after operation in two cases where CEA levels are slightly above normal while CT levels are undetectable.

Stimulation of CT secretion by pentagastrin (Fig. 5) does not affect CEA levels while CT levels are increased. Calcium infusion (Fig. 6) stimulates CT secretion and provokes fluctuations in CEA levels. On the whole CEA tends to decrease.

Levels of CEA in the tissues studies varied from 7 to 207 γ/g of fresh tissue ; levels of CT were 100 to 1 000 times higher.

Multiple dilutions of plasma samples or perchloric extracts of tumours showed identical displacement of tracer as compared to cold CEA. Synthetic human HCT did not displace the labelled antigen in the RIA used nor extractive CEA the labelled CT.

DISCUSSION

Value of CEA in the diagnosis of MCT

The association reported between CEA and CT (7)(8)(9)(11) is confirmed in this larger sample. Moreover, the value of the correlation coefficient and its significance levels are increased (r = 0.6548 versus 0.4146 (9) and P<0.001 versus P<0.05 (9)).

CEA will be certainly helpful in the diagnosis of MCT ; this is apparent in the excellent correlation observed between CEA and CT levels before and after operation, and in members of a family with suspected MCT. However a certain number of cases show patent discripancy : patients with proved MCT and abnormal levels of CT have normal levels of CEA ; the reverse, i.e. abnormal levels of CEA in the presence of normal levels of CT, is less frequent, and elevation in CEA levels tends to be restricted.

Cases with normal levels of CEA may constitute a different type of MCT or the low level of antigen reported may be due to the presence of homologuous antibodies against CEA. Such antibodies have been described in pregnant women and in certain cases of cancer of the colon (12). Alternately the presence of a CEA immunochemicaly not reacting with the antibody used can also be responsible (13). In the few cases in which abnormal levels of CEA are associated with normal levels of CT, the absence of clinical signs of cancer was in favour of a remission but this does not exclude the possibility of a dedifferenciation of the tumour (either accompanied by a loss of the capacity to synthetize CT or by the synthesis of abnormal forms of the hormone not reactive in RIA used). Of course, non specific causes of the elevation of CEA cannot be excluded, i.e. tobacco (14), alcohol (15) or the presence of occult benign or malignant lesions of other types associated with MCT.

CONCLUSION

Raised levels of CEA are a biochemical characteristic of MCT. Assay of the antigen can be used for the diagnosis of MCT with certain restrictions :
- For the detection of sporadic MCT in presence of a cold nodule, both CEA and CT must be assayed.
- For the monitoring of MCT, the assay of antigen or hormone is suitable when both are high ; if not, CT assay must be used.
- When both CEA and CT levels lie within the normal range or slightly exceed it (detection of recurrences, members of families) stimulation test of CT and its assay are mandatory.

REFERENCES

(1) Milhaud, G., Tubiana, M., Parmentier, C. and Coutris, G. (1968) : C. R. Acad. Sc. Paris (série D), 266, 608.
(2) Meyer, J.S. and Abdel-Bari, W. (1968) : New Engl. J. Med., 278, 523.
(3) Cunliffe, W.J., Black, M.M., Hall, R., Johnston, I.D.A., Hudgson, P., Shuster, S., Gudmundsson, T.V., Joplin, G.F., Williams, E.D., Woodhouse, N.J.Y., Galante, L. and Mac Intyre, I. (1968) : Lancet, ii, 63.
(4) Tashjian, A.H. and Melvin, K.E.W. (1968) : New Engl. J. Med., 279, 279.
(5) Milhaud, G., Calmettes, C., Taboulet, J., Jullienne, A. and Moukhtar, M.S. (1974) : Lancet, i, 462.

391

(6) Melvin, K.E.W., Tashjian, A.H. and Miller, H.H. (1972) : Rec. Prog. in Hormone Res., 28, 399, Academic Press, New York and London.

(7) Ishikawa, N. and Hamada, S. (1976) : Br. J. Cancer, 34, 111.

(8) Hamada, S., Ishikawa, N., Yoshii, M., Morita, R., Fukunaga, M., Torizuka, K. and Fukase, M. (1976) : Endocrinol. Japon., 23, 505

(9) Calmettes, C., Moukhtar, M.S. and Milhaud, G. (1977) : Biomedicine, 27, 52.

(10) Moukhtar, M.S., Jullienne, A., Rivaille, P. and Milhaud, G. (1973) :"Radioimmunoassay and related procedures in medicine", Proc. Symp. on Radioimmunoassay and Related Procedures in Clinical Medicine and Research (Istanbul 1973), vol. I, International Atomic Energy Agency, Vienne, p. 381.

(11) Calmettes, C., Cressent, M., Moukhtar, M.S. and Milhaud, G. (1977) : Acta Endocrin., suppl. 212, 198.

(12) Gold, P. (1967) : Cancer, 20, 1663.

(13) Vrba, R., Alpert, E. and Isselbacher, K.J. (1975) : Proc. Nat. Acad. Sci. U.S.A., 72, 4602

(14) Meriadec de Byans, B., Ducimetierre, P., Salard, J.P., Richard, J.L. and Henry, R. (1976) : Bull. Cancer, 63, 639.

(15) Massart, J.P., Meriadec, B., Klepping, C. and Martin, F. (1976) : Bull. Cancer, 63, 639.

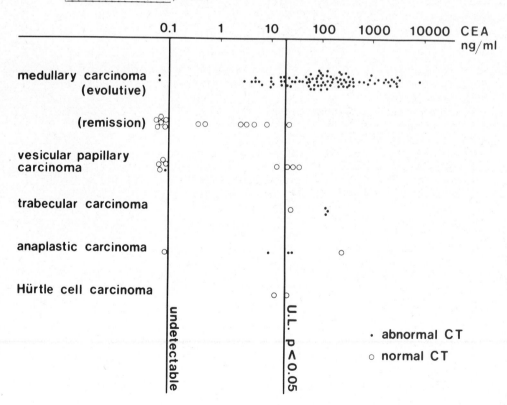

Fig. 1 CEA levels in thyroid tumours (plasma).

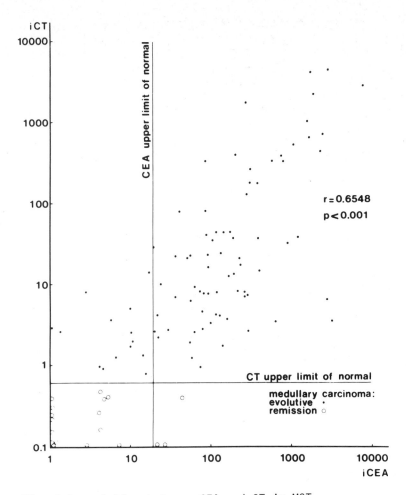

Fig. 2 Correlation between CEA and CT in MCT.

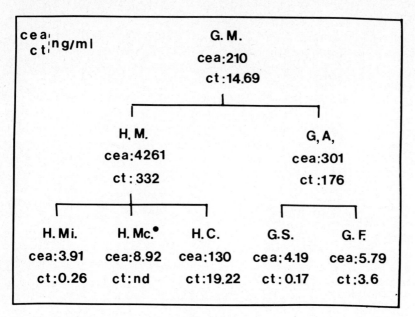

Fig. 3 Familial MCT. H.M.C.•: initial case, diagnosis of MCT on operation, post-operative levels of CEA and CT.

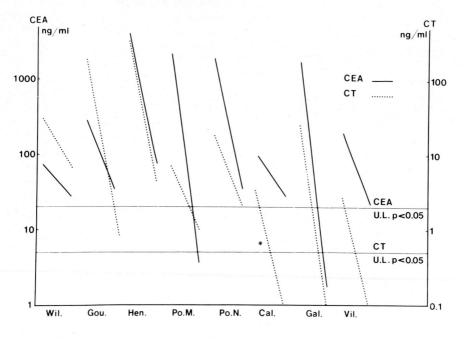

Fig. 4 Pre and post-operative levels of CEA and CT in MCT.

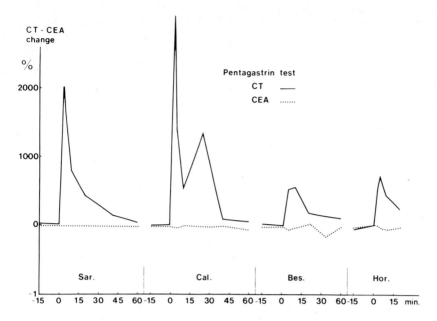

Fig. 5 Changes in CEA and CT after pentagastrin injection.

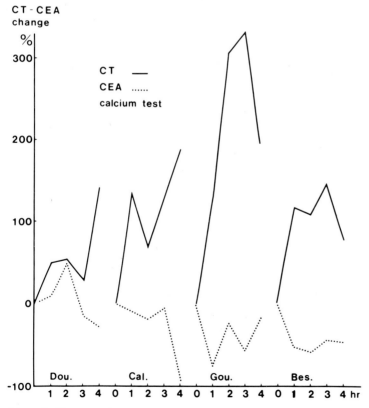

Fig. 6 Changes in CEA and CT during calcium infusion.

DISCUSSION

COUETTE J.E. (Caen): Did you perform systematically TCT assay before lobectomy for thyroid cancer.

CALMETTES C.(Paris): No, but in my opinion, this could be interesting for carcinoma diagnosis.

TALERMAN A.(Rotterdam): We have also been studying CEA both preoperatively and in the follow-up, but unfortunately we do not have as many cases.Our results are not the same. From the pathological point of view, I cannot accept some of your comments concerning the classification of thyroid tumours. I would like to ask whether you have studied CEA and TCT in siblings of patients with tumours and in the families with the Sipple syndrome. We have managed to obtain sera from patients as well as from their families, who did not have any evidence of disease. We have found that in all these cases both the calcitonin and the CEA were within normal limits, indicating that neither of these tests is useful for discovering the presence of a pre-neoplastic state, and the CEA is not raised unless a tumour is already present. Therefore there is no evidence that raised levels of CEA or TCT are present in relatives of patients with medullary carcinoma of the thyroid, unless they are already affected by a tumour.

CALMETTES C.(Paris): To answer the first question, we have studied tissue with an immunofluorescence method, and, in a trabecular cancer of the thyroid, we have found a positive immunofluorescence with anti-calcitonine antibodies. In one case of poorly differentiated follicular cancer, we found effectively follicules inside the tumour. But, these follicules were not fluorescent with our method, only the cells around these follicules were fluorescent. It seems that follicules were enclosed by the tumour as it grew.

MACH J.P. (Lausanne): It is very interesting to see such a good correlation between CEA and a very specific tumour marker TCT. In your series, did you have more metastases than small primary cancers.

CALMETTES C.(Paris): No, there is no close relationship between tumour mass and tumour marker levels; grossly metastases have higher levels.

ROCHMAN H.(Chicago): In a paper published last year in Cancer Research we also found normal CEA levels with adenomata, and elevated levels in medullary carcinoma of the thyroid. There are other papers from Japanese workers, that show all cases of medullary thyroid cancer have elevated CEA.

TALERMAN A.(Rotterdam): We found in 26 cases, that the medullary carcinoma has raised CEA while other tumours both follicular and papillary as well as anaplastic showed normal values of CEA.

BIOCHEMICAL MONITORING OF CANCER TREATMENT *

E.H. Cooper

Department of Experimental Pathology and Cancer Research, School
of Medicine, University of Leeds, Leeds LS2 9NL

The biochemical monitoring of cancer treatment, with a few rare
exceptions, notably hormone producing tumours (1), cannot be expected
to be based on a single test.   There are several reasons why this is
true.   There are differences in the production and destruction of
tumour marker substances that reflect the individual nature of the
host and tumour as well as disturbances in these parameters produced
by treatment and the lack of stoichiometry between the number of
cancer cells and the level of the marker in the blood and urine.
Even the more promising markers when they are judged from the point
of view of their tumour specificity fail to reflect differences in
the general biochemical status of the patient which may play an
overriding part in the evolution of the disease, response to therapy
and hence clinical decision making.

The history of biochemical monitoring of cancer has seen a great
deal of efforts studying a variety of "tests" such as serum enzymes,
serum proteins and more recently the so-called tumour related
antigens and a variety of excretion products in the urine (see 1 for
review).   These have, in the main, been conducted as a series of
vertical studies with varying degrees of sophistication in the
staging of the disease, though more often naive than sophisticated.
Frequently the objective of the investigators has been to try to
find cancer specific markers as their hope was to produce a test
that would revolutionize the detection of asymptomatic cancer.
Nowadays we are not surprised that this quest has, so far, failed to
reach its goal; a consideration of the CEA test shows some of the

* Supported by a grant from the Yorkshire Cancer Research Campaign

causes for failure.   CEA lacks specificity and has an unacceptable
level of false positive and false negative values that have
precluded its widespread application to population screening (2).

      Opinions on the value of CEA as an aid to decision making
therapy vary : some investigators extole its virtues, others are
exhibiting signs of growing scepticism.   My remarks will be confined
to large bowel cancer which is the obvious disease for any large
scale evaluation.   All the major series have shown that the serial
measurement of plasma CEA after "curative resection" of Dukes A, B
and C lesions can by virtue of its rise indicate recurrence and this
may occur when the patient is asymptomatic and give a lead time of
several months over routine clinical surveillance, the duration of
the lead time being strongly influenced by the frequency of CEA
determination.   If the clinician considers this information
important, then 2-3 monthly testing may be required and will be
needed for as long as 5 years in the A and B cases, though most of
the C cases will have recurred before this time.   As yet there is
too little information to assess whether second look surgery
performed because of a rising CEA will significantly alter the
evolution of the disease;   this practice has not roused much interest
in Europe.   Likewise, using a rising CEA as an indication to
commence chemotherapy has some protagonists.   However, the low
efficacy of contemporary chemotherapy in large bowel cancer means
that very large numbers of patients would be required in a trial to
show any significant prolongation of survival.   Consequently it
would need a multicentre trial with high reproducibility of CEA
results.

      Our experience in Leeds (3) of CEA monitoring in the chemo-
therapy of large bowel cancer indicates it can give warning that
therapy for minimal residual disease is failing to restrain tumour
growth prior to its detection clinically.   On the other hand in
advanced disease with indicator lesions, the behaviour of the level
of CEA does not appear to have any relation to survival.   The median
levels and the range of CEA values during the last year of life of

treated and untreated metastatic large bowel cancer are shown in
Table I.

TABLE I   Evolution of plasma CEA in metastatic colorectal cancer

	Time before death		
	1 year	6 months	3 months
Untreated	36*	100	128
	5 - 10,000	5 - 8,000	10 - 25,000
Chemotherapy	35	125	142
	4 - 12,000	6 - 20,000	8 - 12,000

* Median value µg/l.   Ludwig Institute assays upper limit of
normal 30 µg/l (4).
All patients survived at least one year after resection of the
primary lesion.

Clearly the values show a high variance which must contribute
to the lack of relationship to survival.   Patients with high values
of CEA immediately after surgery are Dukes D cases and the fact that
they tend to die within a year adds little to the surgeons'
assessment of the prognosis when making a laparotomy to attempt some
form of palliative surgery.   The lesson that emerges clearly from
the CEA experience is the value of longitudinal studies in any
cancer marker research and the immense difficulties in the
interpretation of isolated measurements in the grey zone of 1-2
standard deviations above the 95% confidence limits of normal.
Indeed this point seems to polarize the US and UK experience on CEA.
British investigators appear to be more conservative in their
assessment of the significance of minor changes of CEA values than
some Americans.
    This experience suggests that what was once regarded as non-
specific change in cancer may still have an information content that
is valuable.   In practice this means studying whether the sum total
of the information in a group of tests run simultaneously is greater
than any single tests in the array and which bits of information are
redundant.   The objective is to produce a logical sequence of tests
that can help the doctor in his decision making, similar to those

established for liver, renal and respiratory diseases.

The initial problem lies in the choice of elements in the array and there seems to be no short cut to this apart from the clues already in the literature relating to measurements made in the past and discarded because they would not fit with the investigators' preconceived ideas of what was wanted, the other approach is keeping a high state of general awareness during an investigation aided by the laws of serendipidy.

Structured systems

The α and β globulin fraction of the plasma proteins are emerging as a highly structured series whose values in health strongly reflect the subject's uniqueness.   In health there is little or no correlation between many of the individual α_1 and α_2 globulins.   They comprise the acute phase reactant proteins (APRPs); each protein tending to remain at a stable level.   On the other hand in disease there is often correlation between changes in groups of the APRPs to give rise to reproducible protein profiles. A typical response in cancer is shown in Fig. 1.   Such changes have been seen in tumours of a wide variety of tissues of origin, stomach, large bowel, bladder, kidney, prostate and lymphomas (5,6).   The general change in the levels of the proteins in metastatic cancer progress with increasing tumour load and although all the APRPs are synthesized in the liver their disturbance in cancer is independent of any direct invasion of the liver.

Current experience suggests it is those APRPs that have a normal distribution in a healthy population and do not exhibit phenotypic variation that are the most useful indicators in cancer. Ceruloplasmin (Cp), α_1 acid glycoprotein (AGP) and antichymotrypsin (ACT) fulfil these criteria, whilst haptoglobin and antitrypsin suffer from the disadvantages of phenotypic variation and a wide variance in health.   Chemotherapy, unless it is hepatotoxic, does not appear to have a direct influence on the levels of these proteins.   On the other hand, it can be shown to exhibit strongly divergent responses to oestrogen with a rise in Cp, a fall in AGP whilst the ACT level remains relatively unaffected by the oestrogen.

400

Discontinuous variates

The C-reactive protein (C-RP) is a good example of a
discontinuous variate as it may be absent in normal sera or present
in low amount ($<$10 mg/l).   In common with other APRPs it responds
to acute injury and infection.   Its behaviour in metastatic or
invasive cancer is of some interest as it tends to relate to the
prognosis.   The level usually rises slowly to about 40-50 mg/l
during the later part of the evolution of metastatic cancer but
can still rise to much higher values when acute incidents complicate
the disease.   The sensitivity to the signals produced by the growth
of a tumour appears to stimulate the production of C-RP at a later
stage than other APRPs.   Hence a chronic rise in the level of C-RP
may be used as an element in a system attempting to give a
biochemical equivalent to performance status prior to the onset of
the gross biochemical disorders consequent upon bilary, urinary or
intestinal obstruction or following haemorrhage.   Evidence is
growing that C-RP can modify cellular immunity and like alpha
fetoprotein may be one of the natural regulators of immunity, a
property that has received little attention so far in cancer research
but should not be neglected.

Serum albumin

The fall of serum albumin is a classical observation in
advanced cancer, values below 20 g/l usually coincide with obvious
hypoproteinaemic syndromes.   However, the fall of values between
30 g/l, held as the lowest limit of normality, and 25 g/l are often
incidious in cancer.   Yet the position on the albumin slope seems
to play a key role in predicting the probability of encountering a
wide variety of biochemical disorders in cancer.   As the value falls
so the cascade of associated disorders increases in number and
severity, as has been well established in studies of tropical calorie
and protein deficiency.   The relation of C-RP and albumin in bladder
cancer illustrates this thesis (Fig. 2).

The multivariate concept

The objective is to provide information about the overall biochemical status and the way in which the host and tumour are interacting in ambulant patients. In other words to try to find factors that may account for the well known phenomena of the ability of some patients to sustain a large load of metastatic cancer for long periods of time whilst others succumb comparatively soon. Such a system could introduce a biochemical index comparable to performance status that may have important prognostic significance or possibly account for some of the conflicting evidence coming from chemotherapy trials in common forms of solid tumours.

In this approach the tumour specific markers CEA, βHCG etc. have a major role when they are produced in cancer but they need to be associated with other appropriate tests in order to reveal the full information content. A few examples at this stage can serve to illustrate this concept.

In gastrointestinal cancer the monitoring of CEA in conjunction with markers of hepatic function such as gamma glutamyltranspeptidase (8) help to identify recurrence and progression of disease but also organ site involvement; a similar logic can be applied to breast cancer where CEA, casein or βHCG may be the tumour marker of choice in a particular patient and non-specific indicators of growing involvement such as hydroxyproline excretion and alkaline phosphatase for bone involvement and the liver function enzyme help to draw attention to involvement and progression in a particular site.

Carcinoma of the prostate provides a special challenge as the routine serum acid phosphatase (SAP) measurements do not fulfil the requirement of an ideal marker. In this instance oestrogens are the anchor of any treatment plan so the first question is 'are the oestrogens producing a pharmacological effect?' or indeed 'is the patient taking the therapy?'. This can readily be answered by measurement of the serum SP2 protein level and the level of Cp (A. Milford Ward - personal communication). The effect of the therapy on the tumour can be decided from the SAP and the level of ACT which are unaffected by oestrogens per se. Finally the general

402

biochemical status of the patient may be indicated by creatinine clearance, serum albumin and C-reactive protein. Once it has been established that the treatment is pharmacologically active and having a beneficial effect on the tumour subsequent monitoring can be maintained with a simple combination of ACT and SAP until any deviation is observed and then the full array used to try to identify the reasons for the change.

The array for each main class of tumours will depend upon the probabilities of different patterns of invasion and referential sites for metastases as well as the predilection of the tumour to produce specific marker substances.

Data analysis

The analysis of a specific tumour marker must still rely upon the examination of its false positive and false negative rates. However, the cut off level for normality seems to be the major difficulty, though it tends to resolve when the test is used to monitor the patient longitudinally. As with most other forms of medicine a value in the grey zone of interpretation can only carry a probability of being a positive indication of active disease, though the clinical context in which it is measured may well be able to weight the probability.

The analysis of multivariate data at a single point in time can be handled by discriminant analysis particularly stepwise analysis which is a powerful technique to identify redundant data. Careful inspection of the data is needed to decide whether parametric methods dependent on normal distribution are applicable. Frequently laboratory data in cancer has complex non-normal distribution and non-parametric discriminant analysis not pre-supposing any special form of the data may be required (9).

There is a growing need for more detailed study of the patterns of evolution of the variables that can be potentially useful as markers in cancer. As yet there is no clearly defined approach to this problem, the clinicians want systems to provide accurate prediction of the longer term behaviour of the patient, as well as knowledge about the particular subset to which they belong.

However, it may be some time before appropriate mathematical models can be set up and tested to handle the type of data that we are currently generating with our contemporary cancer monitoring systems. The remedy would seem to lie in closer liaison with mathematicians.

REFERENCES

(1)   Munro Neville, A. and Cooper, E.H. (1976) : <u>Ann. Clin. Biochem.</u> <u>13</u>, 283.

(2)   <u>Brit. Med. Journal</u> (1977) <u>3</u>, 535 : Leading article.

(3)   Bullen, B.R., Cooper, E.H., Turner, R., Neville, A.M., Giles, G.R. and Hall, R. (1977) : <u>Med. & Ped. Oncology, 3</u>, 289.

(4)   Laurence, D.J.R., Stevens, U., Bettelheim, R., Darcy, D., Leese, C., Tuberville, C., Alexander, P., Johns, E.W. and Neville, A.M. (1972) : <u>Brit. Med. Journal, 3</u>, 605.

(5)   Milford Ward, A., Cooper, E.H., Turner, R., Anderson, J.A. and Neville, A.M. (1977) : <u>Brit. J. Cancer, 35</u>, 170.

(6)   Milford Ward, A., Cooper, E.H. and Houghton, A.L. (1977) : <u>Brit. J. Urol., in press</u>.

(7)   Whitehead, R.G., Coward, W.A., Lunn, P.G. (1973) : <u>Lancet, 1</u>, 63.

(8)   Steele, L., Cooper, E.H., Mackay, A.M., Losowsky, M.S. and Goligher, J.C. (1974) : <u>Brit. J. Cancer, 30</u>, 319.

(9)   Cooper, E.H. and Kenny, T.E. (1977) : <u>Proc. Roy. Soc. Med.,</u> <u>in press</u>.

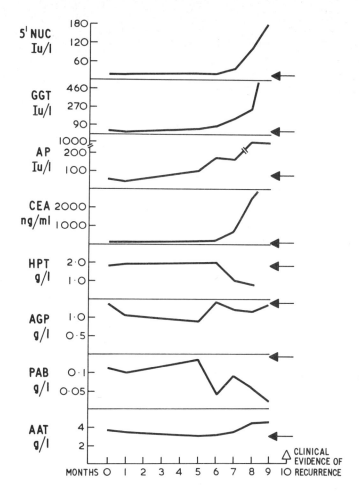

Fig. 1   The biochemical profile of a patient with untreated residual
colon cancer commencing one month after surgery until the disease
became detectable 10 months cancer.   From Bullen et al., Med. & Ped.
Oncology, 3, 289 (1977).

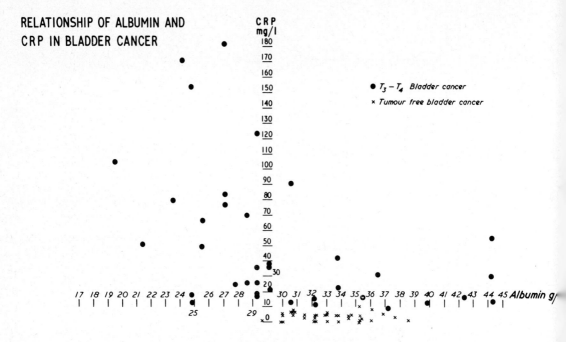

RELATIONSHIP OF ALBUMIN AND
CRP IN BLADDER CANCER

Fig. 2   Interrelation of levels of serum albumin and C-RP in bladder
cancer :   O = T2 - T4 active disease
              x = T1 patients 3 - 12 months after treatment of the
              primary and with no residual tumour.

DISCUSSION

MARTIN E.W. (Columbus): I would like to make a comment. First of
all, I am enjoying the presentation and I want to reinforce
everything said by Dr. Cooper. I think that CEA is a non specific
tumour marker. I think chemotherapy in colonic cancer and colorectal cancer does not exist at this point.

LALANNE C.M. (Nice): Chemotherapy is not as efficient as we would
like it to be in colorectal cancer, but I do not agree with the
negative assessment of Dr. Martin in other cancers, for example
breast cancer. Anyway the panel of assays, presented by Dr. Cooper
is surely useful because chemotherapy is efficient.

COOPER E.H. (Leeds): Yes, I think that if you believe the change of
therapy could be beneficial then the moment of change may be very
decisive. But in that situation where you are not convinced that
the change is important, then the close monitoring is more academic
than practical. Nevertheless, our job is to understand the academic
basis of medicine, even if there is no immediate practical application, if we do not studied scientifically and objectively, there
will be no progress.

ZAMCHECK N. (Boston): I cannot resist to congratulate this group, because his conceptual work is a main basis for much of new developments and a practical comment: it was not possible to really evaluate any chemotherapy based upon the old clinical standard; and in most controlled studies, death is considered as the end point. With the use of monitors, we now know that we detect change in the patients course which were never detectable before, so the tumour markers are enabling us to evaluate the therapy. And I think that this is the new development and hope.

SIMULTANEOUS ASSAYS OF THREE MARKERS IN CLINICAL ONCOLOGY

R. Bugat, P. Canal, G. Soula, P. F. Combes.

Centre Claudius Regaud and University Paul Sabatier , School of Medicine , Toulouse, FRANCE

1 - INTRODUCTION

The ectopic production of hormones and the production of compounds characteristic of fetal life are among the well recognized characteristics of neoplasms in man. The development of specific and sensitive methods for the assay of these products led to their clinical use in the diagnosis of cancer and the monitoring of the effects of cancer treatment. However , this theorical helpful procedure is still neither absolute nor specific (1) . In order to try to improve this fact , we evaluated the role of simultaneous assays of 3 markers in patients with neoplasms. Two are fetal and embryonic antigens, namely carcinoembryonic antigen (CEA) and α -fetoprotein (AFP). The third one, part of a placental hormone , is the beta-glycoprotein chain of human chorionic gonadotrophin (β-HCG), which was reported to be measurable in plasma of patients with non trophoblastic neoplasms (2). We report our practical attempt dealing with 4 different groups of cancers:

                    -breast adenocarcinomas,
                    -head and neck neoplasms ,
                    -colo-rectal adenocarcinomas ,
                    -cancers of the female reproductive system.

2 - METHODS and MATERIAL

2.1 We used the polyethylene glycol method for assaying AFP *
and the double antibody technique for CEA and β-HCG determinations**. The sensitivity was 1 ng/ml , both for CEA and AFP assays and 0.1 ng/ml for β-HCG assay.

Cancer - related markers were measured in the serum of 30 healthy donors of different ages (18 - 45 years). Normal value for each marker was determined by adding twice the standard error to the calculated mean of the group, that gave the following upper limits :

---

* Dainabot Radioisotope Lab. , LTD, Tokyo,Japan
** Kits provided by CEA, Saclay, France

- AFP : 10 ng/ml
- CEA : 10 ng/ml
- β-HCG : 2. 5. ng/ml

2. 2. Blood samples (10ml) were obtained from 325 patients with histologically proven and clinically staged neoplasms other than germinal cell tumors, namely:

      154 breast adenocarcinomas
      44 squamous cell carcinomas of head and neck
      15 carcinomas of the thyroid
      58 colo-rectal adenocarcinomas
      54 cancers of the female reproductive system.

3. RESULTS

3. 1 - Breast cancers

Breast cancers were classified into three groups according to their clinical profile and treatment :

-group I (31 patients) before any treatment in the absence of metastases (T_1 to T_4 , N_1 or N_2, M_0)

-group II (34 patients) during metastatic spread (M+) as shown by clinical examination, chest x-rays, hepatic enzymology, skull and liver scintigraphies.

-group III (84 patients) , following removal of the tumor, during clinical remission phase as proven by the same clinical examination, biological, radiological and isotopical determinations. In this group , 45 patients were receiving adjuvant chemotherapy. Periods of follow-up ranged from 2 months to 6 years.

The incidence of finding at least one marker at a pathological level in the whole serie was 34% - individual incidence for each marker showed that CEA was the most frequently found.

TABLE 1 - Breast Cancer : incidence of positivity of markers

Group	N	Incidence of at least 1 positive marker N	%	AFP	CEA	β-HCG
I	31	16	52	1	12 $\bar{m} = 25 ng/ml$	3
II	34	27	79	1	24 $\bar{m} = 90 ng/ml$	2
III	89	12	14	2	10 $\bar{m} = 18 ng/ml$	0

One must emphasize that in group II the mean value for positive CEA was statistically different from group I and group III, which would mean that relative value of positivity should be taken into account. Among group II, the sites of metastases which yielded to the

lower incidence of positivity of markers were the lung and the pleu-
ra (1 case) which however accounted for 14% of the total metastases.
Table 2 shows the increase incidence of positivity allowed by other
markers (AFP and β-HCG) than CEA .

TABLE 2 - Breast cancer : increase incidence of positivity allowed
by other markers than CEA .

		GROUP I	GROUP II	GROUP III
CEA	N	12/31	24/34	10/89
	%	39	70	11
All Markers	N	16/31	27/34	12/89
	%	52	79	14

3. 2 - Cancers of Head and Neck

We investigated (table 3) 44 patients bearing squamous cell
carcinoma of head and neck, with or whithout cervical metastatic
nodes but all staged T_3 (SV_5 $<20\%$)

TABLE 3 - Squamous cell carcinoma of head and neck , incidence
of positivity of markers

N. total	AFP	CEA	β-HCG	
44	0	14	2	15 positive determina - tions = 34 %

One can see that incidence positivity of one marker compared
to CEA incidence was almost null . Besides, the mean of positive
CEA determination was 18ng/ml + 4 which is low in this population
of heavy smokers.

We have detected high values of CEA ($\bar{m}$ =170 ng/ml) in 7 out
of 7 patients suffering from medullary carcinoma of the thyroid.
Furthermore, one man who had one of the highest value was also
positive for β-HCG . In the contrary, none of the sera from anaplastic carcinoma of the thyroid we assayed (N=8) showed any marker positivity.

3. 3. Colo-rectal cancers

Colo-rectal cancers, all proven adenocarcinomas were devi-
ded into 4 groups (table 4) :

- group 1 (19 patients) included pre-operative DUKES A. and
B, as ulteriorly shown by post-surgical pathology examination , and
patients who where radically operated on, during their remission
phase.

-group II (10 patients) all DUKES C at the onset of the disease before any treatment.

-group III (10 patients) loco-regional metastatic spread or
recurrence to the pelvis or patients bearing inoperable tumors
without evidence of hepatic metastase.

-group IV (19 patients) metastatic spread outside the pelvis.

TABLE 4 - Colo-rectal cancers : results.

| Group. | N | Incidence of at least 1 positive marker | | Absolute indicence | | |
		N	%	AFP	CEA	β-HCG
I	19	1	6	0	1	0
Il	10	7	70	0	7	0
II	10	9	90	0	9	0
IV	19	17	90	1	16	0

One must point out that 5 patients with high CEA determinations who and had normal liver scan, hepatic function and enzymes
values were bearing hepatic metastases at surgery. However , incidence of positivity of at least one marker seems to be as frequent
in pelvic-limited that in general metastatic spread.

3. 4. Cancer of the female reproductive system.
The following table summarises the results we obtained.

	N	AFP	ACE	β-HCG
CERVIX squamous cell. carcinomas	24	1	10	3
CORPUS adenocarcinomas	9	3	I	1
OVARY adenocarcinomas	21	1	1	

A tendancy toward higher values in advanced stages was evi-
denced , however, samples are too small to draw any further conclusions.

4- COMMENTS

The incidence of positive values of CEA is quite impressive. It is shown from this study that the likelihood of a patient having a positive value is increased with advancing stage and bulk of disease.

However, our purpose was not to assess the follow-up of patients. We wanted to know whether simultaneous assays of 3 markers improved the positive incidence displays by CEA alone. It appears that, at least for the localisations we were dealing with, AFP and βHCG only cause a very slight increase of incidence of positivity.

REFERENCES

(1) CHU, T.M. , HOLYOKE, E.D. , and MURPHY, G.P.
(1974) Carcinoembryonic antigen - Current clinical status
N.Y. State J. Med. , 74, 1388.

(2) ROSEN , S.W, WEINTRAUB, B.D. , VAITUKAITIS, J.L.,
et al. (1975) Placental proteins and their subunits as tumor markers .
Ann. Intern. Med. , 82, 71 .

(3) FRANCHIMONT , P, , ZANGERLE , P.F. , HENDRICK, J.C
et al (1977). Cancer. 39, 2806.

CARCINOEMBRYONIC ANTIGEN DETERMINATIONS IN PEOPLE SUBMITTED TO CANCER SCREENING.

B.P.Krebs, P.Bernasconi, J.L.Boublil, C.M.Lalanne

Centre Antoine Lacassagne, 36 Voie Romaine, 06054 Nice Cedex,France.

INTRODUCTION

The early recognition of tumours, truly localised, with possibility of curative therapy, is one of the main goals of biologists working on tumour markers.

The general agreement is that we need more specific tumour associated antigen determinations with less false positive results and eventually more true positive results.

The aim of this study is to appreciate the real value of radioimmunoassay of carcinoembryonic antigen for the selection of high risk populations and as a screening test. Our opinion is that CEA measurement could be useful in screening programmes.

SHORT REVIEW OF LITERATURE

The three pilot studies to be quoted are those of WILLIAMS, McINTIRE and co-workers (1), of COSTANZA and co-workers (2) and of STEVENS, CULLEN and McKay (3).

The first study included a vast quantity of persons; 5209 were followed by every two years in a study aimed at the prevention of cardiovascular disease. Unfortunately, the authors limited the investigation to 8 tumours of the digestive tract, 4 gastric and 4 pancreatic cancers. In these cases, CEA was elevated and predictive ten months before diagnosis, twice for the pancreatic carcinomas and three times for the gastric cancers. One may hope that a more complete analysis of this enormous quantity of samples will be performed by this team.

COSTANZA et al. are more encouraging, since, among their 113 positive CEA estimations out of 576 patients without known cancer, 16 were associated with malignant tumours. This produces the interesting result of an incidence of 14.2% of cancers in a CEA positive population.

In the work published by STEVENS, the population submitted to analysis corresponded to all persons who, in 1969 lived in the Shire of Busselton Western Australia. 4400 persons participated in the survey conducted in 1969 by CURNOW, CULLEN and co-workers. 956 sera of persons aged over 60 were available for testing carcinoembryonic antigen in 1973. 912 results are negative, 44 are positive.

During the four years between 1969 and 1973 the occurence of CEA associated cancer is 2% for people without CEA in the blood in 1969 and 14% in the positive population. This difference is significant. Further more, 21 persons positive for CEA in 1969 consented to reexamination and a further two cases of cancer were discovered: at this time, one bronchogenic carcinoma and one adenocarcinoma of the sigmoïd. This increases the cancer incidence up to 18% . Naturally, no significant difference was shown in the frequency of non CEA associated cancers in the two groups.

In Centre Antoine Lacassagne, there is a screening department, at which all those presenting either with or without symptomatology are submitted initially to general clinical , biological and radiological examinations. Among the 1708 cases seen during the past two years, 32 cancers were diagnosed clinically (1.9%). 11 of these were asymptomatic at the time of diagnosis.

RADIOIMMUNOASSAY OF CEA

CEA was measured on plasma obtained from blood taken on EDTA. Reagents used are those commercialized by CIS (4). We have tested the method on more than 200 normal non smoking adults(fig.1). Only 2.8 % of subjects are positive, more than 5 ng CEA per ml. 6 % of cases present a slight but non significant inhibition, 90% of plasma does not interfere in the radioimmunoassay. The normal range is less than 5 ng/ml.

RESULTS

125 out of the 414 blood samples available from the screening department are positive, in other words 30 per cent.Figure 2 shows the incidence of positive values correlated with age : the highest incidence lies between 65-75 years. This high incidence of positivity is directly related to tabacco consumption, especially in men, among whom 50 to 100 per cent are smokers in the different age ranges. Unfortunately, we were not able to establish , in each case, the time interval between the last cigarette and the blood sampling. This will be taken in account from now on. This fact is of great importance as shown in Table I, demonstrating the findings of MERIADEC(5) et al. Only 2% of non smokers or of people who had stopped smoking some months earlier are positive. This frequency is closely related with our data on normal non smokers. In contrast, 26% of people who had smoked the morning of blood sampling and who inhaled the smoke are positive.

TABLE I   Correlation of incidence of positive values (percentage) with tabacco consumption (B.MERIADEC et al.,(4)).

Subjects who had never smoked	2
Subjects who had stopped smoking some months earlier	2
Smokers who had smoked the morning of blood sampling and who inhaled the smoke	26
Smokers who had smoked the morning of blood sampling	20
Smokers who had not smoked since the previous evening	7

The cancer incidence in our four hundred and fourteen cases : 4.8% of cancer if CEA is below 5 ng/ml, 10.4% if CEA is elevated in the blood. In persons aged between 40 and 75 years, the cancer incidence is 6.4% in CEA negative population, 15.3% in CEA positive population.

Three points can be noticed (Table 2): (i) not one single case of cancer occured in men under 40 despite some raised levels; (ii) among men over 60, 16% of positive CEA were in fact due to malignant disease. In women of the same age group, the incidence is rather higher at 19% . This group corresponds to STEVENS group; (iii) however; it is important to notice that among women without CEA in the blood and aged over 60, cancer nevertheless occured in 13% of cases.

TABLE 2 Frequency of cancer patients according to age, sex and CEA level.

Age		21-40	41-60	more than 61years
Less than 5ngCEA/ml	Males	0	0	5.3%
	Females	3.4	2.1	13.3%
More than 5ngCEA/ml	Males	0	11.1	15.8%
	Females	0	5.4	18.8%

CONCLUSIONS

The level of positivity chosen is critical .Figure 2 shows that if one takes a too high level for positivity, the diagnosis of cancer is quite certain but the harvest of cases is low. If the level of positivity is lowered, the number of cases increases but the diagnosis of cancer becomes less certain.

Many publications underline the important role of CEA measurement on samples other than blood. At this meeting, two papers from our Laboratory have presented the interest of estimations of CEA in

415

pancreatic and bronchial secretions. Many other data are available in literature. Here, MOLNAR (5) et al. show the increasing incidence of positive diagnosis when using fluids directly from the suspected tumour environment. (Table 3).

TABLE 3   CEA assay in fluids other than plasma (MOLNAR et al.,(5))

	Plasma	Colonic mucus	Gastric juice	Duodenal drainage
Cancer of Colon	16/23	23/23		
Gastric Cancer	6/17		9/17	
Pancreatic Cancer	4/6			6/6

Among the 46 malignancies in this study, 11 were missed by standard non surgical diagnostic techniques.

Thus, the measurement of CEA can be a useful element in the selection of high risk populations. This test associated with others, may eventually become, under conditions yet to be defined, a pre-requisite necessitating further and more thorough investigations by medical personel.

* Acknowlegements: Work done in collaboration with the Screening Department of the Centre Antoine Lacassagne.

REFERENCES

(1) Williams,R.R., McIntire,K.R., Wadmann,T.A., Feinleib,M., Go,V.L.W Kannel,B., Dawber,T.R., Castelli,W.P., McNamara,P.M. (1977) : J.nat.Cancer Inst.,58, 1547.

(2) Costanza,M.E., Das,S., Nathanson,L., Rule,A., Schwartz,R.S. (1974) : Cancer, 33, 583.

(3) Stevens,D.P., MacKay,I.R., Scullen,K. (1975) : Br. J.Cancer,32, 147.

(4) Meriadec de Byans,B., Ducimetiere,P., Richard,J.L., Salard,J.L., Henry, R. (1976) : Biomedicine, 25, 197.

(5) Molnar,I.G., Vandevoorde,J.P., Gitnick,G.L. (1977): Gastroentero-logy, 70, 513.

416

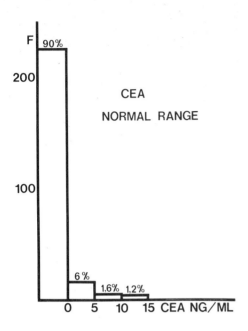

Fig.1 Normal values in non-smoker control group.

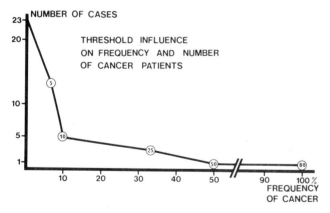

Fig.2 Threshold influence on frequency and number of cancer patients in our population.

417

DISCUSSION

MACH J.P. (Lausanne):Can you give us some information concerning auto-selection of people submitted to screening; it seems that you have a high incidence of cancers.

KREBS B.P. (Nice): There are 2% of cancers in our population with or without symptomatology. If one considers only the population without symptomatology, only one out of thousand presented malignant disease. This is the normal frequence.

MASSEYEFF R. (Nice): Just a comment about what the clinician has to do with positive results. What is the population which is going to undergo this kind of test. Have you calculated the cost of such a screening?

LALANNE C.M. (Nice): The problem of the screening cost is actually worrying for all developped countries. It is a difficult problem . Some light can be drawn from the resuls of cervix carcinoma diagnosis through screening by vaginal smears. This test is well accepted by the majority of women and gives a feeling of security. It is ascertained that the periodic control by vaginal smears has reduced incidence and mortality in cervix carcinoma. But, on the other hand, the cost of screening is already high and thus, it remains to-day questionnable to add CEA for screening purposes. Therefore, some teams must investigate through pilot studies the best and less expensive combination of tests.

USE OF CARCINOEMBRYONIC ANTIGEN IN SCREENING AN UNSELECTED POPULATION.
A FIVE YEAR FOLLOWUP.

I.R. Mackay

The Walter and Eliza Hall Institute of Medical Research, The Royal
Melbourne Hospital, Melbourne, Australia.

It is established that several types of cancer, at the stage
when they are clinically evident, are associated with a high incidence of CEA-positivity in blood, sometimes up to and over 90% (1).
Using the criterion of 50% or greater in incidence, several "CEA-
associated cancers" have been defined: namely, gastro intestinal,
lung, breast. However, such incidences refer to "advanced" cancers
which have already been detected by other means, and hence would be
at a relatively later stage in their evolution. For the purposes of
screening asymptomatic persons for cancer, the test should perform
as well with "early" as with more advanced cancers. Results of low
rates of CEA-positivity in tumours of limited extent in all tumour
types studied are disappointing and have led to the widely-held
opinion that CEA testing as a method of population screening for cancer is not justified in terms of cost - benefit and yield. This opinion was tested in a field survey in a country town of Busselton in
Western Australia (2).

METHODS

This community constitutes a non-transient, predominantly Western European farming population which, since 1966, has been examined
by ongoing health surveys. The survey in 1969 was used for CEA
screening, and the participation rate was almost 90% of the adult
population of 3500. It is the practice for multiple health indices
to be obtained triennially and close followup made. In the study,
coded frozen serum samples were transported by air to Melbourne and
stored at -20° C before being tested for CEA by the double-antibody
radioimmunoassay during 1973-1974. The cut-off level for positivity
was taken as 5 ng per ml. No special investigations were performed
to demonstrate occult cancer, and diseases including cancer were
scored only when these became clinically apparent or were discovered
as the result of investigations performed in the course of local clinical practice. However, in 1974, all persons who had a positive CEA
test in 1969 and were still alive were recalled for symptom enquiry,
physical examination and Xrays of the chest and colon.

RESULTS

The population-prevalence of positive CEA tests in 2372 persons
aged 40 years or over was 73 (3.5%); males numbered 52 (4.5%) and
females 21 (1.7%).

Nine (13%) of the 73 subjects who showed CEA-positivity were found by routine surveillance to have a "CEA-associated cancer" between 1969 and 1974. In 2 further subjects, asymptomatic cancer (colon, 1, and bronchus, 1) was discovered at recall examination prompted by the elevated CEA level. By contrast, 25 (1%) of 2299 subjects whose 1969 CEA level was negative developed "CEA-associated cancer" in the succeeding 5 years. This difference was highly significant (p< 0.001). The influence of smoking habits and sex of the subject was observed. Of the 9 CEA-positive subjects with cancer, 77% were smokers and 77% males. Whereas, the corresponding figures in the 25 CEA-negative subjects were 36% and 52% respectively. Of the 9 patients with cancers associated with CEA-positivity, cancer had been identified before the time of the survey in 2, and during the course of the survey in 7. Elevated CEA levels in 1969 were observed in 6 of 13 subjects who subsequently developed lung cancer, in 3 of 12 who developed gastrointestinal cancer, but in none of 8 who developed breast cancer. However, after 6 years, only one of the 9 CEA-positive subjects is surviving, compared with 6 of the 25 CEA-negative subjects with cancer.

The prevalence of positive results was considerably higher among smokers, and increased progressively with age. Of the 73 subjects with raised CEA levels, 31 were heavy smokers (over 15 cigarettes daily); the levels were raised in 8% of the heavy smokers in contrast to 1% of nonsmokers, and in 8% of male smokers versus 6% of female smokers. However, smokers tended to have only mildly elevated CEA levels, whereas elevated levels in nonsmokers, though rare, tended to be higher. Indeed, the 3 highest levels in the survey - 47, 73 and 97 ng per ml - were all found elderly female nonsmokers.

Variability of CEA levels on serial testing was evident. This retesting during 1972-1974 of subjects whose serum was positive in 1969 showed that some 50% subsequently gave values less than 5 ng per ml. CEA tended to persist more in smokers; of smokers with raised levels in 1969, 63% and 72% still had raised levels in 1972 and 1974 respectively, whereas for the nonsmokers the corresponding figures were lower, 31% and 30%.

CONCLUSION

Despite the statistically significant association between CEA and cancer in this population, the yield of cancers detected was notably low. Only 13% of subjects whose CEA was elevated in 1969 developed a CEA-associated cancer in the next 5 years (87% "false positive") and only 9 of 25 such cancers were predicted by CEA assay (64% "false negative"). When corrected for age, sex and smoking habit, the relative risk of developing a "CEA-associated" cancer was 6.4 for subjects whose serum CEA level exceeded 5 ng per ml. These findings clearly limit the practical applications of the CEA assay in its present form for population screening. Cigarette smoking was identified as the major cause of positive CEA results in subjects without cancer. However, we await the results of the second survey on the same population 6 years later and information on the followup of subjects with persisting CEA-positivity.

REFERENCES

(1)   Hansen H.J., Snyder, J.J., Miller, E., Vandevoorde, J.P.,
       Miller, O.N., Hines, L.R., and Burns, J.J. (1974): Human
       Path., 5: 139.
(2)   Cullen, K.J., Stevens, D.P., Frost, M.A., and Mackay, I.R.,
       (1976): Aust. N.Z.J. Med., 6: 279.

DIAGNOSTIC VALUE OF CARCINOEMBRYONIC ANTIGEN

Walter Hordynsky, Ph.D.

St. Mary's Hospital, 135 So.Center St., Orange, N.J., U.S.A.

The disparity of the reports on CEA from the different groups results from the lack of specificity of the CEA itself (1) and from methodological imperfections.

The present investigation was undertaken to correlate CEA levels and various malignant states with the Hemagglutination Inhibition Method (2) and with RIA Method. (3)

A total of 103 tests were performed by both methods. When 34 patients with clinically and histologically proven malignancy were tested, the Hemagglutination Inhibitition Method results showed 22 positives and the RIA Method 32. With 69 non malignant cases, the Hemagglutination Inhibitition Method results showed 6 positives and the RIA Method only one.

After these experiments, over 2000 CEA tests were performed in 1975 and 1976 by only the RIA Method. Approximately 17% of these tests were positive (above 2.5 ng/ml), with clinical diagnoses confirmed by pathological examination of tissues.

Results revealed elevated levels of CEA in the following neoplasms: lungs, breast, colon, renal, prostate, liver, cervix, lymphosarcoma, stomach, esophagus, thyroid gland, ovary, and uterus.

Seventy eight patients were detected only because of increased CEA levels. The most interesting case was a 69 year old patient with lymphosarcoma. His WBC count was 90,000 and CEA level 5.9 ng/ml. Immunological studies discovered the absence of I_gM in his blood. The patient, a biochemist by profession, separated Immunoglobulins and started to inject himself with pure I_gM. His WBC level dropped to 6,700 and the CEA to 1.8 ng/ml. For 6 months the patient was asymptomatic. Unfortunately, a further follow up was not possible because of his death by heart infarct.

After taking into consideration that CEA appears to be a surface constituent of cells which is released and gains access to lymph spaces, sinusoids and finally blood, an additional investigation was undertaken. Eleven patients with malignant tumors of the lungs were tested for CEA in plasma and in pleural fluid. The CEA levels in the pleural fluid were from 1.4 to 12.0 ng/ml higher than in plasma, despite much lower total protein content of pleural fluid.

On three patients without neoplastic disease the levels of CEA in plasma and in pleural fluid were identical. On five patients with ovarian carcinoma, the CEA level in peritoneal fluid was 2.3 - 8.3 ng/ml higher than in plasma. In one of those patients ovarian cyst fluid was 7.4 ng/ml peritoneal fluid 4.3 ng/ml and plasma 3.3 ng/ml. The body cavities in the intermediate contact with neoplastic cells have undiluted content of CEA. Plasma level is lowered by dilution factor.

All patient material utilized in this study was obtained from St.Mary's Hospital and Orange Memorial Hospital, both located in Orange, New Jersey, U.S.A. Blood, pleural, peritoneal and ovarian cyst fluid were collected in chilled EDTA vacuum tubes centrifuged at $0^{o}C$. and frozen at $20^{o}C$., until used for testing. The precipitation temperature of proteins with percholoric acid was $0^{o}C$. At higher temperatures the precipitation was incomplete. Dialysis bags were checked for their permeability with radioactive CEA. Some brands of dialysis bags had inconsistent molecular weight cut off. Any contact with metal during dialysis decreases the accuracy of the test. The timing for the addition of radioactive CEA and of zirconyl phosphate gel for each tube was individual. By those precautions it was possible to achieve the average one standard deviation of 0.27 and coefficient of variation of 7.6 for RIA Method.

From this study it became apparent that correlations of the Hemagglutination Inhibition and RIA Methods were obtained only in the levels above 8 ng/ml. For the lower levels, the Hemagglutination Inhibition Method in our hands was not sufficiently sensitive. Postoperative observation in the majority of the cancer patients reveals a drop in CEA level. After that any tendency upward was the sign of bad prognosis.

The difficulty in a distinguishing of atypical mesothelial cells from neoplastic cells microscopically in body fluids is a well established fact and considerably minimizes the value of cytologic examinations. The measurement of CEA in body fluids in the combination with cytologic examination and measurement of plasma CEA in the selected patients proved to give better diagnostic yield than the use of either individual test alone (4).

The carcinoembryonic antigen test presently is being employed mainly for its prognostic value. Together with systemic clinical research, by the application of scientific criteria, CEA test is also useful in the diagnosis of cancer.

REFERENCES

(1) Neville, A.M. and Laurence, D.J.R., (1974): Int. J. Cancer 14, 1, 18.
(2) Lange, R.D., et. al, (1971): National Techn.Inform.Service U.S.Department of Commerce pp 379-386.
(3) Hansen, H.J., et. al. (1977): Clinical Res. 19, 143. -
(4) Pschibul, F. and Hordynsky, W. (1977): J. Med. Soc. N.J. 74, 6, pp 535-539

424

CARCINOEMBRYONIC ANTIGEN: THE MOST ACCURATE NONINVASIVE
DIAGNOSTIC TEST FOR PREDICTING MALIGNANCY IN THE JAUNDICED
PATIENT

T.E. Lobe, M. Cooperman, L.C. Carey, E.W. Martin, Jr.

The Department of Surgery, The Ohio State University,
Columbus, Ohio U. S. A.

Jaundiced patients in whom the etiology is unclear
remain a major diagnostic problem. Common hematologic,
metabolic, pharmacologic, infectious, and hepatic disorders can often be diagnosed, but the distinction between benignancy and malignancy as the cause is essential
for proper management. Many combinations of diagnostic
procedures have been suggested, including liver function
tests, liver biopsy, diagnostic radiography, abdominal
ultrasound, radionuclide scans, various forms of
cholangiography, laparoscopy, and minilaparotomy (1-10).
Varying levels of success have been reported with these
studies.
   Diagnosis of the jaundiced patient can be costly.
Unnecessary diagnostic procedures which are expensive,
intricate, unpleasant, and potentially dangerous are
highly undesirable. Excluding the per diem cost of
hospitalization, a patient may pay well over $1000 for
evaluation, yet the physician may still be unsure of the
diagnosis. The addition of carcinoembryonic antigen (CEA)
determination adds little to the patient cost, incon-
venience, length of hospital stay, or risk.
   The diagnostic value of CEA in the presence of
jaundice has been questioned. Lurie et al (10) evaluated
29 jaundiced patients with extrahepatic biliary obstruction and inflammation. The position of the stones
and the presence of cholangitis resulted in some variation
of the CEA level, but 52% of the patients had CEA levels
above the commonly accepted upper limit of normal
(2.5 ng/ml), and 24% had CEA levels greater than 4 ng/ml.
This represents a significant number of patients with
benign disease exhibiting elevated serum levels of CEA.
   Forty jaundiced patients were evaluated at The Ohio
State University Hospitals, using CEA determinations
(Fig. 1). Liver function tests, standard diagnostic
radiography, ultrasound, radionuclide scans, and endoscopic retrograde cholangiopancreatography proved inadequate for differentiating between benignancy and
malignancy. All patients were subjected to laparotomy.
   Of 12 patients with benign disease, including 7 with
concomitant cholangitis, 11 (92%) had CEA levels lower
than 4 ng/ml. Of 27 patients with malignancy proved by

425

metastases on biopsy, 21 (77%) had CEA levels greater
than 4 ng/ml. One patient with benign disease associated
with active inflammation had CEA levels elevated above
4 ng/ml initially; however, as the inflammation subsided,
jaundice decreased and serial CEA determinations returned
toward normal levels. Of those patients in the series
with CEA levels greater than 4 ng/ml, 96% had proved
malignancy.

All patients were tested for total bilirubin on
admission. The mean bilirubin in the group with benign
disease was 10.2 mg/dl compared with 12.6 mg/dl in the
group with malignant disease (Fig. 2). Alkaline
phosphatase and serum glutamate oxaloacetate transaminase
tests were also performed on all patients. Because of
the wide range of values, no significance was established
for the difference between the benign and malignant
groups, and these liver function tests were of no value
in predicting malignancy (Fig. 3).

Radionuclide liver scans were performed in 24 of 27
patients with proved malignancy. There were 33% false
positive scans for metastases, and of those patients
with normal liver scans, 13% had liver metastases proved
at laparotomy. The liver scan therefore proved to be
misleading in evaluating these patients.

The data demonstrate that in differentiating between
benign and malignant causes of jaundice, patients with
CEA levels greater than 4 ng/ml have a high probability
of malignancy. It is clear that CEA determinations may
be of as much value in the presence of jaundice as in its
absence. It is important, however, to emphasize the use
of repeated or serial determinations in complicated or
equivocal cases.

CEA determinations in patients with jaundice in whom
no obvious cause of CEA elevation is known or can be found
provide a simple tool to aid in diagnosis and management.

REFERENCES

(1) Cohn I, Jr. (1976): Cancer 37:582.

(2) Kaplan A. A. and Ludwig W. M. (1976): Hospital
    Medicine, April, p. 111.

(3) Katon R.M. et al. (1975): Western Journal Medicine
    122:206.

(4) Koch H. and Classen M. (1973): Acta Gastroenterologica
    Belgica 36:6.

(5) Stein H. D. (1975): Annals of Surgery 181:386.

(6) Taylor K. J. W. et al. (1974): Journal Clinical Ultra-
    sound 2:105.

(7) Tylen V. et al. (1976): Surgery, Gynecology, Obstetrics 142:737.

(8) Weill F. et al. (1975): J Clinical Ultrasound 3:23.

(9) White, T. T. and Silverstein F. E. (1976): Cancer 37:449.

(10)Lurie B. B. et al. (1975): Journal American Medical Association 233:326.

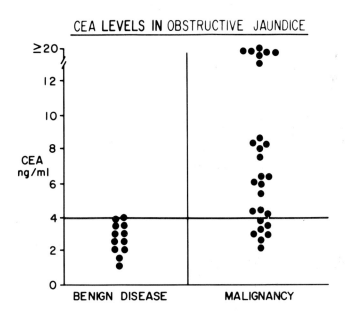

Fig. 1 CEA levels in jaundiced patients.

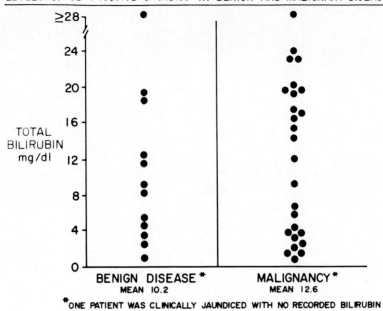

Fig. 2 Levels of jaundice in patients with benign and malignant disease.

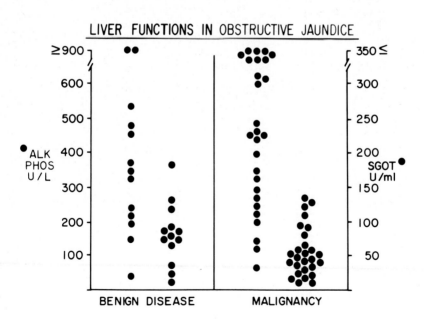

Fig. 3 Liver function tests in jaundiced patients.

DISCUSSION

ZAMCHECK N. (Boston): The risk of misinterpretation of this presentation must be avoided. The authors are concerned merely with obstructive jaundice and not with "medical" jaundice due to liver disease such as especially hepatitis and cirrhosis. We and others have pointed out that one may have elevations of in excess of 4 ng both in benign obstructive disease and in liver disease. We have observed levels as high as 10 ng in patients with cholangitis with or without liver abscesses and levels of the same or greater magnitude in patients with liver disease. I agree with the authors' viewpoint that the CEA test may be useful in this regard, but I fear that selection of a "cut-off" level such as 4 ng/ml to distinguish benign from malignant obstruction is needless and possibly dangerous. To say that patients with CEA levels greater than 4 ng/ml have a high "probability of malignancy" may be correct. But Dr. Martin is correct in saying that the selection of patients is key : and this entails complete work-up and clinical judgment. Much more investigation is necessary on the role of the liver in regulating CEA levels and its clinical application.

CIRCULATING CEA IN CHRONIC FAMILIAL DERMATOSES

H. Rochman, N. Esterly, M. Cooper and K. Soltani

Departments of Pathology, Pediatrics, Nuclear Medicine and
Dermatology, University of Chicago, Chicago, U.S.A.

Striking elevations in CEA levels were observed in some
patients with familial dermatoses. These findings may assist in
diagnosis. It is suggested that the elevated CEA may reflect
involvement of other systems in addition to skin.

Except for multiple polyposis where some elevation in
circulating CEA levels may be observed, there has been little
published on CEA in familial conditions where some tendency to
malignancy may exist.
It is known that epitheliomata may develop in lesions of
chronic dermatosis; the resulting tumor being either a basal cell
or squamous cell carcinoma. Therefore, the present study was of
patients with chronic dermatological pathologies whose genetic
origin had been established.

METHODS

Circulating and tissue CEA were measured by the Hansen-Z-
gel technique (1). To prepare the tissue extract, skin obtained at
operation was weighed (wet), immersed in liquid nitrogen and
shattered in a Thermovac Autopulverizer. The residual tissue
powder was homogenized with efficient cooling in four volumes of
10 mM tris buffer, pH 7.4 using a Polytron PT-10 tissue
disintegrator with 2 or 3 10-second homogenization periods. The
homogenate was centrifuged at 2° C for 30 minutes at 210,000 g
and the resulting supernatant examined for CEA.

RESULTS

The major findings in this study were the striking elevations
in circulating CEA in some patients with epidermolysis bullosa
(Table 1).

TABLE 1 Circulating CEA in Epidermolysis Bullosa

Controls (orthopedic patients; < 10 yr. n = 12)
Mean + 2 S. D. = 3. 54 ng per ml.

Epidermolysis bullosa	Dermatopathology and clinical subclassification	Age years	CEA (ng per ml.)
Males:			
Bin	dystrophic (mild)	22/12	7. 8
Hos	letalis	16. 5	104
Cat	dystrophic (mild)	9	29
Females:			
Cam	dystrophic (mild)	35	0. 3
Bar	dystrophic (mild)	3	0. 8

The highest level, a CEA of 104 ng per ml was obtained on the patient with epidermolysis bullosa letalis but two of the four patients with the dystrophic type also had markedly elevated levels. Since only five patients were studied no conclusions can be made as to whether the CEA levels reflect the severity of the disease or the sex of the patients. The remaining patient with a familial dermatosis examined suffered from keratosis follicularis spinulosa decalvans (Table 2), a sex-linked disorder and he also showed

TABLE 2 Keratosis Follicularis Spinulosa Decalvans

X-linked dominant disorder

Clinical:	generalized hyperkeratosis spiny follicular papular lesions universal alopecia hypoplastic nails	
	May also include	growth retardation absence of eyelids deafness
Patient:		
	Black, male - hospitalized at 10 months	
	at 24 months	CEA 6. 4 ng per ml.
	at 29 months	CEA 36. 0 ng per ml.

markedly elevated CEA levels. Controls in this study were patients with non-congenital dermatoses including skin cancer (Table 3).

TABLE 3 Circulating CEA in Various Skin Pathologies, Adult Patients

Dermatopathological diagnosis	CEA (ng per ml.)
Cicatricial pemphigoid	3. 6
Actinic keratosis	2. 2
Basal cell carcinoma	3. 6
Basal cell carcinoma	2. 4
Basal cell carcinoma + active keratosis	5. 2
Bowen's disease	5. 2
Bowenoid keratosis	4. 2
Kaposi sarcoma	0. 8

Controls:
    a) 892 volunteer subjects*

        0 - 2. 5 ng per ml   97. 0%
    2. 6 - 5. 0 ng per ml   2. 8%
       >   5. 0 ng per ml   0. 2%

    b)   <   4. 94 ng per ml[†]

*See reference (1).

†See reference (3).

No striking increases in CEA levels were observed although one patient with a basal cell carcinoma and active keratosis and another with Bowen's disease did show some increase in circulating CEA. These latter findings are consistent with a published report (2) although comparisons with the published data are difficult since the individual values were not stated.

The source of the elevated CEA in the patients with congenital dermatoses is unclear. Despite the rarity of epidermolysis bullosa, a number of cases (4, 5, 6) have been described in which multifocal squamous cell carcinomata have developed later, during adulthood. Although skin from the affected patients were not examined, the extremely low levels of CEA found with normal skin (Table 4) suggests that the origin of the elevated CEA may be from

TABLE 4 CEA in Extracts of Skin

Source	Age of patient	CEA ng per g tissue (wet weight)
Sample 1. Prepuce (circumcision)	9 yr.	14. 4
Sample 2. Breast (female)	13 yr.	1. 6

other sources; if so, it would indicate that in these congenital skin disorders other systems may also be involved.

REFERENCES

(1) Hansen, H. J., Snyder, J. J., Miller, E. et al. (1974): Hum. Pathol., 5, 139.

(2) Ahmed, A. R. and Chu, T. M. (1976): Lancet, 1, 309.

(3) Alexander, J. C., Silverman, N. A. and Chretien, P. B. (1976): JAMA, 235, 1975.

(4) Halpern, L. K. (1947): Arch. Dermatology and Syphilology, 56, 517.

(5) Rasponi, L. (1950): Archivio Ital. di Dermatologia, 23, 19.

(6) Edland, R. (1969): Birth Defects, 105, 644.

CONTRIBUTION OF CARCINOEMBRYONIC ANTIGEN DETERMINATION IN CSF TO THE DIAGNOSIS AND FOLLOW-UP OF CEREBRAL TUMORS

C. Ardiet, B. Fontanière, M. Clavel, M. Faucon, M. Brunat-Mentigny, M. Mayer, B. Lahneche.

Centre Léon Bérard, 28, rue Laënnec - 69373 - Lyon Cedex 2 France -

Introduction

Since the original work by Gold and Freedman (1) extensive studies aiming at research and quantitative determination of carcinoembryonic antigen (CEA) in the serum of cancer patients have been performed either for diagnostic purposes or for monitoring the disease. The presence of CEA has also been investigated, although to a lesser extent, in different media such as urine (2), faeces (3), pancreatic juice (4), bronchial washing fluid (6). However, to our knowledge, cerebrospinal fluid (CSF) has not hitherto been studied with a view to detecting CEA. The aim of the present work is to evaluate the potential usefulness of CEA assay in CSF as a simple diagnostic test for primary or metastatic brain tumors.

Patients and methods

14 hospitalised patients suffering from non-neoplastic disease (most of them had meningitis) served as control. A single CSF sample was obtained in each patient by lumbar puncture, and simultaneously a blood sample was taken.

105 tumor patients were studied : 39 had brain tumors and 66 had extracerebral tumors. From these patients, 184 CSF samples were collected : in 35 patients, more than one CSF sample was drawn (up to 8 in two patients receiving intrathecal therapy).

In some instances, a blood sample could be obtained simultaneously with the CSF sample. In the patients studied, the reasons for undertaking the lumbar puncture were mainly suspicion of brain metastases, monitoring of brain tumors, or systematic study with intrathecal treatment with methotrexate in acute lymphoblastic leukemia. The histological pattern of the patients studied is listed in table 1.

TABLE 1   Histological pattern of the patients group

Brain Tumors		Extracerebral primary tumor	
Medulloblastoma	16	Adenocarcinoma : mammary	26
Glioblastoma	5	others	3
Retinoblastoma	4	Squamous cell carcinoma	5
N.H. Malignant Lymphoma	2	N.H. Malignant Lymphoma	8
Ependymoma	1	Hodgkin's disease	1
Sarcoma	1	Acute lymphoblastic	
Without biopsy	10	leukemia	5
		Seminoma	2
		Chorioepithelioma	2
		Malignant Melanoma	5
		Osteogenic Sarcoma	1
		Sarcoma	3
		Hepatoma	1
		Malignant tumors	2
		Non malignant diseases	2
Total	39		66

All patients studied were submitted to clinical examination, and to routine paraclinical investigation. A cytological study was systematically performed after filtration of CSF on millipore filter RAWP 304 F1 and Papanico-
laou staining. CEA determination was performed by radioimmunoassay according to the technic described by Mériadec
et al (7) using kits purchased from Commissariat à l'Energie Atomique. CSF samples were tested by the same technic
as sera ,the standard curve being derived from values obtained by addition of standard CEA to a normal human plasma. In all cases 100 microliters of fluid were sufficient
for duplicate measurements.

Results -

In the control group, serum CEA levels ranged from
0 to 16 nanograms /ml, i.e. within the normal range of the
method used. CEA levels in CSF were all found to be
0 ng / ml ; thus in subsequent studies CEA levels higher
than 0 ng / ml in CSF were considered as abnormal ("positive").

In the patients group, CEA levels in CSF ranged from
0 to 3600 ng / ml, the vast majority of "positive" levels

being lesser than 100 ng / ml. Serum levels were found from the normal range up to 970 ng / ml.

Since CSF samples were taken from patients before, during or after surgery, radiotherapy and/or chemotherapy, patients were classified according to clinical and para-clinical criteria into three classes : patients with evolutive cerebral disease, with stabilized disease, and pa-tients with no evidence of cerebral disease (NED) at the time CSF samples were taken. Patients in which the disease was in an active phase at the time of CSF sampling were considered as "clinically positive" : when CEA level in CSF was found positive in a clinically positive patient, the case was recorded as "concordant". Similarly, NED or stabilized patients with negative CEA determination in the CSF were also recorded as "concordant". The patterns of concordances in the patients studied are given in Table 2.

TABLE 2 Concordances between clinical features and CEA levels in CSF

Brain Tumors (39)			Extra cerebral tumors (66)		
	CEA -	CEA +		CEA -	CEA +
Glioblastoma	1	2	Adenocarcinoma :		
Medulloblastoma	3	2	mammary	12	7
Retinoblastoma	2	0	Others	0	2
N.H. Malignant			Squamous cell		
Lymphoma	1	0	carcinoma	4	0
Without biopsy	4	2	N.H. Malignant		
			Lymphoma	4	4
			Hodgkin's disease	1	0
			Osteogenic sarcoma	1	0
			Sarcoma	1	1
			Malignant Melanoma	2	0
			Hepatoma	1	0
			Malignant Tumors	2	0
Total	11	6		28	14
	17/39 : 44 %			42/66 : 63,5 %	

436

When the CEA determination in CSF was found to be negative in a patient with clinically proven evolutive cerebral lesion, the case was recorded as discordant. Cases escaping biological detection were found more frequently amongst patients with brain tumors than amongst patients with brain metastases of extracerebral tumors (Table 3).

TABLE 3   Discrepancies between clinical findings and CEA level in CSF : "False-negatives" of CEA

Brain tumors	(39)	CEA -	Metastases to brain	(66)	CEA -
Medulloblastoma		2	Mammary adenocarcinoma		4
Glioblastoma		2	Seminoma		2
Retinoblastoma		1	Malignant Melanoma		2
Primitive Sarcoma		1	Ovarian choriocarcinoma		1
Unknown		4			
Total		10			9
10/39 : 26 %			9/66 : 14 %		

Discrepancy appears also in patients found without clinical cerebral lesion (stabilized or N.E.D.) and showing a positive level of CEA in CSF, the mean follow up brain tumors being 15 months. These "false-positive" cases for CEA assay are listed in Table 4.

TABLE 4   Absence of brain tumor or metastases with CEA in CSF positive

Medulloblastoma	6	Mammary adenocarcinoma	1
Glioblastoma	1	Acute lymphoblastoid	
Ependymoma	1	leukemia	2
Retinoblastoma	1	Post-operative meningitis	
N.H.Malignant lymphoma	1	(mammary carcinoma)	1
Unknown	1	Non-malignant pathology	1
		Noclinical interpretation possible	5

Table 5 lists 5 cases that were classified NED at the time of the lumbar puncture. A positive level of CEA was found in the assay. Clinical history showed later the appearance of an evolutive lesion. For these cases, biological findings preceded clinical ones.

TABLE 5   Precession of CEA level in CSF with clinical disease

		time
Medulloblastoma	1	6 months
Adenocarcinoma : mammary	2	1 month
ethmoïdal	1	1 month
Malignant Melanoma	1	2 months

Discussion

Our results show clearly that there is a good concordance between the level of CEA in CSF and clinical data. One can note that the concordance is better in cases of extracerebral primary tumors than in cases of cerebral primary tumors. This could be due to our choice of patients and perhaps too, to the fact that Gold's CEA and similar molecular species isolated later have been isolated from hepatic metastases of colic tumors.

It seems logical that tumors known to secrete CEA, such as adenocarcinoma of the breast, secrete it also in CSF in measurable quantities when there is a cerebral metastasis. One of the unexpected results of our study is the discovery of a positive level of CEA in a case of metastatic malignant melanoma : as a matter of fact, in our experience, the blood level of CEA in patients with malignant melanoma, disseminated or not disseminated, has always been normal.

The casesof "negative" concordance, i.e. CEA normal in CSF and no cerebral tumors, have but a poor diagnostic value. On the other hand, "positive" concordances i.e. high level of CEA and cerebral tumoral lesion are a very conforting corroboration of our starting hypothesis i.e. the possibility for intra-cerebral metastases to secrete CEA. The ectopic secretion of the antigen has therefore a diagnostic value. It has too a value in the follow up of intra cranial metastases treated by systemic or intrathecal way. We have in fact observed in several cases a variation of CEA levels in CSF in the same direction as the clinical status, the cytologic status, and the treatment. The decrease of CEA level in CSF seems a good sign of therapeutic efficacy.

Some progress remains to be achieved along two lines : the first concerns the problem of the assay of a biological fluid with hardly any protein (CSF) by means of a method used for plasma or serum, the normal reference plasma being a pool containing in fact slight quantities of CEA. This fact explains,in part at least,that the binding capacity of the antibody for the radioantigen in our control CSF series is higher than this capacity measured in a nil concentration of standard CEA added to the standard plasma. The second concerns a question that has been raised in view of certain CSF dilution curves which are not closely parallel to the standard curves. These statements compel us to be prudent in the assessment of the nature of the CEA found in CSF.

The cases of recurrence or intracerebral metastases with clinical symptoms whereas CSF levels of CEA is nil are somewhat discouraging. Probably a better method, better adapted, currently under study, could diminish the number of these discordant cases. At present the absence of biological expression in malignant tumors is frequent in many cases and well known to clinicians and biologists.

The cases of discordance with presence of CEA in CSF and no clinical sign of intracerebral lesion must be considered from different points of view : the possibility of a biological reaction in advance on the clinical and paraclinical signs is clearly demonstrated in this study, as is the case for recurrences or visceral metastases discovered by plasmatic CEA assay. One must wait some time before assessing that there is a discordance. The blood level of CEA must be known to eliminate a contamination of CSF by blood during the lumbar puncture. One cannot exclude the disappearance of a cerebral metastasis by a systemic or an intrathecal treatment.
Lastly Buffe and Rimbaut (8) have shown that in children the blood level is not reliable : increased levels can be found in the course of many diseases, even neurological diseases. One cannot exclude that in the cases of children with primary brain tumors, in our study, the presence of CEA may not be evidence of a recurrence. We are carrying out a prospective study of these facts.

We think the assay of CEA is of interest in the search for recurrences and for the followup of patients with intracranial primary or secondary tumors. It is only of value if compared with the clinical symptoms and with the blood CEA level which must be known.

Acknowledgments

We wish to thank Pr Garde (Hôpital de l'Antiquaille) who gifted our check series, and J.F. Doré who helped to translation of the text.

REFERENCES

(1) Gold,P. and Freedman, S.O. (1965) : Specific carcino-
    embryonic antigens of the human digestive system.
    J. Exp. Med. 122, 467-481.
(2) Zimmerman, R., Wahren, B., and Edsmyr, F. (1976) :
    Measurement of urinary CEA-Like substance. An aid in
    the management of patients with bladder carcinoma.
    Bull. Cancer 63 (4), 563-574.
(3) Elias, E.G., Holyoke, E.D., Chu, T.M., (1974) : Carci-
    noembryonic antigen (CEA) in feces and plasma of nor-
    mal subjects and patients with colorectal carcinoma.
    Dis. Colon Rectum 17 (1), 38-41.
(4) Rey, J.F., Krebs, B.P., Julien, H., Mondet, M., Del-
    mont, J., (1977) : Intérêt du dosage de l'ACE dans le
    suc pancréatique pur. Symposium on clinical Applica-
    tions of Carcinoembryonic antigen and Others Antigenic
    Markers Assays, Nice, 7-9 October 1977.
(5) Blair, O.M., Goldenberg, D.M., (1974) : A correlative
    study of bronchial cytology, bronchial washing carci-
    noembryonic antigen, and plasma carcinoembryonic anti-
    gen in the diagnosis of bronchogenic cancer. Acta
    Cytologica 18 (6), 510-514.
(6) Lamerz, R., Ruider, H., (1976) : Significance of CEA
    determinations in patients with cancer of the colon-
    rectum and the mammary gland in comparison to physio-
    logical status in connection with pregnancy. Bull.
    Cancer 63 (4), 575-586.
(7) Meriadec, B., Martin, F., Guerin, J., Henry, R.,
    Klepping, C., (1973) : Description d'une méthode de
    dosage de l'antigène carcino-embryonnaire. Bull.
    Cancer 60, 403-410.
(8) Buffe, D., Rimbaut, C., Rudant, C., (1977) : Etude de
    l'intérêt des trois marqueurs : Alpha 1 FP, Alpha 2 H
    isoferritine et CEA en oncologie pédiatrique. Sympo-
    sium on Clinical Applications of Carcinoembryonic
    Antigen and Others Antigenic Markers Assays, Nice
    7-9 October 1977.

440

FREQUENCY OF ELEVATED AFP AND CEA LEVELS IN CHILDREN WITH NON MALIGNANT DISEASES.

J.L.Boublil, B.P.Krebs, R.Mariani, C.Bonet, M.Namer, M.Schneider, C.M.Lalanne, R.Masseyeff

Centre Antoine Lacassagne, 36 Voie Romaine, 06054 Nice, Cedex,France

Plasma levels of CARCINOEMBRYONIC ANTIGEN (CEA) and alpha-feto-protein (AFP) were measured in a non-selected children population treated in the pediatric department. The goal of this study was to dertermine the influence of non-malignant diseases on the frequency of false positive results in children.

MATERIAL AND METHODS

Blood samples were taken on admission to the pediatric depart-ment in children, aged between 1 day (cord blood) and 15 years. AFP was measured in 655 blood samples with the Enzyme immuno method of MAIOLINI and MASSEYEFF (1), the upper limit in normal adults is 5 ng/ml. Out of these ,643 samples were available for radioimmunoassay of CEA, with CIS method (2), in our hand, the cut off level is 5ng/ml in normal non smoking adults. The statistical presentation chosen was that of the median percentiles (10th, 25th, 75th and 90th).

RESULTS

1) Alpha-fetoprotein

The AFP decreases in the first year of life (fig.1) and presents the following characteristics : the 10th percentile reached the normal adult levels, between the first and the third month, the median between 6 months and 12 months, in contrast the 90th is still elevated : 28 ng/ml.
These data are closely related to those of MASSEYEFF et al (3), in the normal infant. After the first year (fig.2), there exists a remarkable stability of AFP levels, since the 90th percentile lies below the detection limit of the method. Nevertheless, after the age of 12 years an elevation of the 90th percentile can be noticed, this elevation does not occur in normal children during puberty (3).
Out of 554 children aged over one year, 10% (53 cases) present a raised AFP level, more than 5ng/ml. The frequency of values higher than 5 ng/ml, correlated with age appears in the figure 3 :
one finds between the ages of 1 and 2 years a percentage of positivity at 27%, between 2 and 12 years from 6-7%, the percentage of positivity subsequently rises to 19% during puberty.
The analysis of the 53 cases presenting abnormal levels of AFP excluding those with showed hepatitis, well known to increase AFP levels, demonstrated that the group of pathology giving rise to the

greatest incidence of positive levels was that of neurological disease : meningitis, encephalitis, convulsions. We have included in this group , patients with head injury. In fact 26 out of the 53 cases had neurological affections. 6 of the 18 cases of head injury had positive levels (33%).

When one compares the incidence of raised levels in all the patients with non-malignant diseases with those presenting neurological affections one sees that the incidence of positivity is increased by 2-3 fold. For example between the ages of 1 to 2 years the level rises from 22% to 61.5%, and from 19% to 36% during puberty. Analysis of the highest abnormal levels attained showed that among the 10 highest estimations 7 were taken in cases of neurological disease (70%).

It seems thus that neurological affections increased not only the incidence but also the absolute levels achieved.

2) Carcinoembryonic antigen

As for AFP, we have used the percentile method. Raised levels are seen in cord blood. Our highest level was 245 ng/ml and 80% of our levels were above 5ng/ml (fig.3). These results differ from those found by TROUPEL, VON KLEIST, BURTIN, who measured serum levels in neonates by   radioimmunossay and found only 46% of values above 5 ng/ml : their highest value was 60 ng/ml (4).

After birth there is a rapid fall in CEA levels. The 10th percentile regains the normal adult level, at about 1 month, the median oscillates in the region of 8 ng/ml. The 90th percentile remains raised (25 ng/ml). After the first year of life CEA levels may be highly variable. Only the two lowest percentiles (10th + 25th) remain within adult levels (fig.4).

On the other hand, during puberty all the percentiles, with the exception of the 90th, regain normal adult values. As for AFP we have attempted to distinguish the pathological groups giving the most false positive values. The main groups became apparent:

A- Those with as many normal values as false positives;
B- Those with few false positive results;
C- Those frequently associated with devoted levels of CEA.

The following three tables resume these results. As with AFP the diseases giving the highest number of false positives are hepatitis and neurological affections. In our series the highest percentage of false positives was seen in rheumatismal diseases.

TABLE 1 : Diseases with symetric repartition of CEA level around 50 percentile.

Pathology	Epilepsy	Eruptive fevers	Acute Gastro-enteritis	Asthma
Above 50 percentile	50%	51%	52%	55%
Below	50%	49%	48%	45%

TABLE 2 : Diseases with asymetric repartition - Predominance of low CEA levels

Pathology	Laryngeal diseases	Meningitis	Renal diseases
Above 50 percentile	40%	35%	20%
Below	60%	65%	80%

TABLE 3 : Diseases with asymetric repartition - Predominance of high CEA levels

Pathology	ENT diseases	Urothelial diseases	Acute pulmonary diseases	Hepatitis	Encephalitis and chronic encephalopathy	Rhuma. diseas.
Above 50 percent.	67%	67%	68%	71%	71%	86%
Below	33%	33%	32%	29%	29%	14%

CONCLUSION

A comparative study of the serum levels of these two proteins during the first 15 years of life demonstrates many similarities but also certain differences. The absolute values seen in cord blood samples are much higher than those seen in normal adults.
The AFP is much more elevated, attaining a level of thousands of ng/ml, than the CEA which attains levels in the hundreds.
After birth, there is a rapid fall in levels of both proteins. However, this fall is more rapid for CEA (around 3 months) than for AFP (between 6 + 12 months).
Non-malignant pathology is reflected differently by the two antigens. After 2 years a remarkable stability of AFP is seen, little influenced by non-malignant disease. Although there are many conditions which may give rise to abnormal levels, hepatitis and as has not hitherto been described neurological affections most commonly give rise abnormal levels. This incidence is significant.
On the contrary after the first year of life CEA levels seem greatly affected by non-malignant diseases. More than 50% of our children had CEA levels higher than 5 ng/ml. Nevertheless as for AFP certain groups are more frequently ACE positive than others, for example patients with hepatitis, neurological affections or rheumatismal conditons.
These facts are important to bear in mind since the monitoring of these proteins is used as a guide to diagnosis and above all for the control of treatment in certain cancers : - for example, the monitoring of AFP in childhood hepatoma and yolk sac tumours.
CEA estimations are of less value in children since CEA secreting tumours are rare or even non-existant.

REFERENCES

(1) Masseyeff,R., Maiolini,R., Bouron,Y. (1973):
    Biomedicine, 19, 314-317.
(2) Meriadec,B., Martin,F., Guerin,J., Henry,R., Klepping,C.(1973):
    Bull.Cancer, 60, 403-410.
(3) Masseyeff,R., Gilli, J., Krebs,B.P., Bonet,C., Zrihen,H. (1974):
    Biomedicine 21, 353-357.
(4) Troupel,S., VonKleist, S., Burtin, P. (1976): Bull.Cancer 63,
    655-660.

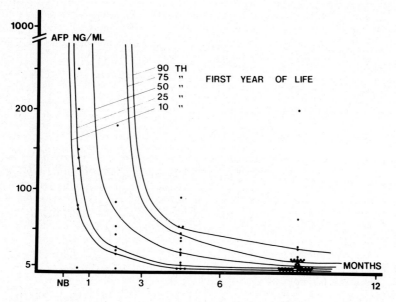

Fig. 1 : Evolution of Alpha-fetoprotein levels during the first
year of life.

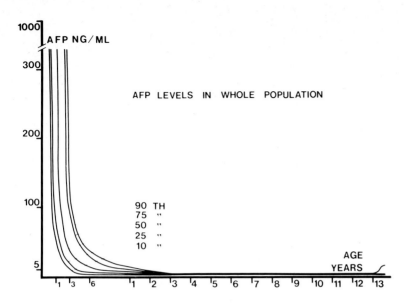

Fig. 2 : Evolution of Alpha-fetoprotein levels between age 0 (cord blood) and age 15 .

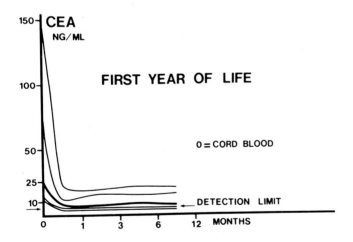

Fig. 3 : Evolution of CEA levels during the first year of life.

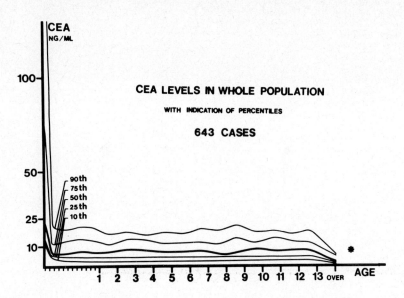

Fig. 4 : Evolution of CEA levels between age 0 (cord blood) and age 15.

446

CLINICAL INTEREST OF THREE MARKERS: α1FP, α2H-ISOFERRITIN AND CEA
IN PEDIATRIC ONCOLOGY.

D. Buffe, C. Rimbaut, C. Rudant.

Institut de Recherches Scientifiques sur le Cancer, Villejuif, BP 8.

Since 1968, in a work realized with the Pediatric department of
Institut Gustave Roussy(Dr O.Schweisguth), we have followed up the e-
volution of the α1FP and α2H-isoferritin level in the sera of tumor
bearing children.Our first studies (1) done by immunodiffusion techniques let only detect protein-amounts above 200-250 ng/ml; however,the
obtained results, allowed us to demonstrate or confirm the clinical
value of these tests as it was shown in table 1 and 2.

TABLE I- α1FP in children's sera tested by immunodiffusion technic
between january 1968 and october 1973.

Malignant Tumor:	Number	Positive for α1FP	% +
Hepatoblastoma	49	45	91
Teratoma	78	44	57
Teratoma in acute phase	48	44	91
Other malignant tumors	416	3	0,7
Benign tumors	45	0	0
Non malignant diseases:			
Hepatitis	153	25	16,2
Metabolic diseases	34	5+	14,6

+Tyrosinosis only (5 of 6)

TABLE 2- α2H-Isoferritin in children's serum

	Number	α2HF +	% +
Healthy or benign diseased children	177	16	9
Malignant Tumors	452	362	80
Hepatoma	41	37	90
Teratoma	43	23	53
Neuroblastoma	87	68	78
Nephroblastoma	88	77	87,5
Embryonic Sarcoma	41	33	80
Lympho-Reticulo-Sarcoma	35	30	85
Brain tumors	34	29	80
Various tumors	83	65	78

The radioimmunoassays have increased the interest of these evaluations in the post-therapeutic survey of children with malignant diseases. In order to add to the probability of an early detection, we
have associated the carcinoembryonic antigen (CEA) dosage with the
alpha-foetoproteine (α1FP) and alpha-2H-isoferritin's (α2HF) one.
If α1FP and CEA are two well known tumor associated antigens, a

few details about α 2H-isoferritin could be necessary.

We have shown in tumor extracts and in the serum of patients with malignant disease the presence of a protein immunologically identical to ferritin (2,3): the alpha 2H globuline (α 2 for electrophoretic mobility and "H" for hepatic origin).So, this protein that we have extracted and purified from foetal and tumoral liver is an "isoferritin.It is different from normal adult ferritin in a few physico-chemical characteristics: its instability in aqueous medium, its lower isoelectric point, its polymeric forms and its carbohydrate components.

Although several teams, american(4), japaneese(5) and french(6) had reported the α 2H-isoferritin modifications during the tumoral evolution, this protein was not considered as a marker because from the first publication ,we have mentioned that it was not specific for tumor.As it could be seen in table 2, the α 2H-isoferritin presence is not correlated with one type of tumor and its level can be increased in serious diseases without known malignancies.

These characters are now also recognized for CEA and make good that it is tried to increase the number of markers in order to enlarge the clinical value of the assays.

I- ALPHA FOETO-PROTEINE "α 1FP".

The use of the radioimmunoassays, even if it increases the sensibility of the detection,does not modify the specificity of the test. α 1FP levels above to 200 ng/ml have been observed only in the two well known types of tumors: hepatoblastoma and some teratoma, the yolk Sac tumor (table 3) (7,8).

TABLE 3- α 1FP in Germ Cell Tumors: 155 cases. 60 YST= 54 +.

Localisation	Number of cases	Yolk Sac T.	Positive
Vagina	15	8	7
Sacro-coccygeal area	30	18	18
Testis	42	16	12
Ovarian	51	13	13
Others localisation	17	5	4

This level could be observed normally in minus two months aged infants. In these cases the repetition of the test, 5 days later, and the comparative dosages evaluated in the same experiment are a good diagnostical argument (fig. 1 and 2).

In order to follow up the evolution after surgery and therapeutic it is also essential to repeat the test and to compare them in one assay. (fig. 3,4 and 5).

Let remember the two non malignant diseases in which high α 1FP levels could be observed: the hepatitis and tyrosinosis (9). This congenital disease could lend itself to a diagnostical error with hepatoblastoma, especially as a young child is concerned and as the α 1FP level is very high and remains high as long as the metabolic disorder is not well cured. The tyrosinemia, methioninemia and the knowledge of serious disorders of the coagulation will give the diagnosis.

II- CARCINO-EMBRYONIC-ANTIGEN "CEA".

In our knowledge not many dosages have been done in children for this antigen, and the clinical value in pediatrics has been estimated With regard to the adult level. Our studies with 150 tumors bearing children and 70 healthy or benign diseased children, have shown excep-

tionaly an increased level: 10 out of 150 tumor bearing children and
6 out of 70 benign diseased children(2 hepatitis,1 fibro-angiomatosis,
1 pleural effusion,1 kidney infection and 1 erythematous pharyngitis:

TABLE 4- 220 children tested with the 3 markers: α 1FP, α 2H-isoferri-
tin and CEA(150 tumors and 70 controls).
Pathological levels:α 1FP, more than 2 years aged children $>$ 20 ng/ml,
3 months to 2 years aged child $>$ 30 ng/ml;α 2HF 80ng/ml;CEA$>$30ng/ml.

Number		Abnormal levels		
		α 1FP	α 2HF	CEA
7	Hepatoma	7	5	3 +
47	Germ Cell tumor	38	31	4
25	Neuroblastoma	2°°	23	2°°
31	Nephroblastoma	0	24	1
26	Sarcoma (LBS, RMS, FS, OS)	0	16	0
14	Brain tumors	0	8	0
70	Healthy or with benign diseases	3	13	6

°°Pepper Syndrom. + Late in the evolution.

III- ALPHA 2H-ISOFERRITIN "α 2HF"
     In pediatrics this protein likes to be a marker more interesting
than CEA; 107 out of 150 children with tumor(70%) had an abnormal level and 13 out 70(18,5%) healthy or benign diseased children.
     The increase of the α 2H-isoferritin level is not dependant of
the type of the tumor. The most important percentage of positivity and
the highest level have been observed in Neuroblastoma and in tumor
with hepatic metastasis.
     Serially dosages during the pathologic evolution show that the
α 2H-isoferritin level can increase several weeks before recurrence or
metastasis (fig.5).The α 2H-isoferritin is synthetized by the liver
and not by the tumor. So, the tumor exeresis is not follow with a sharp
decrease as it is observed for α 1FP and CEA in the adult differenciated tumors.After therapeutic the normal level is reached gradually and
slowly; a sharp decrease indicates a worst prognostic.
     In α 1FP synthetizing hepatoblastoma and germ cells tumors, the
seric α 2H-isoferritin increases always before α 1FP and when the synthesis of this one is important, a diminution of α 2HF is observed.The
cutting of the curves has always been seen in the cases with a bad
prognosis. If a normal level has been choosed after studies one must
keep in mind that variations could be observed in any child and in some non malignant pathological cases as an acute pulmonary infection.
For these reasons it is necessary to repeat the tests and to compare
them in one same radioimmunoassay. It is only in these conditions that
the best benefit will be got with these different markers.

IN SUMMARY AND CONCLUSIONS
     Only α 1FP is a specific marker with a prognostical and diagnos-
tical value for primary liver carcinoma and Yolk sac tumor. A diminution of the level, below 10 ng/ml, in less than 7 days is a good argument for complete exeresis. If α 1FP increases, even slightly, look
for recurrence !
     CEA and α 2H-Isoferritin are not specific markers; they incite
to fuller investigations.
     α 2H-Isoferritin increases even in case of small local recurren-
ce. During the evolution, a plateau and a slow decrease in several

months is a good prognosis; a sharp decrease is a reserve prognosis and let be afraid of a recurrence.

CEA is only related to well differentiated tumor and hepatic metastasis. It increases early, except in case of small local metastasis After surgery a quick decrease and a level below 10 ng/ml in less than 1 month is a good prognosis: probably complete exeresis. If CEA increases again, let weed out an hepatic or pulmonary disease and look for recurrence or metastasis !

REFERENCES :

(1)Buffe, D. (1973): GANN Monograph on Cancer Research,14,117-128.
(2)Buffe, D., Rimbaut, C., Burtin, P. (1968): Int J. Cancer,3,850-856
(3)Buffe, D., Rimbaut, C. (1975) Ann. NY Acad. Sc., 259, 417-426
(4)Alpert, E., Coston, RL., Drysdale, JW. (1973) Nature, 242, 194-195
(5)Wada, T., Anzai. T., Yachi, A., Sakamoto, S. (1970) Prot. of Biological Fluids: H. Peeters Ed. Pergamon Press. 18, 221-226
(6)Martin, JP., Charlionnet, R., Ropartz, Cl. (1971) Presse Med., 79 2.313-2316
(7)Norgaard-Pedersen, B., Albrechtsen, R., Teilum, G. (1975) Acta Pathol. Microbiol. Scand., 83, 573-579.
(8)Rimbaut, C., Caillaud, JM., Caillou, B., Carlu, C., Rudant, C., Buffe, D. (1977) International Res. Carcino.Emb.Prot. Copenhagen.
(9)Buffe, D., Rimbaut, C. (1973) Biomedicine, 19, 172-176

FIGURES: the α 1FP amounts are expressed in international units according to OMS nomenclature.

Acknowledgment.
We are grateful to the Département des radio isotopes du CEA Marcoulle for labelling of α 2H-isoferritin.

The α 1FP and CEA radioimmunoassays have been done with the kits of Commissariat à l'Energie Atomique C.I.S., Saclay, France

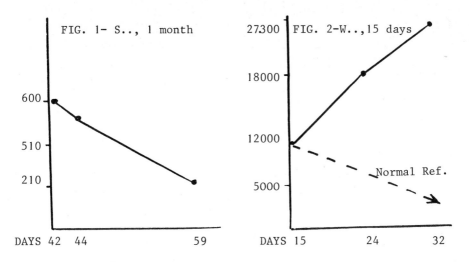

Fig. 1-Abdominal tumor. 1st sample = α 1FP normal for age; α 1FP decreases in the other samples. It is not a teratoma, it is a rhabdomyosarcoma.

Fig. 2-Hepatomegaly. 1st sample = α 1FP slightly increased; the following samples show the α 1FP increase. Surgery = Hepatoma.

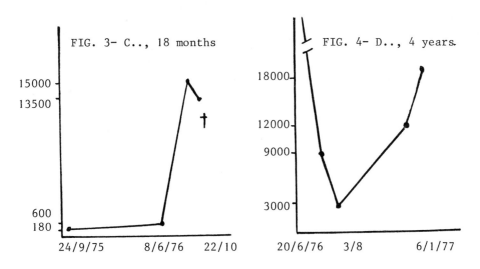

Fig. 3-Testis teratoma. Normal level after surgery. 6 months later very slight increase of α 1FP confirmed by an other sample. Clinical and radiological examinations do not reveale the tumor. α 1FP always increase and an exploring laparatomy show a metastatic para-aortic node.

Fig. 4-Sacro-coccygeal teratoma. Incomplete exeresis. The α 1FP level does not decrease sufficiently after surgery and in spite of chemotherapy, α 1FP rises again = recurrence of the tumor.

451

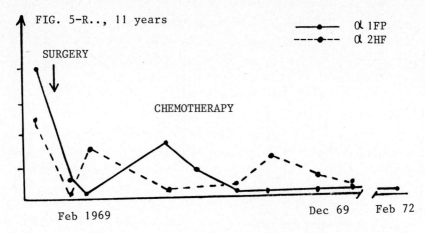

FIG. 5-R.., 11 years

SURGERY

CHEMOTHERAPY

α 1FP
α 2HF

Feb 1969   Dec 69   Feb 72

Fig. 5-Ovarian teratoma. Evolution of the level of α 1FP and α 2H-iso-ferritin after surgery and chemotherapy. After one year the level are normal and remains normal.The child is always well three years later.

DISCUSSION

MILANO G. (Nice): May I have some data concerning cross-reaction of normal feritin in your radioimmunoassay for isoferitin.

BUFFE D.(Villejuif): With reagents now available, it is impossible to make any difference between normal feritin and feritin from neoplastic tissues.

452

BETA 2 MICROGLOBULIN in LYMPHOPROLIFERATIVE DISORDERS with SPECIAL REFERENCE to GAMMOPATHIES

J.P. Cassuto*, B.P. Krebs**, J. Giacchero*,
M.V. Joyner*, P. Dujardin*, P. Audoly* and
R. Masseyeff***

Clinique Médicale*, Centre Antoine Lacassagne**,
Laboratoire d'Immunologie***,
U.E.R. de Médecine, Nice - FRANCE.

Beta 2 microglobulin (β2 m) is a low molecular weight protein (11,800) originally isolated by Berggärd in 1968 (1) from the urine of patients with renal tubular disorders. A striking homology between this molecule and the constant domain C_H3 of IgG has been demonstrated (2). Originally shown to be present on the surface of lymphocytes (3) it has since been found on the cytoplasmic membrane of most nucleated cells (4) as are HL-A antigens. Normal plasma levels are between 0.8 and 2.4 μg/ml (5). Measurements of urinary and serum β2 m levels have proved useful in assessment both of renal glomerular and tubular functions (6,7). In addition β2 m levels have been studied in a variety of malignant diseases (8,9,10,11) including lymphoproliferative disorders. That raised levels of plasma β2 m may be due to the renal insufficiency often accompanying such malignant disease, has led to the exclusion of such patients from various studies (8,10). However Revillard and Vincent have shown in 400 measurements performed in 20 renal transplanted patients a correlation between the plasma concentration of β2 m and creatinine (12). Therefore we have taken into consideration the following ratio :

$$\frac{\text{measured plasma } \beta 2 \text{ m}}{\text{theoretical plasma } \beta 2 \text{ m}} = \frac{M}{Th}$$

which a priori enables all patients to be studied regardless of renal status. We undertook a study of patients with lymphoproliferative disorders which on the one hand have been shown to have very high levels of β2 m (9,10) and on the other hand have a very high incidence of renal impairment. This group of disorders was compared with controls, patients with solid tumours, and other blood diseases.

MATERIALS and METHODS

Measurements were performed in 85 patients with a variety of lymphoproliferative disorders : 27 with myeloma, comprising 10 IgG, 13 IgA, 3 light chain and 1 non-excretory ; 30 with non-myelomatous dysglobulinae-

mias ; 5 with Waldenström's macroglobulinaemia ; 23 with
chronic lymphatic leukaemia (C.L.L.) or non-Hodgkin's
lymphoma (L.S.). Diagnosis of non-myelomatous dysglobulinaemia was made on the basis of two or more normal
bone-marrow aspirations, one or more normal bone-marrow
biopsies, negative skeletal surveys, normal plasma cell
acid phosphatase scores (13) and bioclinical follow-up
from one to twelve years. When several β 2 m assays were
performed, the highest level was used for this study.
Measurements were made in 245 controls. Mean age for the
various groups of patients was as follows : myeloma 75
yrs ; non-myelomatous dysglobulinaemia 76 yrs ; Waldenström's macroglobulinaemia 68 yrs ; C.L.L. + L.S. 66 yrs.
β 2 m was measured by a radio-immunoassay method (Phadebas β 2 microtest). The theoretical plasma β 2 m level
was calculated according to the following formula :

$$\log \beta 2 \text{ m } (\mu g/1) = 0.65 \log \text{ plasma creatinine } (mg/ 1) +$$
2.74 (r = 0.70) (12).

A conversion table was prepared for differing plasma creatinine values. The ratio :

$$\frac{\text{measured } \beta 2 \text{ m } (M)}{\text{theoretical } \beta 2 \text{ m } (Th)}$$

was calculated for each patient.

RESULTS

1925 assays were performed on 1029 patients : 245
controls, 675 solid tumours and 109 blood disorders of
wich 85 were lymphoproliferations. Highest ratios were
found in those with neoplastic blood diseases. In this
group the most elevated values were in myeloma (fig 1).
In controls the measured β 2 m level range was from 0.3
to 3 μ g/ml and the 95 th percentile was 1.5 for the $\frac{M}{Th}$
ratio.

Ratio results for the various lymphoproliferative
disorders are shown in figure 2. Most myelomas (17/27),
all Waldenström's macroglobulinaemia 5/5 and 13/23 C.L.L.
+ L.S. showed ratios above 1.5 the maximum normal value.
9 out of 30 non-myelomatous dysglobulinaemias also gave
ratios above 1.5 but they never exceeded 2.5, whereas 7
myelomas exceeded this figure reaching a maximum ratio
of 13. A correlation between myeloma staging (according
to Durie and Salmon) (14) and $\frac{M}{Th}$ ratio values was observed (fig 3), and in addition the three most elevated
levels were in patients in the terminal stages of the
disease in whom previous values had been lower.

454

The ratio obtained in the 15 cases of Hodgkin's diseases ranged from 0.25 to a maximum of 2.

DISCUSSION

Our results indicate that raised plasma levels of $\beta2$ m and more specifically $\frac{M}{Th}$ ratios are most characteristic of haematological malignant diseases and are in agreement with previous data (9,10). Further, the results suggest that this investigation may be particularly useful in multiple myeloma : i) in the rapid differentiation from non-myelomatous dysglobulinaemias, ii) as an indication of the stage and hence prognosis, and iii) as a disease monitoring criterion.

A similar correlation between $\beta2$ m levels and the staging of malignant disease has been demonstrated by Teasdale et al (11) in relation to carcinoma of the breast. Like Evrin et al (5) these same authors drew attention to the increase in 2 m levels with age (0.24 μ g/ml per decade) although no correction for renal function was mentioned. However in our myeloma and non-myelomatous dysglobulinaemia groups the mean ages were almost identical ie, 76 years and 75 years respectively.

It is worthy of note in relation to the molecular homology already referred to that no correlation was noted between IgG myeloma and excessively high $\frac{M}{Th}$ $\beta2$ m ratios.

Thus, from this and other studies it is clear that lymphoproliferative disorders are often associated with raised $\beta2$ m levels. It must be pointed out however that the patients studied both in this and other series are almost invariably those with B cell lymphoproliferations, and no data on T cell malignant proliferations has been published. Nevertheless, studies in Hodgkin's disease, considered by some as a T cell disorder, have shown almost invariably low levels of $\beta2$ m (9,10), as was the case in this study. In addition we have studied an advanced Sezary's syndrome and a T cell lymphoblastic lymphoma and have found only marginally elevated ratios. Thus although it has not been possible to differentiate between normal T and B lymphocytes on the basis of the amount of membrane $\beta2$ m (15) further studies are required to determine whether $\beta2$ m levels have any discriminitive value in malignant T and B cell proliferations. Similar further studies are required in haematological malignancy to assess the usefulness of this investigation as a tumour monitoring device. It is worth noting in this context that, in contrast to other tumour markers we have studied α.fetoprotein (16), carcino-embryonic A_3(17), myeloma protein (18), β 2 m possesses a negligible half-life which might enable considerably more frequent assessements of tumour mass, and hence an indication, over a short-term period, as to the efficacy of therapy.

Finally, no previous studies other than in renal disease have formally taken into account renal function status, and we feel that such consideration, by use of the $\frac{M}{Th}$ ratio described, is mandatory in the investigation of these patients.

REFERENCES

(1) Berggärd,I., Bearn,A.G. (1968):
J. Biol. Chem., 213, 4095.
(2) Poulik, M., Bernoco, M., Bernoco, D., Ceppellini, R. (1973) :
Science, 182, 1352.
(3) Bernier, G., Fanger, M. (1973) :
J. Immunol., 109, 407.
(4) Evrin, P.E., Pertoft, H. (1973) :
J. Immunol., 111, 1147.
(5) Evrin, P., Wibell, L. (1972) :
Scand. J. Clin. Lab. Invest., 29, 69.
(6) Wibell, L., Evrin, P., Berggärd, I. (1973) :
Nephron, 10, 320.
(7) Hall, P., Vasiljevic, M. (1973) :
J. Lab. Clin. Med., 81, 897.
(8) Evrin, P., Wibell, L., (1973) :
Clin. Chim. Acta, 43, 183.
(9) Kithier, K., Cejka, J., Belamaric, J., Al-Sarraf, M., Peterson, W., Vaitkevicius, V., Poulik, M. (1974) :
Clin. Chim. Acta, 52, 293.
(10) Shuster, J., Gold, P., Poulik, M.D. (1976) :
Clin. Chim. Acta, 67, 307.
(11) Teasdale, C., Mander, A., Fifield, R., Keyser, J., Newcombe, R., Hughs, L. (1977) :
Clin. Chim. Acta, 78, 135.
(12) Revillard, J.P., Vincent, C. (1976) :
Nouv. Presse Med., 40, 2707.
(13) Cassuto, J.P., Hammou, J.C., Pastorelli, E., Dujardin, P., Masseyeff, R. (1977) :
Biomed., 27, 1977.
(14) Durie, B., Salmon, S. (1975) :
Cancer, 36, 842.
(15) Nilsson, K., Evrin, P., Welsh, K. (1974) :
Transplant. Rev., 21, 53.
(16) Delmont, J., Kermarec, J., Lafon, J., Bonet, C., Cassuto, J.P., Masseyeff, R. (1974):
Digestion, 10, 29.

(17) Krebs, B.P., Turchi, B., Bonet, C., Schneider, M.,
     Lalane, C.M., Namer, M. (1977) :
     Europ. J. Cancer, 13, 375.
(18) Dujardin, P., Schneider, M., Cassuto, J.P., Joyner,
     M., Ziegler, G., Audoly, P. (in press) :
     Europ. J. Cancer,

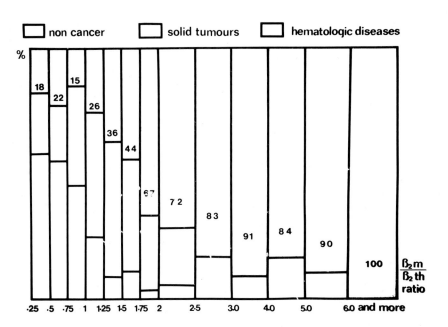

Fig. 1 Increasing percentage of haematological malignancy with the degree of elevation of the M ratio.
                                         Th

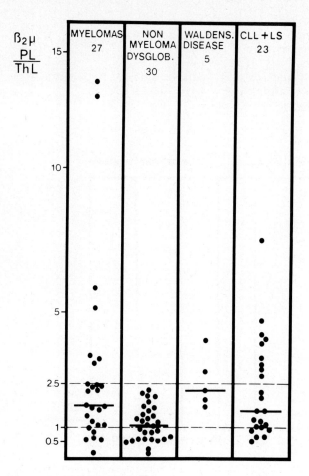

Fig. 2 Observed $\frac{M}{Th}$ ratios in the different lymphoproliferative disorders.

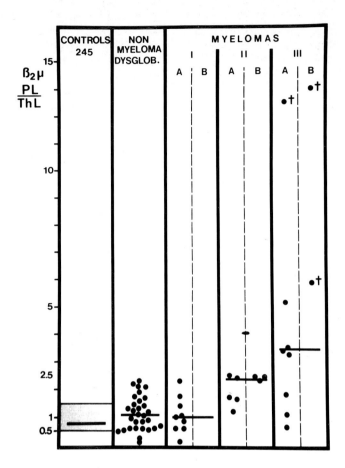

Fig. 3 Correlation between $\dfrac{M}{Th}$ ratios and myeloma staging.

DISCUSSION

KADOUCHE J. (Paris): Is there a relation between blood level of beta2 microglobulin and bone-marrow plasmocytosis cases of myelomas.

CASSUTO J.P. (Nice): There is no relationship between these two parameters because the plasmocytic involvement of bone-marrow is not a good parameter to evaluate the tumour mass in myelomas. The staging from DURIE and SALMON is more accurate and there is a good relation between beta 2 microglobulin and staging.

β_2-MICROGLOBULIN (β_2-MICRO) AND CARCINOEMBRYONIC ANTIGEN (CEA) IN INTESTINAL CANCERS - A CORRELATION WITH STAGE OF DISEASE

A. Daver, J. Wafflart, A. Ben Boueli, J.F. Minier, F. Larra

Laboratoire de Radioimmunologie, Center anticancereux Paul Papin, 2, rue Moll, 49036 Angers, France

and

Bengt Ågerup

Clinical Research, Pharmacia Diagnostics AB, Box 17, 751 03 Uppsala, Sweden.

INTRODUCTION

β_2-microglobulin is a small polypeptide (MW $\simeq$ 12000) present in all body fluids. It is synthesized by all nucleated cells. The function of the protein is as yet unknown but the association with the histocompatibility antigens indicates a role in the mechanisms of cellular immune recognition.

Increasing quantities of β_2-micro in serum have mainly been attributed to impaired renal function, but in recent years much attention has been paid to the high prevalence of elevated serum β_2-micro levels in malignancy.

The purpose of the present study was to investigate if the serum β_2-micro concentration correlates with the stage of intestinal solid tumors. For comparison, an established tumor marker (CEA) was assayed in the same serum samples.

MATERIALS AND METHODS

CEA was assayed by the CEA-IRE-SORIN test where values above 10 ng/ml were considered as pathological. β_2-micro was assayed by the Phadebas β_2-micro Test (Pharmacia Diagnostics AB). Values above 2.4 µg/ml were considered as pathological. Renal function was checked by serum creatinine measurements. Sera with values above 12 mg/l were neglected due to suspicion of renal impairment.

RESULTS

A total of 173 untreated patients were employed in the study. As seen from Fig. 1. the highest values for CEA and β_2-micro were found in colorectal cancers and hepatomas. When analyzing 168 patients with at least two consecutive measurements of CEA and β_2-micro before treatment almost 90 % of them showed increasing values of at least one of the markers as the disease progressed (Fig. 2.). A notable contribution by the β_2-micro assay is evident.

In 31 patients with pancreatic cancer CEA and β_2-micro levels were correlated with stage of disease. The results are shown in Fig. 3. With advancement of disease the proportion of patients with elevated serum levels is increased.

Another correlation with stage of disease was obtained from 60 patients with colorectal cancer. When analyzed according to the TNM

460

system 19 patients had a solid tumor without ganglionary invasion. Of those 47 % and 42 % had elevated levels of β_2-micro and CEA respectively. In 7 patients with solid tumor with ganglionary involvement (N+) 6 and 4 had elevated levels of β_2-micro and CEA respectively. Finally in 34 patients with metastasis (M+) 88 % and 82 % had elevated levels of β_2-micro and CEA respectively.

The degree of extension of solid tumors correlates well with the measured increase in β_2-micro and CEA.

Staging according to Duke was done on 30 patients with colorectal cancer. Two were considered to belong to Group A and had no elevated levels of β_2-micro and CEA. Of 12 patients classified as Dukes B, 2 had elevated β_2-micro levels and one had elevated CEA levels. In Dukes C, 12 and 10 of the 16 patients had elevated β_2-micro and CEA levels respectively.

Benign Diseases

From 38 patients with ethylic cirrhosis or chronic pancreatitis the serum levels of β_2-micro and CEA are presented in Fig. 4. Of the 24 patients with cirrhosis, 20 had elevated CEA levels and 9 had elevated β_2-micro levels. Of 14 patients with chronic pancreatitis 5 had elevated β_2-micro levels whereas 8 had elevated levels of CEA. These findings necessitate further investigation of the influence of benign disease on the levels of β_2-micro and CEA.

Detailed Presentation of Three Patients with Intestinal Cancer

Of the 140 patients studied in the course of disease three typical examples are given.

Patient 1: A.E., 49 years of age, is found to have adenocarcinoma of the pancreas. Upon laparotomy an inextirpatable tumor with local ganglionary invasion is found. No hepatic metastasia is found. Radiotherapy is started. Radiography reveals pulmonary metastasis and shortly thereafter the patient dies of biliary peritonitis (Fig. 5.).

Patient 2: M.A., 76 years of age, was admitted with a local recidive from a tumor in the rectum operated on already 1972. Radiotherapy is started. However, a surgical intervention is carried out due to defect cicatrization and a colostomy is performed. Six months later, a regional metastasis is found in the anal region (Fig. 6.).

Patient 3: S.B., 44 years of age, is found to have an adenocarcinoma in the anal region of the rectum. Successful curietherapy (Ir^{192}) causes resorption of the tumor. Three months later a local recidive is found which is treated surgically (Fig. 7.).

SUMMARY

It has been shown that β_2-micro and CEA are both closely related to tumor growth. The evidences given are firstly that almost 90 % of the cases studied were associated with an increase in at least one of the two markers as the disease progressed. Secondly, colorectal as well as pancreatic cancers had increasing incidences of elevated β_2-micro and CEA values with advances in the stage of disease. Thirdly, in a significant number of patients the serum levels of markers responded adequately to the clinical evolution of disease when studied longitudinally.

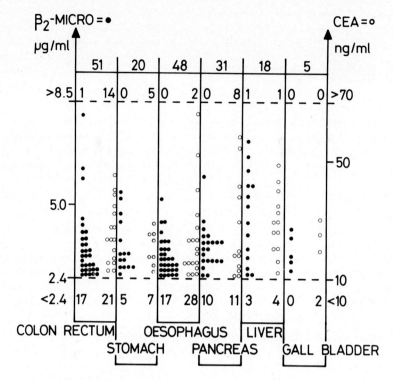

Fig. 1.: The concentration of β_2-micro (o) (left) and CEA (o) (right). The figures indicate from the top to the bottom - total number of patients; number of patients with values above 8.5 µg/ml and 70 ng/ml; number of patients with values below 2.4 µg/ml and 10 ng/ml.

THE PERCENTAGE OF CANCER PATIENTS WITH RISING CEA AND β_2-MICRO VALUES BEFORE TREATMENT

LOCALIZATION	COLON	RECTUM	OESOPHAGUS	STOMACH	PANCREAS	LIVER
NO OF PATIENTS	9	42	45	23	31	18
% CEA	78	60	40	61	71	78
% β_2-MICRO	78	67	60	78	71	78
% COMBINED	89	88	82	86	87	95

Fig. 2

THE RATIO OF ELEVATED LEVELS OF CEA AND β_2-MICRO
AT DIFFERENT STAGES[X] OF PANCREATIC CANCER

	STAGE			
	I	II	III	IV
CEA	1/2	3/4	3/6	15/17
β_2-MICRO	0/2	1/4	4/6	14/17

[X] STAGING ACCORDING TO HERMRECK, THOMAS AND FRIESEN

Fig. 3

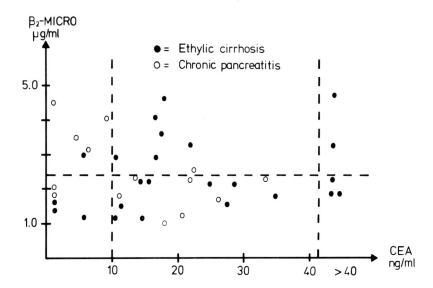

Fig. 4.: β_2-micro and CEA in benign diseases.

463

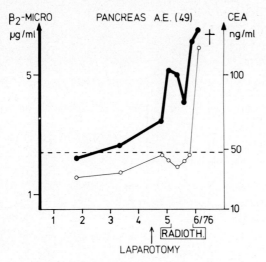

Fig. 5.: A longitudinal study on a patient with adenocarcinoma of the pancreas. Thick line indicates β_2-micro and thin line CEA.

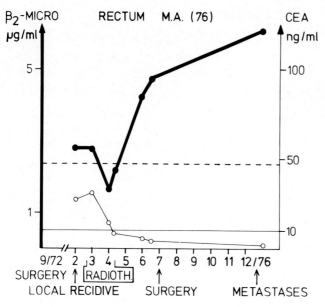

Fig. 6.: A longitudinal study on a patient with rectal cancer. Thick line indicates β_2-micro and thin line CEA.

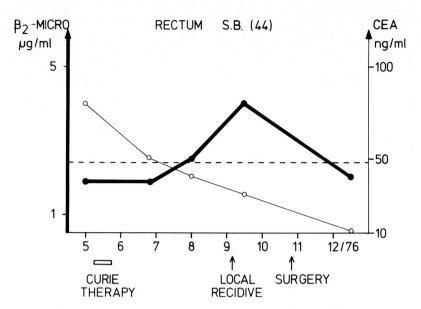

Fig. 7.: A longitudinal study on a patient with adenocarcinoma of the rectum.   Thick line indicates β_2-micro and thin line CEA.

CORRELATION BETWEEN THE SERUM VALUE OF β_2-MICROGLOBULIN AND CARCINOEMBRYONIC ANTIGEN IN PULMONARY DISEASES

J.P. Kleisbauer[+], R. Poirier[+], F. Roux[++], R. Sauvan[++], G. Baldocchi[+], J.P. Bisset[++]

+ Pneumology Department, Pr P. Laval, Michel Levy Hospital, Marseilles , France

++ Nuclear Medicine, Pr H. Roux, C.H.U. Timone, Marseilles France

Human β_2-microglobulin (β_2-m), isolated and characterized by Beggard (1), is a low molecular weight protein (m.w. = 11,800) producted by lymphocytes ; this protein of which the function is unknown is one of the two HLA polypeptide chains ; it is linked on the cell surface.

At first, β_2-m was used to study the renal function (2), then in immunology and in cancerology (3),(4),(5).

The object of this investigation was to study the serum β_2-m levels in healthy subjects and patients hospitalised in a Department of Pneumology and to compare them to the serum CEA values.

PATIENTS AND METHODS

The reagents for β_2-m assays used in this study were prepared by Phadebas.

The serum β_2-m and CEA levels were performed in 3 groups of subjects without renal disease : healthy subjects patients with benign pulmonary disease, patients with bronchogenic carcinoma.

RESULTS

Healthy subjects,from 20 to 60 years old, had the results shown in Table 1.

TABLE 1   Control

	number of subjects n	mean value	limits	units
β_2-m	29	1.3	1-2.4	mg/l
CEA	49	2.9	0-17	ng/ml

Our normal mean value of β_2-m is 1.3 mg/l with limits 1-2.4 mg/l ; these values are similar to normal mean values recently reported (3),(4),(5).

Tuberculosis : 3 series according to treatment were investigated : before, during and after (Table 2).

TABLE 2 β_2-m in tuberculosis (mg/l)

Antituberculous treatment	n	mean value	limits
During	76	1.9	1.0-3.0
Before	15	2.8	1.3-5.5
After	10	2.6	1.3-4.4
	101	2.1	1.0-5.5

These data indicated that β_2-m mean values and limits are greater in tuberculous patients than in healthy subjects.

Figure 1 shows that the minimum β_2-m level of discrimination between tubercular patients and patients with malignant disease should be 2.8 mg/l if we consider only chronic tuberculosis (A) and 3.2 mg/l if we consider the group of tuberculous patients (B).

In Table 3, we studied the correlation between CEA and β_2-m levels in the group of tuberculous patients.

TABLE 3   Number of tuberculous patients with different β_2-m and CEA levels

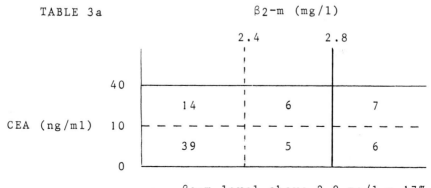

TABLE 3a

β_2-m level above 2.8 mg/l = 17%

467

TABLE 3b

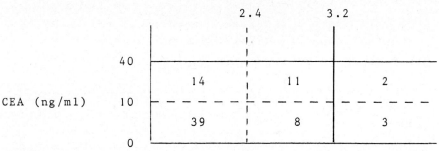

β_2-m level above 3.2 mg/l = 6 %

83 % of tuberculous patients have a β_2-m level below 2.8 mg/l (Table 3a), 94 % have a β_2-m level below 3.2 mg/l; this account four our choice of 3.2 mg/l as the point of discrimination.
In a precedent publication (6) we had proposed 40 ng/ml for CEA level of discrimination between malignant and non malignant pulmonary disease.

Lung carcinoma : in Figure 2 and Table 4 we showed there was no correlation between high CEA value (11 % of subjects) and high β_2-m value (28 % of subjects).

TABLE 4 Correlation between CEA and β_2-m levels in patients with bronchogenic carcinoma

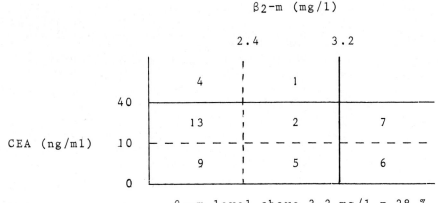

β_2-m level above 3.2 mg/l = 28 %

CEA level above 40 ng/ml = 11 %

CONCLUSIONS

At first sight, it seems that the β_2-m test could be used in the diagnosis of lung carcinoma in 28 % of the cases. However, if we studied patients with acute pulmonary disease, we obtaind the results shown in Table 5.

TABLE 5   Correlation between CEA and β_2-m levels in acute pulmonary disease

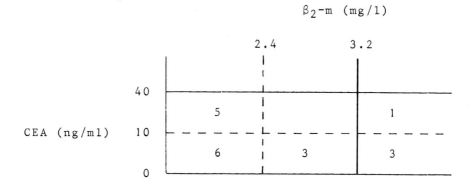

In this case, there were 22 % of high β_2-m value (0 % for CEA). These first results seem to show that the β_2-m assay can't be used for lung carcinoma diagnosis ; concerning the follow-up of the patients with cancer, further prolonged studies are being done ; only this research may permit us to reach definite conclusions.

REFERENCES

(1) Berggard, I. and Bearn, A.G. (1968) : J. Biol. Chem., 243, 4095.
(2) Revillard,J.P. and Vincent, C. (1976) : Nouv. Pres. Med., 5, 2707.
(3) Kindt, T.R. and Van Vaerenbergh, P.M. (1976) : Acta Clin. Belg., 31, 33.
(4) Shuster, J., Gold, P. and Poulik, M.D. (1976) : Clin. Med. Acta, 67, 307.
(5) Evrin, P.E. and Wibell, L.B. (1973) : Clin. Chim. Acta 43, 183.
(6) Poirier, R., Kleisbauer, J.P. and Laval, P. (1976) : Rev. Fr. Mal. Resp., 4, 589.

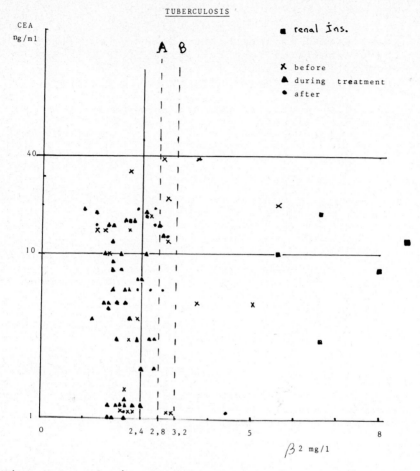

Fig. 1 Correlation between CEA and β_2-m levels in pulmonary disease (β_2-m - linear scale - , CEA - logarithmic scale). A is β_2-m significant limit for chronic tuberculosis, B is β_2-m significant limit for group of tuberculous patients.

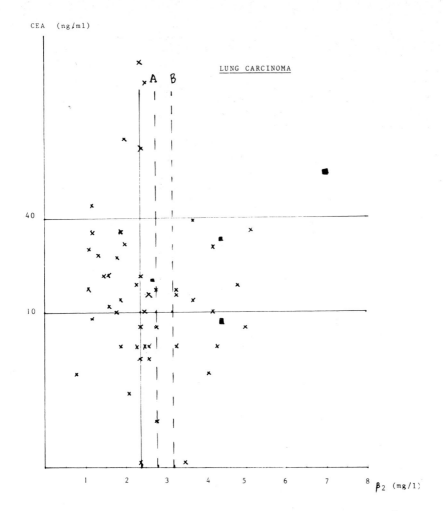

Fig. 2 Correlation between CEA and β_2-m levels in bronchogenic carcinoma.

DISCUSSION

KREBS B.P. (Nice) : A point of clarification. If results of
Beta 2 microglobulin are given as a ratio between actual level of
Beta 2 on theoretical level of Beta 2, calculated according to the
creatininemia, it is possible to take care of results obtained in
patients with nephrotic complications.

THE VALUE OF QUANTITATIVE DETERMINATION OF β_2-MICROGLOBULIN IN MAMMARY CANCER

C. Pourny, J.C. Jardillier, G. Deltour, P. Coninx and A. Cattan

Institut Jean-Godinot, Reims Cedex, France

β_2-Microglobulin was discovered in 1968 in the urine of patients suffering from tubulopathy. In 1972 the complete determination of the sequence of the 100 amino acids of which it consists was published (Peterson et al., 1972), and two different teams were able to demonstrate that this is related very closely to a fragment of the IgG globulins (Peterson et al., 1972; Smithies and Poulik, 1972). It is also a fragment of the HL-A antigen, a fact that was confirmed with almost complete certainty in 1974 (Peterson et al., 1974; Nakamuro et al., 1973; Creswell et al., 1974; Peterson et al., 1975).

Accordingly, in all probability β_2-microglobulin is a polypeptide with a molecular weight around 12,000 (Berggard and Peterson, 1969). Its level in the blood of normal subjects amounts to 1.7 ± 0.5 μg/ml. This level rises with advancing age and high concentrations have been encountered in cancer patients, in patients with renal failure or inflammatory syndromes and in patients with a protracted or otherwise abnormal immune response (Evrin and Wibell, 1972).

The purpose of the present study was to assess the value of the quantitative determination of β_2-microglobulin in patients with breast cancer from the point of view not of diagnosis but rather of detection of residual malignancy and of monitoring therapy, and to compare it in this sense with other markers.

MATERIAL AND METHODS

Fifty-three patients with mammary cancer were examined (Table 1): 20 of them were in a state of seemingly complete remission, and these varied in age between 31 and 72 years (median age 58 years); the 33 others, aged from 27 to 74 years (median age 56 years) were in a phase of demonstrable disease. Of the latter group 8 had liver metastases, 3 had bone metastases and 12 had both liver and bone metastases, all of them confirmed, while 10 showed only local recurrence, skin, lung or lymphnode metastases (Table 2).

Table 1. Cancer of the breast

Patients tested	53
Demonstrable disease	33
Complete remission	20
Total	53

Table 2. Patients with demonstrable disease: main localizations

Metastases	Number of patients
Liver	8
Bone	3
Liver + bone	12
Miscellaneous	10
Total	33

Throughout the period of observation all the patients were subjected to chemotherapy, as an adjuvant or for 'curative' purposes.

All patients were subjected to the simultaneous quantitative determination of β2-microglobulin, α-foetoprotein, carcino-embryonic antigen (CEA) phospho-hexose isomerase and alkaline phosphatase; these determinations were repeated at intervals to (4 to 6 weeks)

Serum was used for the determinations. The β2-microglobulin was determined by a solid-phase radio-immunological assay method using an anti-β2-micro-globulin bound to Sephadex * particles; with this method, normal levels are less than or equal to 2.5 μg/ml^{-1} (mean 1.7 μg; S.D. 0.5).

The alpha-foetoprotein was determined by a method of precipitating the antigen-antibody phase with poly-ethylene glycol **. The initial technique was modified so as to obtain a range from 0 to 544 mg/ml^{-1} by dilution of the antibody and of the alpha-foetoprotein: 95% of normal values lie between 0 and 10 ng.ml^{-1} (mean 3.2; S.D. 0.8).

The CEA was determined by a radio-immunological assay method rendered more sensitive by the sequential addition of a second antibody in the solid phase ***: by this technique, 98% of normal subjects show values of 10 ng.ml^{-1}.

* Société Phadebas; ** Ria Gnost alpha-foetoprotein, Behringwerke; *** Kit CEA-K from CIS

In women, an occasional concentration between 10 and 25 ng may be observed.

Phosphohexose isomerase (PHI) was determined in serum by the technique of Bueding-Mac Kinnon (1955) [*] : normal values amount to 53 ± 24 mU/ml.

Alkaline phosphatase was determined by the optimized technique at 25° [**] , with which the normal levels range from 60 to 170 mU/ml. Table 3 lists the values which we have considered as normal, pathological or doubtful.

Table 3. Levels of markers observed, classified as normal, doubtful (intermediate) or clearly pathological

	Normal	Intermediate	Pathological
β_2M (μg.ml^{-1})	2.5	2.6 - 3	3
CEA (ng.ml^{-1})	10	11 - 20	20
αFP (ng.ml^{-1})	10	11 - 20	20
PHI (mU.ml^{-1})	100	101 -150	150
Alkaline phosph. (mU.opt.ml^{-1})	170	171 -250	250

RESULTS

Examination of the results from the 80 determinations carried out in patients in complete remission showed that 16 of them were clearly pathological for β2-microglobulin as against 5 for PHI and 3 for alkaline phosphatase (Table 4)

In the patients with demonstrable malignancy, β2-microglobulin and alkaline phosphatase appear to be the two most sensitive indicators of the presence of bone metastases (Table 5) and at least equally sensitive for the presence of liver metastases for which, however, PHI may be regarded as equally useful (Table 7).

---

[*] Kit Behringwerke Labs
[**] Boehringer reagent

Table 4. Patients in complete remission

80 tests	20 Patients		
	Normal	Intermediate	Pathological
β_2M	51	13	16
CEA	78	2	0
αFP	78	2	0
PHI *	66	6	5
Alk.phosph.**	57	18	3

* 3 tests not performed
** 2 tests not performed

Table 5. Patients with bone metastases with or without other localizations but free from liver metastases

48 tests	12 Patients		
	Normal	Intermediate	Pathological
β_2M	21	10	17
CEA	38	2	8
αFP	45	3	0
PHI *	30	6	7
Alk.phosph. **	12	12	21

* 5 tests not performed
** 3 tests not performed

Table 6. Patients with liver metastases with or without other localizations but free from bone metastases.

12 tests	3 Patients		
	Normal	Intermediate	Pathological
β_2M	4	5	3
CEA	7	1	4
αFP	12	0	0
PHI *	1	3	7
Alk.phosph.	3	4	5

* 1 test not performed

Table 7. Patients with bone and liver metastases
(with or without other localizations)

32 tests	8 Patients		
	Normal	Intermediate	Pathological
$_2$M	7	9	16
CEA	11	5	16
XFP	32	0	0
PHI$^+$	18	5	6*
Alk.phosph.	7	5	20

* 3 tests not performed.

To conclude, in patients without either liver or
bone metastases, β2-microglobulin is pathological in
1 out of 2 cases; in these cases it is the only marker
of real value (Table 8).

Table 9 contains the comparison of the marker levels
in complete remission cases and in demonstrable disease
cases and suggests that, taking the numbers of tests
performed into account, β2-microglobulin, CEA and alkaline phosphatase are the most interesting markers.

Evaluation of the markers in pairs brings to light
a significant correlation between β2-microglobulin and
CEA on the one hand and between alkaline phosphatase
and PHI on the other (Table 10). Finally, it is only
the variations in the levels of β2-microglobulin and of
alkaline phosphatase, which are correlated with the
extent of clinically demonstrable malignancy (Table 11).

Table 8. Patients with metastases not localized in
either liver or bone

40 tests	10 Patients		
	Normal	Intermediate	Pathological
β_2M	16	6	18
CEA	31	5	4
αFP	30	9	1
PHI *	33	4	2
Alk. phosph.	27	9	4

* 1 test not performed

Table 9. Comparison of marker levels in patients in complete remission (CR) and with demonstrable disease (DD)

	CR	DD	Statistical significance
β_2M	2.53 ± 0.55	3.05 ± 0.73	$p < 0.01$
CEA	5.44 ± 1.33	84.08 ± 286.93	$p < 0.001$
αFP	5.64 ± 0.88	6.60 ± 2.60	NS
Alk. phosph.	147.17 ± 40.21	241.78 ± 113.89	$p < 0.001$
PHI	75.08 ± 25.57	113.98 ± 108.81	NS

mean ± 2 S.D.

Table 10. Correlations between the levels of the various markers in patients with demonstrable disease (calculated on the basis of the absolute values of the markers)

	β_2M	CEA	αFP	PHI	Alk.phosph.
β_2M	1	0.37 *	0.11	0.06	0.15
CEA		1	-0.04	0.02	0.01
αFP			1	-0.23	-0.25
PHI				1	0.48 **
Alk.phosph.					1

* $0.02 < p < 0.05$
** $p < 0.01$

Table 11. Correlation between the variations of the clinical condition and the variations of marker levels

	β_2M	CEA	αFP	PHI	Alk.phosph.
clinical condition	0.38 *	0.22	-0.09	0.21	0.35 *

* $p < 0.05$

DISCUSSION

We may conclude from this investigation that quantitative determination of β2-microglobulin is of definite interest not as a diagnostic element but as an aid in the follow-up of patients with cancer of the breast: of the 4 markers studied it is the only one that is really changed in patients with demonstrable disease but free from liver and bone metastases.

Conversely, its level is too frequently abnormal in the absence of demonstrable disease. In this respect, however, it may be argued that alterations of other markers often precede clinical demonstrability of the disease by several months, so that the numer of 'false-positives' may well decrease in the course of a longer follow-up. β2-microglobulin shows no correlation with the serum alkaline phosphatase level which is an excellent indicator of liver or bone metastasization. Consequently, systematic determination of both these parameters seems a reasonable proposal. To the extent CEA is indeed secreted by the tumor cell itself (referring to CEA-producing cells), CEA is theoretically a better indicator of tumor size than β2-microglobulin, but only in those cases in which its level is altered and this level is, in any case, correlated with that of β2-microglobulin, so that, as matters stand at present, the respective roles of these two markers in the follow-up of breastcancer patients cannot be defined. The value of PHI (Leroux et al., 1976; Pourny et al., 1977) on the other hand, has not been confirmed by the present investigation.

CONCLUSION

In 53 patients with mammary cancer, β2-microglobulin was determined quantitatively together with 4 other markers, and these determinations were repeated at regular intervals. At present it looks as if β2-microglobulin fulfils most of the requirements of a good marker and deserves a place in the standard follow-up of women with cancer of the breast.

REFERENCES

Berggard, I. and Peterson, P.A. (1969): J. Biol. Chem., 244, 4299.

Bueding,E. and Mackinnon, J. (1955) : J. Biol. Chem., 215, 507.

Cresswell, P., Springer, T., Strominger, J.L. et al. (1974): Proc. nat. Acad. Sci. (Wash.), 71, 2123.

Evrin, P.E. and Wibell, L. (1972): Scand. J. Clin. lab. Invest., 29, 69.

Leroux, D., Pourny, C. and Jardillier, J.C. (1976) : Paper presented at the 2nd European Congress on Clinical Chemistry, Prague 3-10 October 1976.

Nakamuro, K., Tamgaki, N. and Pressman, D. (1973) : Proc. nat. Acad. Sci. (Wash.), 70, 2863.

Peterson, P.A., Cunningham, B.A. and Berggard, I. (1972) :
Proc. nat. Acad. Sci. (Wash), 69, 1697.

Peterson, P.A., Rask, L. and Lindblom, J.B. (1974):
Proc. nat. Acad. Sci. (Wash.), 71, 35.

Peterson, P.A., Rask, L. and Sege, K. (1975) :
Proc. nat. Acad. Sci. (Wash.), 72, 1612.

Pourny, C., Cattan, A., Coninx, P., Deltour, G.,
Jardillier, J.C. and Leroux, D. (1977) : Paper presented
at Journées dakaroises de Cancérologie, Dakar, 28,29,30
march 1977.

Smithies, O. and Poulik, M.D. (1972) : Science, 175, 187.

CEA AND β^2MICROGLOBULIN ASSAYS IN 263 BREAST CANCER PATIENTS

A.F.Bertrand, A.Daver, F.Larra, C.Chapoy, C.Deroche, J.Wafflart

Centre Anticancéreux, Angers, France

I - CEA AND BREAST CANCER

The carcino-embryonic antigen (CEA) discovered by GOLD and FREED MAN in 1965, was isolated from sera from patients with cancers of various types, but more particularly those of the breast (LOGERFO, PUSZ TASZERI, MACH).Since 1975, we have assayed this antigen in breast cancer patients according to the technique established by the French Atomic Energy Commission. We consider concentrations of 10 ng/ml and above to be pathological.

A) - CEA titers as criteria in diagnosis

In 51 cases, the concentration of CEA was measured before treatment (table 1). It is clear that the titer cannot be used as a cancer detection test since 34 patients out of 51 show CEA concentrations within normal limits.

TABLE 1   CEA titers before treatment : 51 cases

	Number of cases	Meta +	Meta −
CEA −	34	2	32
CEA +	17	6	11

B) - CEA titers in pre-treatment evaluation

1. Table 2 shows the absence of any relationship between tumor size and CEA titers.

TABLE 2   Tumor size and pre-treatment CEA titers : 51 cases

	T1 - T2	T3 - T4	Bilateral
CEA −	19	14	1
CEA +	8	9	

2. In 36 cases, with histological control after ganglion cleansing, a significant relationship is found between CEA titers before treatment and ganglion involvement even single ganglion involvement in phase Mo patients. Table 3 shows 10 cases N+ as against 2 cases N- with high CEA titers. This does not concord with the general view in current literature but the discrepancy may be due to the fact that our reference threshold level is 10 ng/ml rather than 15 ng/ml used by other authors.

TABLE 3   Ganglion infection and CEA titers before treatment: 36 cases

	N −	N +
CEA −	14	10
CEA +	2	10

3. In the case of extra-ganglionic metastases, the CEA **+**
titer is even higher as seen in Table 1 : increased CEA concentrations
in 6 patients out of 8.

C) CEA titers in prognostic evaluation

A high CEA titer is thus an important element in determining
the prognosis. Table 4 analyses CEA curves plotted for patients at the
beginning of treatment.

TABLE 4 CEA curves in prognosis evaluation : 92 cases

92	28 CEA **+**	11 metastases.
		13 curves return to normal after initial treatment.
		4 (cirrhosis, causes unknown).
	64 CEA **–**	8 **+** 5 metastases / 3 without metastases
		56 **–** 53 without metastases / 3 metastases

Out of 92 patients, 19 showed metastases : 16 of these cases
had CEA **+**titers, 11 right from the start and 5 secondarily; while the
remaining 3 cases showed negative CEA values.

A high CEA titer right from the beginning suggests an eventual
metastasis with a probability of about 40%. A CEA titer lower than nor
mal brings this probability down to about 12,5%.

D) CEA titers in patient follow-up

CEA titers and curves are very useful in patient follow-up.
CEA curves plotted for 263 patients. Table 5 shows good agreement between high CEA titers in 66 cases, out of 86 with metastases. The 13
patients with high CEA titers but without metastases are under close
observation since it was noticed that the increase of CEA could precede the appearance of metastase by 1 - 6 months.

TABLE 5 CEA titers and patient follow-up : 263 cases.

	Number of cases	CEA –	CEA +
Metastases –	177	164	13
Metastases +	86	20	66
Total ...	263	184	79

Moreover, CEA titers vary with the location of metastases as
shown in Table 6.

TABLE 6 CEA titers and location of metastases : 88 cases.

Location	Number of cases	CEA +	Mean CEA titer ng/ml	CEA –
Liver	21	20	377	1
Brain	8	8	122	0
Bone	45	35	81	10
Lung	14	12	35	2

- patients with hepatic metastase show the highest CEA titers,
the maximum being 1800 ng/ml.

- pleural metastases are associated with the lowest CEA titers
and the curves are generally flat.

- bone metastases are found to have the highest number of CEA –
values. In the case of single bone metastasis, CEA titers are low at
about 20 ng/ml.

Another advantage of the CEA titer is the possibility evaluating

the effectiveness of the treatment after radiotherapy or surgery :in
13 cases, high initial CEA titers were seen to normalize with cure.
Besides, CEA **+** variation curves were plotted for 55 patients with metastases under radiotherapy or chemotherapy. In 51 of these cases, a
good agreement was found between the CEA curves and the clinical state
of the patient as illustrated in Table 8.

TABLE 8 :

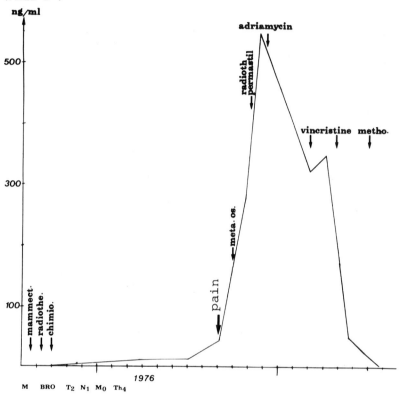

II - COMPARISON OF β^2MICROGLOBULIN TITERS WITH CEA TITERS.

An attempt was made to compare CEA titers with another biological
marker β^2microglobulin, the normal concentration of which is inferior
to 2,4 ng/ml. Patients with high creatininemia were not included in
this comparison.

A) Diagnostical value.

Table 9 shows that before treatment β^2microglobulin alone is
positive in 5 cases while CEA alone is positive in 7 cases.

TABLE 9 Pre-treatment titers : β^2microglobulin and CEA

β^2 \ CEA	+	−
+	0	5
−	7	13

B) Pre-treatment evaluation.
1. The examination of 25 patients before treatment suggests some relationship between tumor size and one or the other of the two markers.

TABLE 10 Relation between tumor size and β^2 or CEA titers.

	T1 - T2 (15 cases)		T3 - T4 (10 cases)	
β^2 \ CEA	+	−	+	−
+	0	3	0	2
−	5	7	2	6

2. 22 of the 25 cases above had undergone ganglion cleansing. No significant relationship could be established between ganglion involvement and the two biological markers, the number of case being too low : Table 11.

TABLE 11 : Relation between ganglion involvement and β^2 oder CEA titers

	N − (11 cases)		N + (11 cases)	
β^2 \ CEA	+	−	+	−
+	0	2	0	1
−	3	6	4	6

C) Post-treatment follow-up.
Table 12 shows that in cases with extra-ganglionic metastases the β^2microglobulin tiers by itself is positive in 3 patients. The association of the two markers, β^2microglobulin and CEA allows a biological diagnosis in 15 out of 16 cases a considerable gain over the results obtained by using the CEA titer on its own.

TABLE 12 Relationship between extraganglionic metastases and β^2microglobulin and CEA titers : 16 cases

β^2 \ CEA	+	−
+	10	3
−	2	1

β^2microglobulin and CEA curves were plotted in 62 cases of which 16 were in phase M+

TABLE 13 β^2microglobulin and CEA curves : 62 cases

CEA − β^2− 28 cases	CEA + β^2 − 3 cases	CEA − β^2 + 17 cases	CEA + β^2 + 14 cases
1 M + 27 M −	2 M + 1 M −	3 M + 14 M −	10 M + 1 R 3 M −

β^2 \ CEA	+	−
+	14	17
−	3	28

In the 28 CEA $- \beta^2 -$ cases and in the 14 CEA $+ \beta^2 +$ cases, that is, in 42 out of 62 cases the CEA and the β^2microglobulin curves run parallel. Table 13 shows that β^2microglobulin titers are more often positive than CEA titers, the highest positive titer being found in the CEA $- \beta^2 +$ group : out of 17 patients only 3 had metastases. We have considered the possible influence of chemotherapy but as seen in Table 14, 10 patients out of 17 underwent no chemotherapy :

TABLE 14 : Chemotherapy and β^2microglobulin titers in 17 CEA $- \beta^2 +$ cases.

3 cases M +	= 2 under chemotherapy	
14 cases M −	= 8 under chemotherapy	{ β^2 increased in 4 cases before treatment and in 4 cases after treatment.
	= 6 whitout chemotherapy.	

However, we do not yet have sufficient experience to evaluate the eventual prognosis of an abnormal increase in β^2microglobulin titers. Table 15 illustrates the good agreement between CEA titers and β^2microglobulin titers.

TABLE 15

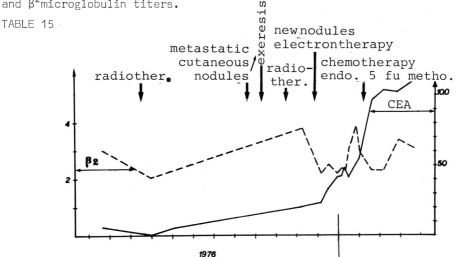

CONCLUSION -

We consider CEA assays of great value in prognosis evaluation in the following-up of initial treatment and in chemotherapy after the appearance of metastases. The addition of a second biological marker β^2microglobulin, improves biological diagnosis by about 20%. The two titers are not exactly superposable, hence the usefulness of their association. However, we cannot yet satisfactorily evaluate the prognosis of high β^2microglobulin titers for lack of adequate experience. The preliminary results reported above encourage further work in the same direction so as to obtain statistical significant information on a greater number of cases.

REFERENCES

(1) Borthwick N.M., Wilson D.W., Bell P.A.(1977) : Europ. J.Cancer
    Vol.13, 171 - 176.
(2) Daver A., Wafflart J., Ben Bouali A., Minier J.F., Larra F.
    (1977 = à paraître) : Europ J.Cancer.
(3) Tormey D., Waalkes P., Ahmann D., Gehrke Ch., Zunwatt R.,
    Smyder J., Hansen H.: Cancer, 35, 1095 - 1100.(1975).
(4) Steward A.M., Nixon D.W., Zamcheck N. et al. (1974) : Cancer 33,
    1246 - 1252.

COMPARISON OF THE VARIATIONS IN THE LEVELS OF BETA 2 MICROGLOBULIN AND CARCINOEMBRYONIC ANTIGEN IN CANCER OF THE BREAST AND MALIGNANT MELANOMA

J.Grenier, B.Serrou, P.Suquet, H.Pujol

Centre Paul Lamarque, 34059 Montpellier Cedex, France.

ABSTRACT

A variety of markers have been used in the surveillance of carcinoma of the breast and malignant melanoma, e.g. carcinoembryonic antigen, Beta 2 microglobulin and prolactin. These markers have been studied for two reasons : first, to investigate indicators of eventual relapse or metastatic evolution in the cancer patient and secondly as a therapeutic monitor . 92% of the breast cancer subjects demonstrating bone metastases had an elevated CEA or Beta 2 microglobulin. Two-third of the malignant melanoma patients in relapse had an elevated Beta 2 microglobulin level .

INTRODUCTION

In recent years, the strategy in treatment of the cancer patient has turned from a local focus to the additional consideration of post-therapeutic monitoring of the more hidden aspects of a remaining disease. Most often, biological markers play a part in the more recent approach. In the present study we have made a comparison between the variations in the levels of Beta 2 microglobulin, carcinoembryonic antigen and prolactin in breast cancer and malignant melanoma patients. Beta 2 microglobulin (M.V.11,800) was first isolated in 1968 by Beggard and Bearn. Its structure resembles that of the immunoglobulins and is associated with histo-comatibility antigens found on the surface of most cells. In 1973, Evrinaud Wibell reported elevated Beta 2 microglobulin levels in patients with malignancies. In 1974, Poulik et al. found elevated Beta 2 microglobulin levels in 45% of the advanced cancers studied.

MATERIAL AND METHODS

Our present study involves 51 breast cancer patients (37 of which had bone metastases) and 47 malignant melanoma patients.
CEA was measured by the "Commissariat à l'Energie Atomique" technique (M= 10 ng/ml) while the Beta 2 microglobulin was analysed by the Phadebas microtest method (M= 2,4 ug/ml).

487

RESULTS

I- Breast cancer patients

We have compared the variation over time of markers with the clinical evaluation, radiographies and osteo-scintigraphies.

a) CEA levels
81% of the patients with bone metastases demonstrated elevated CEA levels; 84% with normal CEA levels showed no evidence of bone metastases , 16% of the patients had normal CEA levels in spite of bone metastases.

b) Beta 2 microglolubin levels
55% with an elevated beta 2 microglobulin presented bone metastases; 78% with normal beta 2 microglobulin showed no evidence of bone metastases . 22% of the patients with normal beta 2 microglobulin levels demonstrated bone metastases.

c) Rise in marker levels in relation to the appearance of metastases

1- 63% of the patients studied showed an elevated CEA prior to diagnosis of bone metastses.

2- 32% presented elevated beta 2 microglobulin values prior to bone metastases.

II- Malignant melanoma

Two groups of patients were studied : patients in relapse and those showing no indication of relapse.

a) Beta 2 microglobulin levels
61% of the patients with an elevated Beta 2 microglobulin levels suffered a relapse , 95% of the patients studied who had normal Beta 2 microglobulin levels demonstrated no relapse.

b) Prolactin levels
5 out of the 6 patients with elevated prolactin levels suffered a relapse.

c) CEA levels
Only 1 patient out of 47 demonstrated a high CEA.

d) Rise in marker levels prior to relapse
In 64% of the cases studied, Beta 2 microglobulin levels rose prior to relapse.

DISCUSSION

92% of breast cancer patients with bone metastases had an elevated CEA or Beta 2 microglobulin level. In 2/3 of CEA and 1/3 of the Beta 2 microglobulin analyses, these markers rose prior to the appearance of bone metastases. 2/3 of the relapse patients with malignant melanoma had an elevated Beta 2 microglobulin; 1/3 showing no present relapse have an elevated Beta 2 microglobulin. Elevation of the Beta 2 microglobulin prior to all indications of relapse occurec in 64% of the patients studied. An increased prolactin level is associated with poor prognosis. In two cases we are presently following the variation in marker levels as a function of therapeutic efficacity.

REFERENCES

(1) Berggard, Bearn,H.G. (1968): J.Biol.Chem. 243, 4095.

(2) Evrin,P.E., Wibell,L. (1973): Clin.Chim.Acta 43, 183.

(3) Poulik,M.D.et al(1974): Clin. Chim.Acta 52, 293.

(4) Shuster,J., Gold,P., Poulik,M.D. (1976): Clin. Chim.Acta,67,307.

CARCINOEMBRYONIC ANTIGEN IN UTERINE CANCERS: EVALUATION OF
247 CASES. A COMPARISON WITH β^2 MICROGLOBULIN

F.Larra, A.Daver, C.Deroche, C.Mittler
Centre Paul Papin, Angers, France

This study analyses the results of 719 carcinoembryonic antigen
assays on 247 cases of uterine cancer and reports preliminary work
suggesting the usefulness of associating β microglobulin as a second
biological marker for improved diagnosis.

CARCINOEMBRYONIC ANTIGENS AND UTERINE CANCERS

A) Clinical material

I- Methods.

The radioimmunoassays of CEA were realized by the double antibody method, according to the technique established by the French
Atomic Energy Commission. A level is considered to be normal when it
is less than 10 ng/ml.

II- Cancers of the cervix.

187 patients with uterine neoplasms became the object of 558
assays performed before, or after treatment. The stage-wise distribution was as follows : 55 stage 1, 105 stage 2, 21 stage 3, 6 stage 4
histologically, the neoplasms were all of the squamous-cell carcinoma
type, with the exception of 5 adenocarcinomas.

III- Cancers of the uterine body.

In this regard, our study is smaller : 60 patients, 167 assays;
the distribution includes 44 T1, 8 T2, 4 T3 and 4 vaginal metastases;
the histological diagnosis is that of adenocarcinoma in 58 of the
cases, sarcome in one case, and anaplasia in one case.

B) Diagnostic worth of carcinoembryonic antigens

I- Cancers of the cervix.

70 patients with cancers of the cervix were the object of one
or several assays before treatment (112 assays in total); only 31
cases showed positive CEA levels before the institution of treatment;
the test was deficient in 39 cases.

II- Cancers of the uterine body.

44 assays were performed on 19 patients prior to therapy; only
6 out of 19 patients exhibited positive levels.

III- It follows that :

CEA level is an unreliable test in diagnosis of the primary tumour; this concept is but a further confirmation of data which are now classic.

C) CEA in the evaluation of tumoral expansion

I- CEA and extent of primary tumour.

a) Cancer of the cervix : statistical analysis reveals no significant relation between the stage of disease and CEA results (Table 1)

Table 1

Stages	Cases	Positive levels	Negative levels	Mean levels
St. 1	10	3	7	7,7 ng/ml
St. 2	42	21	21	18,24ng/ml
St. 3	13	6	7	24,85ng/ml
St. 4	5	1	4	10,40ng/ml
	70	31	39	

b) Cancer of the uterine body : there exists no correlation between CEA and extent of the tumour (Table 2)

Table 2

Stages	Cases	Positive levels	Negative levels
T1	9	3	6
T2	4	1	3
T3	2	2	0
Vag. Met.	4	0	4
	19	6	13

II- CEA and lymph node involvement (Table 3)

Table 3

	Cases	Positive levels	Negative levels	Mean levels
No	31	11	20	13,7 ng/ml
N+	11	7	4	20,1 ng/ml
Nx	10	4	6	19,0 ng/ml
	52	22	30	

Lymph node involvement in cervical cancers was determined by histological examination performed after lymphadenectomy, with the exception of those cases classified as Nx, which correspond to patients who did not undergo an operation and for whom, therefore, a histological verification was impossible.

The Table 3 quantifies the observed results : there exists no significant link between lymph node involvement and CEA levels.

D) Value of carcinoembryonic antigens in post-therapeutic follow-up

I- CEA and follow-up of cervical neoplasms.

168 cancers of the cervix were assayed at regular intervals upon completion of therapy (446 assays).

a) CEA and follow-up of patients without recurrence or metastasis:
at the present time, 149 patients are free of recurrence and metastasis. 94% of the CEA levels are negative, coinciding with the clinical data: only 9 cases (6%) are positive; of these, one patient suffers from ulcerous colitis, a condition which is known to be capable of elevating CEA levels; 4 CEA levels fall into a marginal range of values, between 10 ng/ml and 20 ng/ml, which can be considered as a zone of uncertainty; 4 other CEA levels are positive, with no clinical explanation at the present time; these patients are under close observation.

b) CEA and follow-up of patients with local recurrence :
relapses are rare; our statistics contain only 9 such cases , 2 cases witness an increase in CEA level. The existence of a normal CEA level therefore does not imply the absence of local recurrence.

c) CEA in the follow-up of patients with metastases :
metastases were observed in 9 patients: in 4 cases the CEA level remained negative; 5 metastatic patients exhibited extremely elevated, positive CEA level.

It must be stressed that the recurrence or metastases which manifest positive levels of CEA are the result of primary tumours whose initial CEA levels were positive; those cases of recurrence or metastasis whose CEA levels are negative are the result of primary tumours whose CEA levels were negative before treatment.

The delay from the onset of positive CEA levels during follow-up until the eventual clinical detection of a metastasis or recurrence has been variable; in general, the positive CEA level precedes the clinical manifestation by several months. In one of our cases the delay was 12 months.

d) Follow-up of 31 cancers of the cervix whose CEA levels were elevated before treatment:
27 of the files were usable; the other 4 files include one patient whose whereabouts is unknown and three patients who died while treatment was in progress.

These 27 patients exhibiting an elevated CEA level before treatment underwent regularly repeated CEA assays during the post-therapeutic follow-up; an elevation of CEA levels occured for three of them, coinciding with the clinical data; in these three cases the increased CEA levels corresponded respectively to one bone metastasis, one pulmonary metastasis, and one non-sterilization. For the remaining 24 patients, CEA levels returned to normal after treatment and maintained a normal value throughout follow-up.

When curietherapy was combined with surgery, the return to a normal CEA level was unfailingly observed at the time of the first assay performed one month after the completion of treatment. When the therapy limited itself exclusively to irradiation, the delay requisite to a return to normal CEA values increased in varying degrees, extending to as much as 4 months.

II- CEA and post-therapeutic follow-up of cancers of the uterine body.

117 assays were performed at regular intervals upon 52 patients

a) CEA and follow-up patients without recurrence or metastasis: 42 patients, or 86% of the CEA levels are negative, which means they coincide with the clinical data; it would appear that 7 CEA levels are false positive, but only one exceeds 20ng/ml. These patients are under strict observation.

b) CEA and follow-up of patients with local recurrence : only one patient sustained a local recurrence without an increase in CEA level; it is pertinent to stress that the initial level, before any treatment of the primary lesion, was negative.

c) CEA and follow-up of patients with metastases ; 2 patients sustained metastases; their CEA levels were markedly elevated. The primary neoplasm of these patients had exhibited a positive CEA level.

d) Evolution of 6 cancers of the uterine body, positive before treatment; three of these patients witnessed a return to normal CEA levels; the first, one month after surgery, the other 2 and 3 months after radiotherapy, respectively; 2 patients witnessed an increase in their CEA level: they have obvious metastases; one patient died during the course of treatment.

e) In concluding this study,

1) This study of 719 assays confirms that :
a) CEA assays do not constitute a reliable test in the diagnosis of cancers of the cervix or of the body of uterus, due to the incidence of false negatives.
b) Furthermore, there exists no correlation between CEA levels and either the clinical stage or the extent of lymph node involvement.

2) On the contrary, when the CEA level ascertained before treatment of the primary neoplasm is positive, CEA levels are of great prognostic value during the course of follow-up, due to:
a) the low number of false positive results, probably linked to the fact that one is dealing with a feminine population without the use of alcohol and tobacco.
b) Their unfailing elevation upon inception of a metastasis or recurrence (after prior return to a normal level).
c) The early increase of CEA levels which can precede by several months the clinical manifestation of recurrence or metastasis.

β^2 MICROGLOBULIN AND UTERINE CANCERS

In a complementary and preliminary study of 56 uterine cancers, we sought to determine the worth of a second tumoral marker : β^2m., and to define what interest might exist in combining the CEA assays with those of the β^2m.

A) Clinical material

I- Cancers of the cervix :
Assays of β^2m. were performed on 33 patients with cancer of the cervix. The distribution according to stage was the following : 1 T0, 5 T1, 18 T2, 5 T3, 4 T4.

II- Cancers of the uterine body :
β^2 m. assays were performed on 23 patients; the distribution according to stage is the following : 11 T1, 8 T2, 4 T3.

III- Assay method :
A level less than 2,4 ng/ml is considered normal.

B) Diagnostic value of β^2 microglobulin

I- Cancers of the cervix :
a) 26 cancers before treatment became the object of both a β^2m. assay and a CEA assay.

b) The results obtained were the following : 12/26 exhibited positive β^2m. levels, 9/26 exhibited a positive CEA level. When the 2 assays are jointly considered, it becomes apparent that 16 cancers were positive for at least one of the tests.

c) Although the number of cases is not large, the results suggest that : β^2m. assays by themselves have no value in the diagnosis of cancers of the cervix; an increase in the number of positive levels is obtained when the 2 markers are jointly considered; the increase does not permit once to attribute a diagnostic reliability to this method, for there persists 10 false negative levels among the 26 assays effected.

II- Cancers of the uterine body :
Comparative assays of β^2m. and CEA before treatment were performed on 14 patients with cancer of the uterine body. 8 out of 14 cancers exhibited a positive level of β^2m.; as with the cancers of the cervix this assay therefore does not constitute a reliable diagnostic test.

When one employs both markers, β^2m. and CEA, and if one considers those tumours exhibiting a positive level in at least one of the 2 assays, the number of positive levels rise only to a figure of 10 out of 14 cancers.

C) Value of β^2 microglobulin in evaluation of the extent of the tumour

Despite the limited number of cases, it seems that there exists no correlation between the stage and the incidence of positive levels of β^2 m. Nor is it possible to establish a correlation between the stage and combined β^2 m.-CEA assays.

D) Value of β^2 microglobulin in follow-up

I- Up to now, the number of patients observed and the subsequent lapse of time have been too low to appreciate adequately the worth of β^2 m. in post-therapeutic follow-up.

II- For a certain number of patients, however, the curve noting the evolution of β^2 m. levels was traced concomitantly with the curve of CEA levels.

a) In a certain number of cases, the curves parallel each other and coincide with the clinical data.

b) In another group of patients, the CEA values before treatment are negative; in coinciding with the clinical data the β^2 m. level thus becomes significant.

III- A third category of patients exhibits discordant values in the evolution of 2 assays; insufficient observation time of this group precludes analysis of the discordance.

CONCLUSION

It should be emphasized that, in regard to uterine cancers, the CEA assay has proven its excellent value as a test in follow-up when the CEA level, before treatment of the tumour, was positive.

When the CEA test is negative, are the β^2 m. assays capable of compensating for this deficiency. A greater number of patients under longer observation will answer this question; a complementary study is in progress.

REFERENCES

(1) Haegele, P., Petit, J.C., Eber, M. (1976): Bull.Cancer 63, 515.

(2) Khoo, S.K., McKay, E.V. (1973): Aust.N.Z.Obstet.Gynaec. 13, 1.

(3) Larra, F., Herve, C., Daver, A., Tigori, J. (1976): Bull.Cancer 63, 505.

(4) Seppala, M., Pihko, H., Ruoslahti, E. (   ): Tract Cancer 35, 1377 .

DISCUSSION

MACH J.P. (Lausanne): In some cases of successful chemo or radiotherapy , when there is an important destruction of tumour cells, did you observe an increase in plasma beta 2 microglobulin?

LARRA F. (Angers): Yes, this phenomenon was observed, but our analysis is not yet conclusive.

VIOT G. (Nice): One must say that the renal excretion of beta 2 microglobulin is fast and important, so an increase in the 24 hours urinary eliminations of beta 2 microglobulin will be more interesting for this kind of study.

LALANNE C.M. (Nice): Discrepancies between beta 2 microglobulin and CEA might be an advantage if measured simultaneously, they will enhance the total positive results.

LARRA F. (Angers): I agree with you but in several occasions, there were no correlation between Beta 2 microglobulin, CEA and clinical status; in these cases, it is very difficult to know what is required for the patient.

SYNTHESIS AND CONCLUSION

C.M.Lalanne, B.P.Krebs, M.Schneider

Centre Antoine Lacassagne, 36 Voie Romaine, 06054 NICE Cedex, France

The Nice Symposium was mainly devoted to Clinical Application of Carcinoembryonic Antigen(CEA) radioimmunoassay. Since Gold and Freedman's original work, about ten years ago, there were many disputes about the specificity of radioimmunoassay due to the heterogeneity of CEA and the presence of CEA-like molecules. A great amount of data is already available and was presented at the symposium. It is worthwhile to draw for the practitioner useful conclusions on the methods of radioimmunoassay, on the significance of their results and on their use for the immediate benefit of the patient.

I- Several *methods of radioimmunoassay* were offered, introducing somewhat different normal values and different cut-off levels. Radioimmunoassay of CEA was first performed in perchloric acid extract. This indirect method does not allow a great number of determinations without a large investment in laboratory staff. Nevertheless it is the only one commercially available in the United States(Hoffman-La Roche). Direct methods are used in other countries. They are unexpensive. The difference in methods introduces discrepancies in results, mainly between american and european oncologists. Results of the two methods have been compared by Kadouche and co-workers and Milano and co-workers. Discrepancies are mainly due to technical artefacts. For Zamcheck's group and others there is in indirect measurements, an important jump of CEA values as soon as the level is higher than the endpoint of the calibration curve. In these cases (high level of CEA) the biologist must use the direct assay. CEA loss during the extraction step is quite evident. Dr. Burtin in his communication insists that in radioimmunoassay " the specificity of antisera does not influence the results in a major way. Absorption of antisera by NCA for example will not modify the results". However, if the perchloric acid extract method (indirect) is a pre-requisite for measurement of CEA in biological fluids other than blood as shown in several papers, the direct method is advisable for routine determination in blood. In fact, despite the choice of different methods and different cut-off levels, results presented at the Symposium are in good agreement.

II- Every cancer does not produce and release CEA to the same extent. The rate of cancers positive for CEA in blood and CEA *levels varies widely from one site of cancer to another*. And great variations are also observed between patients within the same site. CEA is a reliable marker only when produced in sufficient amount and released in blood. From the data collected at the Symposium, *COLO -RECTAL*, *LUNG* and *BREAST* cancers are the most often productive and could best benefit from CEA radioimmunoassay and for these cancers , it can be recommanded for daily routine practice. In gynaecological cancer, the situation remains controversial and requires more work, but the outlook seems "promising" for ovarian carcinoma, at least if pretherapeutic levels are high. On the opposite, CEA measurements seem of poor clinical use in urological and head and neck cancers.

III- Variations of CEA *in blood are closely related to clinical status* with a good productive value. Localized tumours do not often increase blood level of CEA in a significant way. CEA radioimmunoassay cannot be accepted as a reliable tool for primary diagnosis. Nevertheless, before treatment, it is useful because it gives the basic level and in a few cases could provide from the start, some information on metastatic disease. High CEA level suggests strongly dissemination even in apparently localized tumours. After treatment, repetition of CEA measurements at two or three months intervals are rewarding. During the post-operative period, normalization of elevated CEA indicates complete resection of the tumour and good prognosis. On the other hand, CEA is a fairly reliable index for early detection of recurrence and metastases before their clinical appearance. In some cases, the biological marker is ahead of other symptoms. The lead time often reaches several months. The slightest increase in CEA must be rapidly controlled and if confirmed, therapeutic decision follows, allowing treatment at a moment of better efficiency. For instance, in colo-rectal cancer, second-look surgery is, when possible, advisable. In other cancer sites, the fact is also of paramount importance since chemotherapy and immunotherapy have proved their ability to destroy pre-clinical metastases. In short, serial CEA determinations are required for follow-up in all CEA producing cancers.

IV- Carcinoembryonic antigen radioimmunoassay appears to be useful in at least three of the more frequent cancer sites : colo-rectal, lung and breast. *Unreliable for primary diagnosis, it is of very good value for follow-up of the patients and monitoring the treatment.* However, some of these cancers do not release significant amounts of CEA. Thus, the search for other markers is welcome. Some have been rapidly reviewed at the Symposium: tissue polypeptide antigen(TPA), Beta 2 Microglobulin, Goblet cell antigen... For the time being, the series of patients are too short to draw any practical conclusions And, none of the molecules studied seems to have the same clinical value as CEA.

AUTHOR INDEX